Tuberculosis: Causes, Clinical Assessment and Treatment

Tuberculosis: Causes, Clinical Assessment and Treatment

Editor: Rupert Condron

AMERICAN
MEDICAL PUBLISHERS
www.americanmedicalpublishers.com

AMERICAN
MEDICAL PUBLISHERS
www.americanmedicalpublishers.com

Cataloging-in-Publication Data

Tuberculosis : causes, clinical assessment and treatment / edited by Rupert Condron.
p. cm.
Includes bibliographical references and index.
ISBN 979-8-88740-537-7
1. Tuberculosis. 2. Tuberculosis--Etiology. 3. Tuberculosis--Diagnosis.
4. Tuberculosis--Treatment. 5. Mycobacterium tuberculosis. 6. Mycobacterial diseases.
I. Condron, Rupert.
RC311 .T83 2023
616.995--dc23

American Medical Publishers,
41 Flatbush Avenue,
1st Floor, New York,
NY 11217, USA

ISBN 979-8-88740-537-7 (Hardback)

Contents

Preface

Tuberculosis (TB) is an infectious disease that usually affects the lungs. It is caused by airborne bacteria named Mycobacterium tuberculosis. There are three stages of TB, namely, primary infection, latent TB, and active TB. Miliary tuberculosis is the most lethal form of TB. Older people, children under the age of four, and people with a weakened immune system are more susceptible to miliary tuberculosis. It can lead to several complications, such as meningitis, Addison's disease, hepatitis, TB lymphadenitis, etc. Mantoux tuberculin skin test (TST) and a blood test, known as the interferon gamma release assay (IGRA) are a few major screening tests for TB. Some other diagnostic tests include chest X-ray, computed tomography (CT) scans, and lab tests on sputum and lung fluid. TB treatments depend on the type of infection and comprise based on medications. This book outlines the causes, clinical assessment and treatment of tuberculosis in detail. It presents researches and studies performed by experts across the globe. The extensive content of this book provides the readers with a thorough understanding of tuberculosis.

The information shared in this book is based on empirical researches made by veterans in this field of study. The elaborative information provided in this book will help the readers further their scope of knowledge leading to advancements in this field.

Finally, I would like to thank my fellow researchers who gave constructive feedback and my family members who supported me at every step of my research.

Editor

1

Tuberculosis Treatment Outcomes and Associated Factors among TB Patients Attending Public Hospitals in Harar Town, Eastern Ethiopia: A Five-Year Retrospective Study

Assefa Tola,[1] **Kirubel Minsamo Minshore**,[2] **Yohanes Ayele**,[2] **and Abraham Nigussie Mekuria**[3]

[1]*Department of Epidemiology and Biostatistics, College of Health and Medical Sciences, Haramaya University, Harar, Ethiopia*
[2]*Department of Clinical Pharmacy, College of Health and Medical Sciences, Haramaya University, Harar, Ethiopia*
[3]*Department of Pharmacology, College of Health and Medical Sciences, Haramaya University, Harar, Ethiopia*

Correspondence should be addressed to Assefa Tola; asseharar@yahoo.com

Academic Editor: Vincent Jarlier

Introduction. Tuberculosis remains a major public health threat throughout the world particularly in developing countries. Evaluating the treatment outcome of tuberculosis and identifying the associated factors should be an integral part of tuberculosis treatment. *Objectives.* The aim of this study was to assess the treatment outcome of tuberculosis and its associated factors among TB patients in the TB clinics of Harar public hospitals, Eastern Ethiopia, 2017. *Methods.* A retrospective document review was conducted in two public hospitals of Harar town, located 516 km east of Addis Ababa. A systematic random sampling technique was used to select the document of TB patients who were registered in the hospitals from 1st of January, 2011, to 30th of December, 2015. The data were collected using a pretested structured data extraction format. SPSS Version 21 for window was used for data processing. Bivariate and multivariate analysis with 95% confidence interval was employed in order to infer the associations between TB treatment outcome and potential predictor variables. *Results.* One thousand two hundred thirty-six registered TB patients' documents were reviewed. Of these, 59.8% were male, 94.2% were urban dwellers, 97% were new cases, 61.2% were presented with pulmonary TB, and 22.8% were HIV positive. Regarding the treatment outcome, 30.4% were cured, 62.1% completed their treatment, 3.9% died, 2.4% were defaulted, and the remaining 1.2% had failed treatment. The overall rate of the treatment success among the patients was 92.5%. In the present study, being female (AOR = 1.89, 95% CI: 1.14 - 3.14), having pretreatment weight of 20 - 29 kg (AOR = 11.03, 95% CI: 1.66 - 73.35), being HIV negative (AOR = 6.50, 95% CI: 3.95 - 10.71), and being new TB patient (AOR = 3.22 95% CI: 1.10 - 9.47) were factors independently associated with successful treatment outcome. On the other hand, being in the age group 54 – 64 years (AOR =10.41, 95% CI: 1.86 - 58.30) and age greater than 65 years (AOR =24.41, 95% CI: 4.19 - 142.33) was associated with unsuccessful TB treatment outcome. *Conclusion.* In the current study, the rate of successful TB treatment outcome was acceptable. This rate should be maintained and further improved by designing appropriate monitoring strategies.

1. Introduction

Tuberculosis [1] remains a major public health threat throughout the world, developing countries shouldering much of the burden. According to the WHO report, TB is the ninth leading cause of death worldwide and it is also a leading cause of death among infectious agents, ranking above HIV/AIDS. In 2016 alone an estimated 10.4 million people fell ill with TB, of whom Africa accounted 74% cases and around 1,674,000 TB deaths were recorded globally.

According to WHO TB report, 20 countries share 85% of all estimated TB cases worldwide and Ethiopia falls under this category indicating high TB burden in the country [2]. Although the incidence of infection with TB is decreasing and there has been a positive move toward its management, more effort is needed to meet End TB Strategy, which aims at reducing the death rate by 90% by the year 2030, compared with 2015 [2, 3].

TB epidemiology is closely connected with social and economic conditions which make its prevention, care, and control more challenging [4, 5]. Many of the TB related morbidities are preventable by early diagnosis and appropriate treatment; however, owing to various reasons, its management is not always that easy [4, 5]. Evaluating the treatment outcome of TB and identifying its associated factors is an integral part of the treatment. Although the rate of the successful treatment outcome of the disease varies from country to country, 83% has been reported globally [2].

Studies conducted in various parts of Ethiopia reported different success rates of the treatment and the associated factors. For instance, a study conducted in the Northern part of the country reported 89.2% [6], but another study in the same region reported only 60.1% [7]. In the prior study, it was indicated that age greater than 40 years, family size greater than five, and being a retreatment case were strongly associated with unsuccessful treatment outcomes whereas coinfection with HIV and being male were associated with unsuccessful treatment outcomes in a later study.

Undoubtedly, the success rate of TB treatment outcome and the associated factors vary from setting to setting. Routine monitoring of the extent of the outcome and its determinants is important, but studies that have focused on TB treatment outcome and associated factors are lacking in Eastern Part of Ethiopia. Therefore, the aim of this study was to assess TB treatment outcome and factors associated among TB patients in Public Hospitals of Harar town, Eastern Ethiopia.

The objective of the study is to assess TB treatment outcome and associated factors among TB patients in Public Hospitals of Harar town, Eastern Ethiopia, 2017.

2. Methods and Materials

2.1. Study Area and Period. This study was conducted in two public hospitals (Hiwot Fana Specialized University Hospital and Jugal Hospital) in Harar town. The data were collected from April 24 to 29, 2017.

2.2. Study Design and Data Collection. A retrospective document review was conducted to assess the treatment outcome of TB patients and the associated factors from TB patients' documents registered from January 1, 2011, to December 31, 2015, at Public hospitals in Harar town.

2.3. Source Population. The documents of all the TB patients who were registered in the two public hospitals from 1st of January, 2011, to December 31st, 2015, were the source population.

2.4. Study Population. The documents of the randomly selected TB patients who were registered in the two public hospitals from 1st of January, 2011, to December 31st, 2015, were the study population.

2.5. Inclusion and Exclusion Criteria. The documents of all the registered TB patients at two public hospitals were included in this study.

However, registries in which treatment outcomes were missing and patients were transferred to other districts were excluded from the study.

2.6. Sample Size Determination. The sample size was determined by using double population proportions formula.

$$n = \frac{\left(z_{\alpha/2} + z_{\beta}\right)^2 x2\overline{P}\left(1 - \overline{P}\right)}{\left(p_1 - p_2\right)^2} \quad (1)$$

where **n**= sample size for each group

$Z_{\alpha/2}$= the desired level of statistical significance: 95% => 1.96

Z_{β} = the desired power: 80% power => 0.84

P_1= proportions of good/poor treatment outcome among the nonexposed

P_2= proportions of good/poor treatment outcome among the exposed

$p_1 - p_2$ = the difference in proportions of good/poor treatment outcome among the nonexposed and exposed

$\overline{P} = (p_1 + p_2)/2$

By using the above formula

(1) cure rate among HIV negative and HIV positive TB patients

$Z\alpha$=95% $Z\beta$= 80%, r=1, P1=85. %, P2=55.7% n=74

(2) cure rate among male and female TB patients

$Z\alpha$=95% $Z\beta$= 80%, r=2, P1=4.3% P2=8.6% n=1026

(3) Cure rate among male and female TB patients

$Z\alpha$=95% $Z\beta$= 80%, r=2, P1=3.6 % P2=7.2 % n=1236

From the above options, the largest sample size (1236) was selected [8].

2.7. Sampling Technique. Totally 3329 TB patients registered during the review period, from January 1st, 2011, to December 31st, 2015, in two public hospitals (1535 in Jugal Hospital and 1794 in Hiwot Fana).

The sample size (1236) was distributed to each clinic using a proportionate allocation. Therefore, a total sample size for each TB clinic was

$$\text{Jugal Hospital TB clinic} = \frac{N_i}{N} \times n = \frac{1535}{3329} \times 1236 = 570$$

$$\text{HiwotFana Specialized University Hospital TB clinic} = \frac{N_i}{N} \times n = \frac{1794}{3329} \times 1236 = 666 \quad (2)$$

From each TB clinic, registry which met the inclusion criteria was selected through a systematic sampling technique. This sampling interval (K) was obtained by dividing the total TB patients in each hospital to its sample size (k =1869/940=1.99 ~2 for Hiwot Fana Hospital and 1460/734=1.99 ~2 for Jugal Hospital). The 1st sample was taken by lottery method from 1 and 2; then the data were collected, every other registration number at both sites.

2.8. Data Collection. The data were collected by using a pretested structured data extraction format. The standard TB registry, laboratory findings, and monthly cohort follow-up form were reviewed to generate the required data. The standardized checklist used included all important sociodemographic data, clinical characteristics (sputum smear, type of TB, patient type, HIV status, drug regimen, and treatment outcomes), laboratory findings, and follow-up data. Data was collected by four BSc. nurses who have had training on comprehensive TB care and experience in data collection.

2.9. Statistical Analysis. Data were entered, cleaned, and analyzed using SPSS Version 21 for windows. Appropriate descriptive statistics such as mean (with standard deviation), median (with inter quartile range [IQR]), and frequencies (with percentages) were used to describe the study population in relation to relevant variables.

Bivariate and multivariate analysis with 95% confidence interval was employed to infer associations between the independent and dependent variables.

Binary logistic regression was used to calculate the crude odds ratio (COR) with 95% confidence interval. Each variable was entered into a logistic regression model so as to determine the presence of statistical significant association with the outcome variable. Multicollinearity among selected independent variables was checked through variance inflation factor (VIF) and none was found. All the explanatory variables with a P value$\leq$ 0.2 in the bivariate analyses were included in the final multivariable logistic model in order to identify the independent predictors of TB treatment outcome. A P value < 0.05 was considered statistically significant. Assumption on fitness of goodness of the final model was checked by Hosmer and Lemeshow test and was found fit.

2.10. Ethical Statement. Ethical approval was obtained from research review technical committee of Harar health Science College. A legal authorization letter was written from Harar health Science College to study settings to get permission before data collection. The information obtained was made anonymous and deidentified prior to analysis to ensure confidentiality.

2.11. Operational Definitions. In this study, treatment outcomes are categorized into successful and unsuccessful treatment outcomes.

Successful treatment outcome included "cured" and "treatment completed" cases.

Unsuccessful treatment outcome included "treatment failure" cases, "defaulter," and patients who "died."

According to the WHO, Treatment Outcomes Were Categorized into the following.

> *Successful outcome*: if the TB patients were cured (negative smear microscopy at the end of the treatment and on at least one previous follow-up test) or completed treatment with resolution of symptoms.
>
> *Unsuccessful outcome:* if the treatment resulted in treatment failure (remaining smear positive after 5 months of treatment), patients are defaulted (patients who interrupted their treatment for two consecutive months or more after registration), or patients died.

According to the standard definitions of the National Tuberculosis and Leprosy Control Program guidelines of Ethiopia (NTLCP)[9], the following definitions were used for treatment outcome.

> *Cured:* if the patients had finished treatment with negative bacteriological result at the end of the treatment.
>
> *Treatment completed:* if the patients had finished treatment, but without bacteriological result at the end of the treatment.
>
> *Treatment failure:* a patient who, while on treatment, remained smeary positive or became again smear positive at the end of the five months or later, after commencing treatment or a patient who was PTB-negative at the beginning and turned out smear positive at the end of the intensive phase.
>
> *Defaulter:* a patient who had been on treatment for at least 4 weeks and whose treatment was interrupted for 8 or more consecutive weeks.
>
> *Died:* if the patient died from any cause during the course of the treatment.
>
> *New case:* a patient who had never had treatment for TB or had been on anti-TB treatment for less than four weeks.

Three types of TB were considered in this study. These were smear positive pulmonary TB (PTB+), smear negative pulmonary TB (PTB-), and extra-pulmonary TB (EPTB).

> *Smear positive pulmonary TB (PTB+):* a patient who had at least 2 initial smear examinations positive for AFB by direct microscopy or one initial smear examination positive and culture positive or one initial smear positive and radiographic abnormalities consistent with TB.
>
> *Smear negative pulmonary TB (PTB-):* a patient who had three initial smear examinations negative for AFB and no response to course of broad-spectrum chemotherapy and again 3 smear examinations negative by direct microscopy and radiographic abnormalities consistent with PTB and three initial smear examinations negative by direct microscopy but positive by culture and decision by a clinician to treat with anti-TB

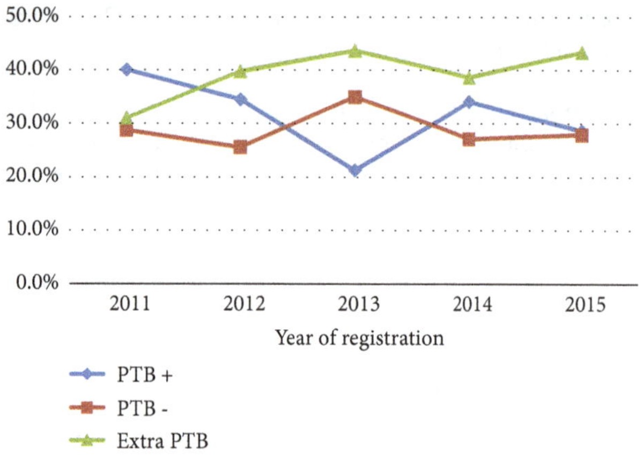

Figure 1: Trends of types of tuberculosis at public hospitals of Harar town, Eastern Ethiopia, 2011 - 2015.

> *Extra-pulmonary TB (EPTB)*: a patient who had TB in organs other than the lungs proven by one culture-positive specimen from extra-pulmonary site or histopathological evidence from a biopsy or TB based on strong clinical evidence with active EPTB and decision by a physician to treat with anti-TB.

3. Results

3.1. Sociodemographic Characteristics. The documents of 1236 TB patients were reviewed in this study. More than half of these TB patients (59.8%) were male, with male-to-female ratio of 1.5 to 1. Their age ranged from 1 to 95 years, with a median of 29 years (IQR: 22 - 40 years). About 363 (29.4%) of the participants were in the age range of 25 – 34 years and 355 (28.7%) were in the age range between 15 and 24 years. The weight of the TB patients ranged from 6 to 89 kg with mean (± SD) weight of 48.9 (±11.3) kg. More than half (59.7%) weighed 38 – 54 kg (Table 1).

3.2. Clinical Characteristics of Patients. Most of the attendants (97%) were new TB cases. Seven hundred fifty-six (61.2%) of the patients were presented with pulmonary TB of whom 400 (52.9%) were smear positive. Significant number of the patients 282 (22.8%) were found to be HIV positive of whom 250 (88.7%) and 258 (91.5%) were on ART and Cotrimoxazole Preventive Treatment (CPT), respectively.

Among smear positive PTB patients at the beginning of the treatment, 10 (2.5%), 7 (1.75%), and 14 (3.56%) were smear positive at second, fifth, and seventh months of the treatment, respectively. Most of the (97%) patients were treated with Rifampicin, Isoniazid, Pyrazinamide, and Ethambutol (RHZE) in intensive phase and 86.4% were on Rifampicin and Isoniazid (RH) during the continuation phase (Table 2).

Concerning the trend of all forms of TB, the proportion of extra-pulmonary TB slightly increased from 31.1% in 2011 to 43.3% in 2015 whereas the proportion of smear positive pulmonary TB decreased in the first three years from 40.1% in 2011 to 21.3% in 2013 (Figure 1).

3.3. Treatment Outcome of TB Patients on Anti-TB Therapy. Among the TB patients included in this study, 376 (30.4%) were cured, 767 (62.1%) had completed their treatment, 48 (3.9%) were dead, 30 (2.4%) were defaulted, and the remaining 15 (1.2%) had failed treatment.

The cure rate was high in the year 2011 (38.1%) and low in the year 2013 (19.8%). The default rate showed slight increment during the review period, 1.3% in the year 2011 to 3.4% in the year 2015. However, the death rate showed a reduction in the first three years (2011 – 2013) from 6.1 % to 2.0% and then started to increase in the final two years of the study period (2014 and 2015) from 3.3 % to 4.4% (Table 3).

3.4. Factors Associated with TB Treatment Outcome. The overall rate of the treatment success (cure and treatment complete) in this study was 92.5%. The rate of treatment success was higher among females (93.8%) than males (91.6%) and patients from rural setting (94.4%) than urban setting (92.4%). The proportion of TB patients with treatment success steadily decreased since 2012 (94.8%), 2013 (93.9%), 2014 (93.0%), and 2015 (90.8%); however, the difference was not statistically significant (P value =0.429). The treatment success rates were 94.3%, 90.7%, and 92.3% among the PTB+, PTB-, and EPTB patients, respectively. In the bivariate analysis, variables with P value of < 0.2 were sex, age, pretreatment weight, HIV status, patient category, and type of TB (Table 4).

In the multivariable logistic regression; sex, age, pretreatment weight, HIV status, and TB patient category were found to be independently and significantly associated with the treatment outcome. The chance of having successful TB treatment outcome was *1.89 times* higher among the female TB patients (AOR = *1.89*, 95% CI: 1.140 - 3.135) compared to the male. The HIV negative patients had 6.50 times higher odds of (AOR = 6.502, 95%CI: 3.947 - 10.712) having treatment success than the HIV positive. Similarly, the odds of treatment success were 3.22 (AOR = 3.222 95%CI: 1.096 - 9.472) times higher among new TB patients than retreatment TB cases (Table 5).

4. Discussion

Monitoring tuberculosis treatment outcomes and analyzing the responsible factors for unsuccessful treatment have paramount importance to evaluate the effectiveness and efficiency of TB intervention programs. In this study, we aimed to assess TB treatment outcomes and the associated factors in Harar public hospitals, Eastern Ethiopia.

In this study, the majority of the TB cases were male (59.8%). This finding was consistent with previous studies conducted in different areas of Ethiopia (Gimbi (59.3%) [10], Debre Tabor (58.1%) [11], Metema (60%) [12], Gambella (60%) [13], Dilla (61.3%) [14], Afar (62.6%) [15], Southern Ethiopia (57%) [16], Gondar (56%) [7], Hossana (55.3%) [17], Sidama Zone (55%) [18], Tigray (54.3%) [6], and Western Ethiopia (54.3%) [19]) and elsewhere in (Egypt (60.4%) [20], Ibadan Nigeria (55%) [21], South West Nigeria (59%) [22], Ebonyi state of Nigeria (57·7%) [23], and Malaysia (65%)

Table 1: Socio-demographic characteristics of TB patients attending public hospitals of Harar town, Eastern Ethiopia, 2017 (n=1236).

Variables	*Frequency*	*Percent*
Sex		
Male	739	59.8
Female	497	40.2
Age		
1 - 14 years	68	5.5
15 - 24 years	355	28.7
25 - 34 years	363	29.4
35 - 44 years	205	16.6
45 - 54 years	119	9.6
55 - 64 years	72	5.8
> 64 years	54	4.4
Place of residence		
Urban	1164	94.2
Rural	72	5.8
Pretreatment Weight		
Less than 20 Kg	22	1.8
20 - 29 Kg	30	2.4
30 - 37 Kg	85	6.9
38 - 54 Kg	738	59.7
Greater than 54 Kg	361	29.2
Year of treatment		
2011	312	25.2
2012	191	15.5
2013	197	15.9
2014	243	19.7
2015	293	23.7

[24]). The higher TB rate among males than the females might be due to the fact that males are more likely either to be exposed to the disease or to utilize health services than the females. Women may also underreport their disease and seek care outside health institutions because of socioeconomic constraints.

The age of the TB patients in this study ranged from 1 to 95 years, with the median age of 29 years and this is also similar to the findings of previous studies [7, 10, 12–14, 16, 18, 19]. Moreover, many of the TB cases we reviewed were between 15 and 34 years of age. This finding indicates that TB affects mainly the productive age group of the society, which can add up on the economic burden of the society particularly in developing countries.

In the present study, 3% of the patients were in the retreatment category. Similar findings were reported in studies conducted in Enfranz (2.4%) [25], Sidama Zone (5%) [18], and Metema (5.7%) [12]. However, it was less than reported from Gimbi (9.9%) [10], Western Ethiopia (8.9%) [19], Debre Tabor (10.9%) [11], Addis Ababa (11.1%) [26], and Gondar (17.5%) [7]. This could be due to the difference in time of the study, study setting, and sample size. Those studies reported the treatment outcome of TB patients before 2013 [7, 11, 19, 26] and were conducted at health centers [11, 19, 26] with smaller sample size [10, 11].

The prevalence of HIV among the patients in this study was 22.8%, which is comparable with the reports from Gambella (26%) [13], Gimbi (23.5) [10], and Metema (20.1%) [12]. However, our finding was higher than previous studies at Hosanna (16.5%) [17], Debre Tabor (12.7%) [11], Enfranz (11.7%) [25], Gondar (13.4%) [7], Iran (2.7%) [27], Dembia (11%) [28], Malaysia (6.6%) [24], Tigray region (8.6%) [6], and Western Ethiopia (17%) [19]. This high TB-HIV coinfection in our study could be due to the higher proportion of patients from urban setting where there is high prevalence of HIV.

More than one-third of the study subjects (38.8%) were presented with extra-pulmonary TB. This finding was comparable with studies from Gimbi (36%) [10], Western Ethiopia (39.7%) [19], Debre Tabor (33.3%) [11], and Addis Ababa (40.1%) [26]. Our finding was also consistent with the report of Ethiopian national population based tuberculosis prevalence survey [29]. This national TB survey stated that the mean (±SD) percentage of extra-pulmonary TB over total notifications from 2000 to 2010 was 34.8% (1.2%). This high proportion of extra-pulmonary TB in Ethiopia might be due high HIV prevalence, over diagnosis or misclassification bias. Furthermore, a similar proportion (32.4%) of TB patients in our study were presented with smear positive pulmonary TB and this is similar with the reports from Metema (30%) [12],

TABLE 2: Clinical characteristics of TB patients attending public hospitals of Harar town, Eastern Ethiopia, 2017 (n=1236).

Variables	*Frequency*	*Percent*
TB clinic		
Hiwot Fana SUH	666	53.9
Jugal Hospital	570	46.1
Category of patient		
New case	1199	97.0
Re treatment	37	3.0
Types of TB		
Pulmonary TB	756	61.2
Extra PTB	480	38.8
Smear result (n=756)		
Smear positive	400	52.9
Smear negative	356	47.1
HIV status		
HIV positive	282	22.8
HIV negative	954	77.2
ART initiated (n=282)		
Yes	250	88.7
No	32	11.3
CPT initiated (n=282)		
Yes	258	91.5
No	24	8.5
Smear result after 2 months (n=400)		
Positive	10	2.5
Negative	390	97.5
Smear result after 5 month (n= 400)		
Positive	7	1.75
Negative	393	98.25
Smear result after 7 months (n=387)		
Positive	9	2.3
Negative	378	97.7
Anti-TB Drug on Intensive phase		
RHZE	1199	97.0
SERHZ	37	3.0
Anti-TB Drug on continuation phase		
RH	1068	86.4
EH	168	13.6

Debre Tabor (28%) [11], Dabat (30%) [30], and Dilla (35.4%) [14].

In the current study, the overall rate of the treatment success of the TB patients was 92.5%, and this is similar to the findings reported from Tigray Region (89%) [6], Dabat (88%) [30], Debre Tabor (87.1%) [11], and Enfraz (95%) [25]. However, it is higher than national report of Ethiopia (84%) [2] and other previous studies in Ethiopia which reported treatment success ranging from 43.3% in Hossana to 85% in Dilla [7, 10, 12–19, 26]. This high treatment success rate in this study might be due to good implementation of DOTs strategy, which was indicated by lower defaulting and treatment failure rates. Another possible explanation could be also due to the exclusion of transfer out patients in this study which was categorized under unsuccessful treatment outcome group in previous studies. In addition, the majority of the TB patients in this study were urban residence; they might have had a better health seeking behavior.

TB associated death rate in present study was 3.9%. This figure was in line with report from Dilla (3.4%) [14], Addis Ababa (3.7%) [26], Afar (4.5%)[15], Enfranz (3.4%) [25], Gambella (3.7%), Dembia (3.3%), Metema (3%), Sidama zone (3.1%), Gimbi (3.7%), Tigray Region (3.9%) [6], Dabat (3.1%) [30], and Hossana (2.9%) [17]. However, some studies reported higher proportion of TB associated death rate, ranging from 5.6% in Debre Tabor and Egypt to 17.7% in Gondar [16, 19, 22, 24, 27, 31].

Defaulting from Anti-TB treatment clinic is one of the main challenges of TB controlling program. The defaulting rate of TB patients from their treatment in this study was

TABLE 3: Distribution of treatment outcome with socio-demographic and clinical characteristics of TB patients attending public hospitals of Harar town, Eastern Ethiopia, 2017 (n=1236).

Characteristics	*Treatment outcome*					*Total*
	Cure	*Completed*	*Died*	*Failure*	*Defaulted*	
Year of registration						
2011	119 (38.1%)	166(53.2%)	19(6.1%)	4(1.3%)	4(1.3%)	*312*
2012	62(32.5%)	119(62.3%)	4(2.1%)	3(1.6%)	3(1.6%)	*191*
2013	39(19.8%)	146(74.1%)	4(2.0%)	3(1.5%)	5(2.5%)	*197*
2014	78(32.1%)	148(60.9%)	8(3.3%)	1(0.4%)	8(3.3%)	*243*
2015	78(26.6%)	188(64.2%)	13(4.4%)	4(1.4%)	10(3.4%)	*293*
Place of residence						
Urban	359 (30.8%)	716 (61.5%)	48 (4.1%)	14 (1.2%)	27 (2.3%)	*1164*
Rural	17 (23.6%)	51 (70.8%)	0 (0.0%)	1 (1.4%)	3 (4.2%)	*72*
Age group						
1 - 14 years	12 (17.6%)	50 (73.5%)	4 (5.9%)	1 (1.5%)	1 (1.5%)	*68*
15 - 24 years	129 (36.3%)	213 (60.0%)	8 (2.3%)	1 (0.3%)	4 (1.1%)	*355*
25 - 34 years	120 (33.1%)	219 (60.3%)	10 (2.8%)	4 (1.1%)	10 (2.8%)	*363*
35 - 44 years	60 (29.3%)	131 (63.9%)	6 (2.9%)	2 (1.0%)	6 (2.9%)	*205*
45 - 54 years	32 (26.9%)	75 (63.0%)	2 (1.7%)	5 (4.2%)	5 (4.2%)	*119*
55 - 64 years	15 (20.8%)	46 (63.9%)	7 (9.7%)	2 (2.8%)	2 (2.8%)	*72*
>64 years	8 (14.8%)	33 (61.1%)	11 (20.4%)	0 (0.0%)	2 (3.7%)	*54*
Sex						
Male	241 (32.6%)	436 (59.0%)	27 (3.7%)	11 (1.5%)	24 (3.2%)	*739*
Female	135 (27.2%)	331 (66.6%)	21 (4.2%)	4 (0.8%)	6 (1.2%)	*497*
Pre-treatment weight						
< 20 Kg	2 (9.1%)	16 (72.7%)	2 (9.1%)	1 (4.5%)	1 (4.5%)	*22*
20 - 29 Kg	3 (10.0%)	24 (80.0%)	2 (6.7%)	1 (3.3%)	0 (0.0%)	*30*
30 - 37 Kg	28 (32.9%)	47 (55.3%)	5 (5.9%)	0 (0.0%)	5 (5.9%)	*85*
38 - 54 Kg	232 (31.4%)	456 (61.8%)	29 (3.9%)	8 (1.1%)	13 (1.8%)	*738*
>55 Kg	111 (30.7%)	224 (62.0%)	10 (2.8%)	5 (1.4%)	11 (3.0%)	*361*
HIV status						
HIV positive	73 (25.9%)	159(56.4%)	25(8.9%)	9(3.2%)	16(5.7%)	*282*
HIV negative	303(31.8%)	608(63.7%)	23(2.4%)	6(0.6%)	14(1.5%)	*954*
Type of TB						
Pulmonary TB	376 (49.7%)	325 (43.0%)	25 (3.3%)	15 (2.0%)	15 (2.0%)	*756*
Extra PTB	0 (0.0%)	442 (92.1%)	23 (4.8%)	0 (0.0%)	15 (3.1%)	*480*
Patient category						
New cases	352 (29.4%)	759 (63.3%)	46 (3.8%)	13 (1.1%)	29 (2.4%)	*1199*
Re treatment	24 (64.9%)	8 (21.6%)	2 (5.4%)	2 (5.4%)	1 (2.7%)	*37*
Total	*376 (30.4%)*	*767 (62.1%)*	*48 (3.9%)*	*15 (1.2%)*	*30 (2.4%)*	*1236*

2.4%, which is in line with the finding in Debre Tabor. However, the majority of previous studies reported that defaulting from TB treatment ranged from 2.8% in Dabat to 30.8% in South West Nigeria [6, 7, 10, 12–16, 18–22, 24, 26, 28, 32]. The lower defaulting rate in our study could be due to better implementation of DOT strategies, including defaulter tracing system, supervision, and health education activities.

The other main problem of TB controlling program is treatment failure. In our study, 1.2% of the TB patients were identified as treatment failure. This figure is lower than the reports from Ibadan Nigeria (8.1%) [21], Egypt (6.25%), Niger delta (4.8%), South West Nigeria (3.8%), Tigray Region (3.7%), and Debre Tabor (3.5%), but it is higher than finding from many studies conducted in different parts of Ethiopia [7, 12–16, 18, 19, 25, 26, 30] which ranged between 0.2% and 0.8%.

Identification of factors associated with treatment outcome of TB patients is very crucial in order to tackle those factors leading to poor treatment outcome. The present study revealed that being female; age greater than 55 years, having

TABLE 4: Bivariate analysis of treatment outcome with socio-demographic and clinical characteristics of TB patients attending public hospitals of Harar town, Eastern Ethiopia, 2017 (n=1236).

Characteristics	*Treatment outcome*			
	Successful Treatment	Unsuccessful treatment	*P. value*	*COR (95%CI)*
Place of residence				
Urban	1075 (92.4%)	89(7.6%)	0.516	1.00
Rural	68 (94.4%)	4(5.6%)		1.407 (0.502 - 3.947)
Sex				
Male	677 (91.6%)	62(8.4%)	0.161	1.00
Female	466(93.8%)	31 (6.2%)		1.377 (0.880 - 2.153)
Age group				
1 - 14 years	62 (91.2%)	69 (8.8%)	*≤ 0.001*	1.00
15 - 24 years	342(96.3%)	13(3.7%)	0.068	0.393 (0.144 - 1.072)
25 - 34 years	339(93.4%)	24(6.6%)	0.512	0.732 (0.287 - 1.863)
35 - 44 years	191(93.2%)	14(6.8%)	0.585	0.757 (0.279 - 2.055)
45 - 54 years	107(89.9%)	12(10.1%)	0.779	1.159 (0.414 - 3.242)
55 - 64 years	61(84.7%)	11(15.3%)	0.248	1.863 (0.648 - 5.355)
>64 years	41(75.9%)	13(24.1%)	*0.026*	*3.276 (1.153 - 9.313)*
Pre-treatment weight				
< 20 Kg	18 (81.8%)	4(18.2%)	0.177	1.00
20 - 29 Kg	27(90.0%)	3(10.0%)	0.074	2.863 (0.902 - 9.084)
30 - 37 Kg	75 (88.2%)	10(11.8%)	0.576	1.432 (0.407 - 5.036)
38 - 54 Kg	688(93.2%)	50(6.8%)	0.169	1.718 (0.795 - 3.714)
>55 Kg	335 (92.8%)	26(7.2%)	0.793	0.936 (0.573 - 1.531)
Year of registration				
2011	285(91.3%)	27 (8.7%)	0.429	1.00
2012	181(94.8%)	10(5.2%)	0.809	0.933 (0.534 - 1.632)
2013	185(93.9%)	12 (6.1%)	0.112	0.544 (0.257 - 1.152)
2014	226 (93.0%)	17 (7.0%)	0.213	0.639 (0.316 - 1.294)
2015	266 (90.8%)	27(9.2%)	0.353	0.741 (0.394 - 1.395)
HIV status				
HIV positive	232 (82.3%)	50(17.7%)	*≤ 0.001*	1.00
HIV negative	911(95.5%)	43(4.5%)		*4.566 (2.963 - 7.036)*
Patient category				
New cases	1111 (92.7%)	88 (7.3%)	0.169	1.00
Re treatment	32 (86.5%)	5(13.5%)		0.507 (0.193 - 1.333)
Type of TB				
PTB +	377 (94.3%)	23 (5.8%)	0.188	1.00
PTB -	323 (90.7%)	33 (9.3%)	0.253	0.730 (0.426 - 1.251)
Extra PTB	443 (92.3%)	37 (7.7%)	0.421	1.223(0.749 - 1.998)

pretreatment weight of 20 – 29 kg and 38 – 54 kg, being HIV negative, and being new TB patient were independently significantly associated with successful treatment outcome.

As reported by many studies [12, 15, 21, 23, 24, 27, 33], females have had bigger chance of successful TB treatment outcome than males. However, the odds of successful treatment outcome were better for males compared to females in studies conducted in Debre Tabor [11], Southern Region [16], and Tigray Region [6]. This difference might have been related to other variables like severity of the disease, timing of the treatment, adherence to the treatment, and behavioral and socioeconomic characteristics. Since almost all of these studies were based on retrospective document review, they did not take into consideration the effect of those important variables.

The HIV status of the TB patients was one of the factors that were associated with the treatment outcome. Not surprisingly, in this study, the HIV negative patients

TABLE 5: Multivariate analysis of treatment outcome with socio-demographic and clinical characteristics of TB patients attending public hospitals of Harar town, Eastern Ethiopia, 2017 (n=1236).

Characteristics	*Treatment outcome*			
	Successful Treatment	Unsuccessful treatment	*P. value*	*AOR (95%CI)*
Sex				
Male	677 (91.6%)	62(8.4%)	0.015	1.00
Female	466(93.8%)	31 (6.2%)		*1.890 (1.140 - 3.135)*
Age group				
1 - 14 years	62 (91.2%)	69 (8.8%)	*≤ 0.001*	1.00
15 - 24 years	342(96.3%)	13(3.7%)	0.367	2.138 (0.411 - 11.126)
25 - 34 years	339(93.4%)	24(6.6%)	0.217	2.617 (0.545 - 14.561)
35 - 44 years	191(93.2%)	14(6.8%)	0.318	2.386 (0.436 - 13.009)
45 - 54 years	107(89.9%)	12(10.1%)	0.098	4.243 (0.766 - 23.520)
55 - 64 years	61(84.7%)	11(15.3%)	0.008	*10.413 (1.860 - 58.298)*
>64 years	41(75.9%)	13(24.1%)	*≤ 0.001*	*24.41 (4.188 - 142.331)*
Pre-treatment weight				
< 20 Kg	18 (81.8%)	4(18.2%)	0.035	1.00
20 - 29 Kg	27(90.0%)	3(10.0%)	0.012	*11.027(1.658 - 73.347)*
30 - 37 Kg	75 (88.2%)	10(11.8%)	0.088	4.053 (0.813 - 20.192)
38 - 54 Kg	688(93.2%)	50(6.8%)	0.022	*2.824 (1.167 - 6.831)*
>55 Kg	335 (92.8%)	26(7.2%)	0.612	1.151 (0.669 - 1.978)
HIV status				
HIV positive	232 (82.3%)	50(17.7%)	≤ 0.001	1.00
HIV negative	911(95.5%)	43(4.5%)		*6.502 (3.947 - 10.712)*
Patient category				
Re treatment	32 (86.5%)	5(13.5%)	0.033	1.00
New cases	1111 (92.7%)	88 (7.3%)		*3.222 (1.096 - 9.472)*
Type of TB				
PTB +	377 (94.3%)	23 (5.8%)	0.415	1.00
PTB -	323 (90.7%)	33 (9.3%)	0.208	0.686 (0.382 - 1.233)
Extra PTB	443 (92.3%)	37 (7.7%)	0.876	0.959 (0.566 - 1.625)

had bigger chance of successful TB treatment than the HIV positive ones. This finding is consistent with several previous studies [7, 10, 12, 19, 22, 24, 27, 28].

5. Conclusion and Recommendation

The treatment outcome of the TB patients who received TB treatment at the study area was satisfactory and in line with the WHO target. The treatment outcome was significantly associated with gender, age, pretreatment weight, HIV status, and TB category. Moreover, it was not significantly affected by place of residence, year of treatment, and types of TB.

Based on the findings of this study, we recommend that frequent supportive supervision and health education programs for patients with a high risk of unsuccessful treatment outcome should be carried out. In addition, further prospective studies are needed to identify other potential sociodemographic and behavioral factors that could affect the treatment outcomes of TB patients.

Authors' Contributions

Assefa Tola, Kirubel Minsamo Minshore, Yohanes Ayele, and Abraham Nigussie Mekuria conceived the study, participated in the design, data analysis, and interpretation of the result. Assefa Tola, Kirubel Minsamo Minshore, Yohanes Ayele, and Abraham Nigussie Mekuria were involved in data acquisition and writing the draft manuscript. Assefa Tola, Kirubel Minsamo Minshore, Yohanes Ayele, and Abraham Nigussie Mekuria critically reviewed the manuscript. All authors read and approved the manuscript.

Acknowledgments

We would like to extend appreciations to the individuals who were involved in data collection and those hospitals that willingly gave us all the information we needed without any reservation.

References

[1] M. T. Baysari, K. Oliver, B. Egan et al., "Audit and feedback of antibiotic use: utilising electronic prescription data," *Applied Clinical Informatics*, vol. 4, pp. 583–595, 2013.

[2] WHO, "Global Tuberculosis Report," *2017*, 2017.

[3] M. Uplekar, D. Weil, K. Lonnroth et al., "WHO's new end TB strategy," *The Lancet*, vol. 385, no. 9979, pp. 1799–1801, 2015.

[4] M. Raviglione and G. Sulis, "Tuberculosis 2015: burden, challenges and strategy for control and elimination," *Infectious Disease Reports*, vol. 8, no. 2, 2016.

[5] P. Glaziou, C. Sismanidis, K. Floyd, and M. Raviglione, "Global epidemiology of tuberculosis," *Cold Spring Harbor Perspectives in Medicine*, vol. 5, no. 2, Article ID a017798, 2015.

[6] G. Berhe, F. Enquselassie, and A. Aseffa, "Treatment outcome of smear-positive pulmonary tuberculosis patients in Tigray Region, Northern Ethiopia," *BMC Public Health*, vol. 12, no. 1, 2012.

[7] M. Biruk, B. Yimam, H. Abrha, S. Biruk, and F. Z. Amdie, "Treatment outcomes of tuberculosis and associated factors in an Ethiopian university hospital," *Advances in Public Health*, vol. 2016, Article ID 8504629, 9 pages, 2016.

[8] T. Abebe, "Treatment outcome of tuberculosis and risk factors for poor treatment outcomes at jimma university specialized hospital and ommo-nada trainin health center, South West Ethiopia," 2013.

[9] Ministry of Health of Ethiopia, *Tuberculosis, Leprosy and TB/HIV Prevention and Control Program*, Ministry of Health of Ethiopia, Addis Ababa, Ethiopia, 6th edition, 2016.

[10] D. Garedew and G. Nemera, "Treatment outcome of tuberculosis and associated factors at gimbi town health facilities Western Oromia, Ethiopia," *Nursing & Care Open Access Journal*, vol. 7, no. 2, 2017.

[11] A. Melese, B. Zeleke, and B. Ewnete, "Treatment outcome and associated factors among tuberculosis patients in Debre Tabor, Northwestern Ethiopia: a retrospective study," *Tuberculosis Research and Treatment*, vol. 2016, no. 8, 2016.

[12] D. Tarekegne, M. Jemal, T. Atanaw et al., "Treatment outcomes of tuberculosis patients in metema hospital, northwest ethiopia: a four years retrospective study," *Mycobacterial Diseases*, vol. 5, no. 4, 2015.

[13] G. Asebe and H. Dissasa, "Treatment outcome of tuberculosis patients at gambella hospital, Southwest Ethiopia: three-year retrospective study," *Journal of Infectious Diseases & Therapy*, vol. 3, no. 2, 2015.

[14] G. Gebrezgabiher, G. Romha, E. Ejeta, G. Asebe, E. Zemene, and G. Ameni, "Treatment outcome of tuberculosis patients under directly observed treatment short course and factors affecting outcome in southern ethiopia: a five-year retrospective study," *PLoS ONE*, vol. 11, no. 2, 2016.

[15] T. Zenebea and E. Teferab, "Tuberculosis treatment outcome and associated factors among smear-positive pulmonary tuberculosis patients in Afar, Eastern Ethiopia: a retrospective study," *The Brazilian Journal of Infectious Diseases*, vol. 2, no. 6, pp. 635-636, 2016.

[16] M. Muñoz-Sellart, L. E. Cuevas, M. Tumato, Y. Merid, and M. A. Yassin, "Factors associated with poor tuberculosis treatment outcome in the Southern Region of Ethiopia," *The International Journal of Tuberculosis and Lung Disease*, vol. 14, no. 8, pp. 973–979, 2010.

[17] T. Mohammed, K. Daniel, D. Helamo, and T. Leta, "Treatment outcomes of tuberculosis patients in nigist Eleni Mohammed general hospital, hosanna, southern nations, nationalities and peoples region, Ethiopia: A five year (June 2009 to August 2014) retrospective study," *Archives of Public Health*, vol. 75, no. 16, 2017.

[18] M. H. Dangisso, D. G. Datiko, and B. Lindtjørn, "Trends of tuberculosis case notification and treatment outcomes in the sidama zone, southern ethiopia: Ten-year retrospective trend analysis in urban-rural settings," *PLoS ONE*, vol. 9, no. 12, 2014.

[19] E. Ejeta, M. Chala, G. Arega et al., "Outcome of tuberculosis patients under directly observed short course treatment in western ethiopia," *The Journal of Infection in Developing Countries*, vol. 9, no. 7, pp. 752–759, 2015.

[20] M. El-Shabrawy and D. A. El-Shafei, "Evaluation of treatment failure outcome and its predictors among pulmonary tuberculosis patients in Sharkia Governorate, 2013–2014," *Egyptian Journal of Chest Diseases and Tuberculosis*, vol. 66, no. 1, pp. 145–152, 2017.

[21] A. A. Fatiregun, A. S. Ojo, and A. E. Bamgboye, "Treatment outcomes among pulmonary tuberculosis patients at treatment centers in Ibadan, Nigeria," *Annals of African Medicine*, vol. 8, no. 2, pp. 100–104, 2009.

[22] O. A. Babatunde, O. E. Elegbede, M. Ayodele, J. O. Fadare, and A. O. Isinjaye, "Factors affecting treatment outcomes of tuberculosis in a tertiary health center in Southwestern Nigeria," *International Review of Social Sciences and Humanities*, vol. 4, no. 2, pp. 209–218, 2013.

[23] S. N. Oshi, I. Alobu, K. N. Ukwaja, and D. C. Oshi, "Investigating gender disparities in the profile and treatment outcomes of tuberculosis in Ebonyi state, Nigeria," *Epidemiology and Infection*, vol. 143, no. 05, pp. 932–942, 2015.

[24] S. M. Liew, E. M. Khoo, B. K. Ho, Y. K. Lee, O. Mimi, and M. Y. Fazlina, "Tuberculosis in Malaysia: predictors of treatment outcomes in a national registry," *International Journal of Tuberculosis and Lung Disease*, vol. 19, no. 7, 2015.

[25] M. Endris, F. Moges, Y. Belyhun, E. Woldehana, A. Esmael, and C. Unakal, "Treatment outcome of tuberculosis patients at enfraz health center, Northwest Ethiopia: a five-year retrospective study," *Tuberculosis Research and Treatment*, vol. 2014, Article ID 726193, 7 pages, 2014.

[26] B. Getahuna, G. Amenia, G. Medhina, and S. Biadgilign, "Treatment outcome of tuberculosis patients under directly observed treatment in Addis Ababa, Ethiopia," *International Journal of Tuberculosis and Lung Disease*, vol. 17, no. 5, pp. 521–528, 2013.

[27] S. Khazaei, J. Hassanzadeh, S. Rezaeian et al., "Treatment outcome of new smear positive pulmonary tuberculosis patients in Hamadan, Iran: A registry-based cross-sectional study," *Egyptian Journal of Chest Diseases and Tuberculosis*, vol. 65, no. 4, pp. 825–830, 2016.

[28] M. G. Beza, M. T. Wubie, M. D. Teferi, Y. S. Getahun, S. M. Bogale, and S. B. Tefera, "A five years tuberculosis treatment outcome at kolla diba health center, Dembia District, Northwest Ethiopia: a retrospective crosssectional analysis," *Infectious Diseases & Therapy*, vol. 1, no. 1, 2013.

[29] FMoH of Ethiopia and Ethiopian Health and Nutrition Research Institute. First Ethiopian National Population Based Tuberculosis Prevalence Survey, Addis Ababa, July 2011.

[30] S. Tadesse and T. Tadesse, "Treatment success rate of tuberculosis patients in Dabat, northwest Ethiopia," *Health*, vol. 6, no. 5, pp. 306–310, 2014.

[31] I. Ebuenyi, P. Ikuabe, and J. Jumbo, "Treatment Outcome of Tuberculosis at One Year: A Single Centre's Experience in Niger Delta, Nigeria," *International Journal of Tropical Disease & Health*, vol. 12, no. 1, pp. 1-6, 2016.

[32] N. A. Ifebunandu and K. N. Ukwaja, "Tuberculosis treatment default in a large tertiary care hospital in urban Nigeria: Prevalence, trend, timing and predictors," *Journal of Infection and Public Health*, vol. 5, no. 5, pp. 340–345, 2012.

[33] D. Demeke, M. Legesse, and J. Bati, "Trend of tuberculosis and treatment outcomes in gambella region with special emphasize on Gambella regional hospital, Western Ethiopia," *Mycobacterial Diseases*, vol. 3, no. 2, 2013.

2

Delay for Tuberculosis Treatment and its Predictors among Adult Tuberculosis Patients at Debremarkos Town Public Health Facilities, North West Ethiopia

Yibeltal Estemech Ayalew,[1] Fikadu Ambaw Yehualashet,[2] Worknesh Akanaw Bogale,[3] and Mengistu Berhanu Gobeza[3]

[1]*Department of Medical Nursing, University of Gondar, Gondar, Ethiopia*
[2]*Department of Community Health Nursing, University of Gondar, Gondar, Ethiopia*
[3]*Department of Pediatrics and Child Health Nursing, University of Gondar, Gondar, Ethiopia*

Correspondence should be addressed to Fikadu Ambaw Yehualashet; fekaduambaw14@gmail.com

Academic Editor: Alexander S. Apt

Background. Delay in the diagnosis and treatment of tuberculosis exacerbates the disease and clinical outcomes. It further enhances transmission of the infection in the society as well as increased the severity of the illness and raised rate of mortality. *Objectives.* The major goal of this study is to determine the magnitude of delays in tuberculosis treatment and factors affecting tuberculosis treatment among adult tuberculosis patients at Debremarkos town, North West Ethiopia, 2018. *Methods.* Institution-based cross-sectional study design was employed. Systematically selected 300 adult TB patients were recruited to the study. The study was conducted at Debremarkos town public health facilities from March 1 to April 30, 2018. Logistic regression models were fitted to identify the predicting variables and control confounder's of the outcome variables. P value ≤ 0.05 with 95% CI was considered as an indicator for the presence of statistically significant association. The result revealed that the median total delay was 23 days (IQR: 19-28 days). The median patient and health system delays were 20 days (IQR: 15-20 days) and 4 days (IQR: 3-5 days), respectively. Tuberculosis patients living in a rural area were 1.14 times more likely to delay for the TB treatment (AOR: 1.141, 95% CI (1.106, 2.608)). Patients who were unable to read and write have almost two times a chance of being delayed (AOR: 2.350, 95% CI (1.630, 2.608)). Monthly income of patients has found another predictor for delay; patients with low monthly income were about six times more likely to delay for TB treatment (AOR: 6.375, 95% CI: (1.733, 23.440)). Those TB patients who had visiting traditional healers before arrival to health facilities were about 2.7 times more likely to delay for TB treatment(AOR: 2.795, 95% CI (1.898, 8.693)). *Conclusion and Recommendation.* The significant proportion of delays in tuberculosis treatment was found in this study. Living in the rural area, unable to read and write, lower monthly income, and visiting traditional healers were found independent predictors of TB treatment delay. The regional and zonal health administrator shall design various awareness creation mechanisms to educate the public about timely initiation of tuberculosis treatment.

1. Introduction

Tuberculosis (TB) is the ninth leading cause of mortality worldwide and the leading cause from a single infectious agent, ranking above HIV/AIDS [1]. Almost one-third of the world populations (about 2 billion) are infected with mycobacterium tuberculosis [2].

Treatment delay leads to more serious illness; as a result, it increased infectivity within the community and increased transmission of TB [3, 4]. Delay in initiation of treatment gratuitously prolongs the period of TB transmission within the community [5]. Delay in the diagnosis and treatment of tuberculosis results in increasing severity of the disease, chance of death, and risk of transmission of the infection in the society particularly among people who have contact with the patient. It is evident that, as delay for TB treatment progress, patients would become more contagious [6]. Delay in TB detection, diagnosis, and early initiation of treatment results in increased rate of infectivity in the society, and it is estimated that untreated smear positive patients can infect on average 10 contacts annually and 20 during the natural history of the disease until death [7].

According to a study conducted in Vietnam, the total median delay was 4 weeks, 3 weeks for patient delay, and health care system was responsible for a delay of 1 week. Nearly 15% of patients with long total delay (≥12 weeks) accounted for 49% of cumulative number of delay weeks [8]. Another study conducted in Tanzania among 639 TB patients showed that patient delay was observed in 35.1% of the patients, with significantly high proportion in females (41%). In addition, diagnosis delay has recorded in 52.9% of the patients, with a high proportion in females (62.1%). In 34.4% of patients, treatment delay was noticed but no significant differences among males and females [9, 10].

Studies conducted at a different setting have showed that different factors contribute for the delay of treatment. For instance, first visit to traditional healers (private clinic), residence, education, severity of illness at first presentation to health facility, patient with good functional status, patients in contact with more than two health providers, not knowing TB symptoms, unemployment, and distance from a health facility were factors associated with TB treatment delays [11–13]. A study conducted in Zambia revealed that, the median diagnostic delay was 8.6 weeks and was significantly associated with sex, education, level of health care encounters, and visiting a private doctor or traditional healer [3]. However, income was found as an independent predictor in a study conducted in Pakistan [4].

Ethiopia has designed various TB diagnosis, treatment, and prevention and control strategies in order to reach at the MDG goals; as a result, it achieved reduction of more than half of most of the MDG targets related to tuberculosis. However, the progress of reduction of the incidence and prevalence has been comparatively slow. Irrespective of all the efforts to achieve early detection of TB and prompt management of cases, significant proportion of TB cases arrived at health facilities after developing serious complications.

In Ethiopia, although there are reports on length of delay to initiate treatment, data regarding proportion of delay among cases and factors associated to delay was scarce. Therefore, this study is aimed at estimating the magnitude of delays in TB treatment and identifying the determinant factors contributing for TB treatment delay.

2. Methods and Materials

A facility-based cross-sectional study was conducted from March 1 to April 30, 2018, at Debremarkos town public health institutions. According to the Central statistics report of Ethiopia, Debremarkos town is located in East Gojjam zone, North West Ethiopia, at 300 km far from Addis Ababa, the capital of Ethiopia, and 265 km from Bahirdar, the regional capital. According to the 2015 population projection of major cities in Ethiopia, Debremarkos town has a total population of around 70,000. There are five governmental health institutions (four health centers and one referral hospital) which have been providing Direct Observed Therapy Service (DOTS) to TB patients for the first two months and continuation phase for a varied period of time accordingly. Simple random sampling technique was employed to select Debremarkos town from other seven zonal administrative towns in the region. TB patients who were attending their anti-TB treatment at Debremarkos Health Center, Gozamin Health Center, and Debremarkos Referral Hospital were included in study based on proportional allocation. Systematic random sampling technique was used to draw a sample of 300 TB patients from a total of 1088 patients. Considering list of registered TB patients as a frame, the calculated K value was 3. Hence, every three patients attending TB clinics of Debremarkos town were recruited in to the study.

2.1. Operational Definitions. *Patient delay* is the time interval between onset of symptoms and the patient's first contact with a healthcare provider [14, 15].

Diagnostic delay is the time interval between the first consultations of healthcare provider to diagnosis. Interval more than 3 days was considered as diagnostic delays [10].

Health care system delay is the time interval between the dates of visiting health care provider to the initiation of anti-tuberculosis treatment [10, 16].

Total delay is time interval from the onset of symptoms to treatment initiation [17].

The patient has *good knowledge about TB*, if the patient can answer correctly the knowledge questions about TB and score equal to and above the median value [11].

The patient has *high perceived stigma about TB*, if the patient scores above and equal to the median value of the questions assessing stigma [11].

2.2. Data Analysis. Data was entered using the EPI-info version 7 and then exported to SPSS version 20 for analysis. Binary logistic regression was made to see the crude significant relation of each independent variable with dependent variables. Then, variables with P value less than 0.25 in binary logistic regression were taken to multivariable logistic regressions [18] to control the effect of confounding and identify the true relationship between variables. Variables having P value of less than 5% with 95% CI were used to declare significant association with the outcome variable. Key descriptive variables were analyzed and presented in texts, tables, figures, and graphs. Ethical clearance letter was obtained from the ethical review committee of the School of Nursing, College of Medicine and Health Science, University of Gondar, with a reference number of C/H/N/U/124/2018. Official letters of permission were taken from zonal health office and respective health institution officers.

The purpose of the study was clearly explained for each study participant, and written verbal consent was taken from participants before interview; besides, they were also informed as participation is on voluntary basis. Patients' name and card number were not taken to assure the privacy and confidentiality of participants.

3. Results

In this study, a total of 300 study participants were enrolled from three public health facilities. The median age of the participants was 30 years (IQR 16 years). Of the total 300 study participants, 144 (48%) were males, 118 (39.3%) lived in the rural areas, and 99 (33%) were illiterate. Regarding the occupational status of participants, 48 (16%) were government employed, nearly one-third of study participants (88 (29.3%)) earn a monthly income of less than 500 birr, and a quarter of the participants (76 (25.3%)) have 1500 birr income per month. More than three-fourth of the study participants (266 (82%)) were HIV negative. Just above half of the participants (156 (53%)) were diagnosed as extrapulmonary tuberculosis (EPTB). One hundred twenty (40%) of the participants were living at 6-10 km radius from the nearby health facility (Table 1).

3.1. Patient's Clinical Presentation. Closer to half (47%) of the study participants diagnosed pulmonary tuberculosis, and of the total subjects, about 16% were screened HIV positive. Regarding their smoking history, only 6% of participates reported as they have a habit of cigarette smoking. Majority of the study participants (88.7%) revealed as they manifest cough as TB symptom, 203 (67.7%) weight loss, and 174 (64.7%) said they had chest pain (Figure 1).

Although majority of TB (71%) patients had consulted health care provider during the onset of the illness, significant proportion of patients (17.7%) had visit traditional healers as a first priority of care center (Figure 2).

3.2. Participant's Knowledge and Perceived Stigma. Almost all the study subjects (99.3%) heard about TB, and more than 92% of the clients are aware about the type of illness they had. About 96% of study subjects know as TB is a contagious illness and curable disease (Table 2). In regard to the source of information, sixty-three percent of participants received information about TB from MOH campaign through media, 16% from formal education, and 12.7% from friends/relatives. The overall knowledge of study subjects showed that above half of the participants had poor knowledge about TB (60%). On the other hand, two-fifth of the participants (40%) perceived that there is high level of stigma for being a TB client. The measure of internal consistency or Cranach's Alpha was 0.744 which showed a better consistency.

3.2.1. Perceived Causes of Delay. Closer to three-fourth of study participants (72.7%) perceived that there is delay for TB treatment. Almost sixty percent of the study subjects explained that their reason of delay to seek medical care was waiting a spontaneous resolution of the symptoms. On the other hand, poor quality of health services delivered in the health facilities account for 13% of study subjects in reason for late presentation to TB treatment.

3.2.2. Proportion of Delay for TB Treatment. About half of the study participants (48%) have shown total delay for TB treatment with a median 23 days (IQR: 19-28 days). The minimum and maximum length of total delays for TB treatment was 13 and 64 days, respectively. Significant proportion of patients (42%) demonstrate patient delay above three weeks of duration with a median value of 20 days (Table 2).

3.3. Determinant Factors of Delay in Tuberculosis Treatment. As the multivariable logistic regression result revealed, rural residency has been identified as a determinant variable for delay in TB treatment. Participants who lived in the rural area have 1.14 times higher chance of delay for TB treatment than urban dweller AOR = 1.141 (95% CI: 1.106, 2.608). Educational status is also another variable which showed a significant association with delay for TB treatment; being illiterate patients were two times more likely to delay for TB treatment than participants with an educational status of college and above AOR = 2.35 (95% CI: 1.63, 2.61). Monthly income of participants has found another determinant factor affecting patients delay for TB treatment; as a result, participants who earn below 500 birr per month were six times more likely to delay for TB treatment as compared to those who got 1500 birr and above AOR = 6.37 (95% CI: 1.733, 23.440). Furthermore, participants who visit traditional healers before they came to health facilities were four times more likely to delay for TB treatment AOR = 4.475 (95% CI: 1.204, 16.633). Consulting health care professionals at health facility was found a protective variable for delay for TB treatment AOR = 0.101 (95% CI: 0.020, 0.508) (Table 3).

4. Discussion

Early detection of disease and prompt initiation of treatment are essential for an effective TB control program [12]. This study focuses on determining the magnitude of delays to start TB treatment and its contributing factors among TB patients attending DOTS clinics of public health facilities. Patients' delay in seeking care during the onset of TB symptoms and health system delay in diagnosing and initiating antituberculosis treatment contribute for total delays in treatment.

In this study, the median patient delay was 20 days (with IQR: 15-20 days). Forty-two percent (42%) of patients experienced delay greater than 21 days. The median patient delay of this study is shorter than other studies done in Nepal (50 days) [12], Uganda (30 days) [19], southern Ethiopia (30 days) [20], and South-east Ethiopia (63 days) [21]. This might be due to a better health care access to the community and health professionals' campaign in finding cases and promotes early initiation of health services. Moreover, it might be also due to the presence of the urban health extension workers who are responsible to work communicable disease in the community. However, this finding is similar with a study done in Afar region, Ethiopia, which is 20 days [22], and it is also closer to a study done in Malawi that was 14 days (IQR: 15-28 days) [23].

The median health system delay of TB patients in the study area was 4 days (IQR: 3-5 days) which is much lower than previous studies done in Southeast Ethiopia which was 34 days [21], Malawi 59 days (IQR 26-108 days) [23], and Afar, Ethiopia, 33.5 days [22]. This discrepancy might be due to a difference in health professional's ability to detect TB symptoms and availability of advanced diagnostic modality.

TABLE 1: Sociodemographic characteristics of tuberculosis patients attending DOTS clinic.

Variables	Category	Frequency	Percent
Sex	Male	144	48
	Female	156	52
Age	≤20	24	8
	21-39	187	62.3
	≥40	89	29.7
Religion	Orthodox	284	94.7
	Muslim	13	4.3
	Other catholic	3	1
Residence	Rural	118	39.3
	Urban	182	60.7
Marital status	Unmarried	136	45.3
	Married	164	54.7
Educational status	No education	99	33
	Read and write only	30	10
	Primary school	30	10
	2ndry school and above	141	47
Occupation	Unemployed	56	18.7
	Self-employed	92	30
	Government employed	48	16.0
	Private employed	33	11.0
	Housewife	71	23.3
Income	≤500	88	29.3
	501-1500	136	45.3
	≥1501	76	25.3
Distance from the nearest health center	1-5 km	115	38.3
	6-10 km	120	40.0
	11-20 km	62	20.7
	≥21 km	3	1.0

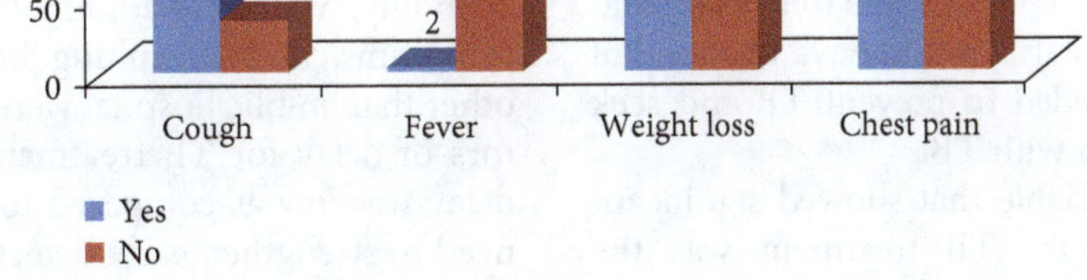

FIGURE 1: A graph showing clinical presentations of TB patients during onset of illness, Debremarkos Health facilities, Ethiopia.

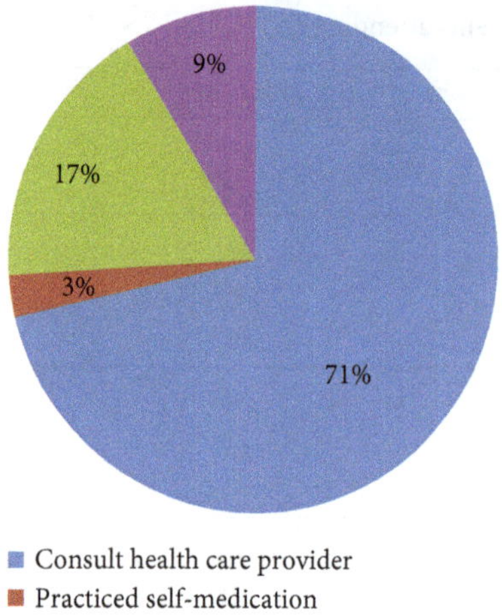

FIGURE 2: Proportions of patient's first action during the onset of TB symptoms at Debremarkos town public health facilities, North West Ethiopia, 2018.

The median total delay for treatment among TB patients in the current study was 23 days with an IQR: 19-28 days which is comparatively lower than other previous studies done in Tanzania (136 days) [13], India (55.5 days) [17], and Zimbabwe (36 days) [24]. This wider variation across nations might be due to a difference in the health policy and TB prevention and control treatment strategy of nations. Besides, the finding was also lower than studies conducted in Ethiopia, Southern Ethiopia (45 days) [20], and Afar region (70.5 days) [22], and this could be due to the sociodemography and the infrastructural differences.

Residence of study participants was significantly associated with total delay in TB treatment. Patients who dwell in the rural areas were more likely to delay for TB treatment than the urban inhabitants. This finding is in line with previous studies done in Nigeria [25] and south west Ethiopia [26]. This may be due to transportation problem, lack of money for transportation, poor access health facilities, and lack of health information about TB.

Educational status was also found as another important predicting variable which showed significant association with total delay for TB treatment. The odds of delay among participants who are illiterate, read and write only, and attend primary school only were higher than participants who attended college level and above of education. Hence, being at a higher level of education is a protective variable for delay in TB treatment. This study finding is supported by other studies done in South Africa [9], Dares salaam Tanzania [10], Nigeria [26], and Norway [27]. This could be due to the fact that patients with low educational status would have low level of comprehensive knowledge needed to prevent TB and seek medical care while got infected with TB.

The other determinant variable that showed significant association with total delay for TB treatment was the monthly income of participants. The odds of delay for TB treatment of participants who got less than 500 ETB per month were six times higher than participants who got 1500 ETB and more per month. This finding is in line with other reports done in North West Ethiopia [28]. Patients who did not have adequate income face difficulty to seek health care facilities at the early stage of the disease due to different reasons like fear of medical expenses and transport costs. Hence, they tend to delay for TB treatment.

The odds of delay in TB treatment among those who visited traditional healers before they start ant TB medication were about four times higher than those who contacted health care providers while they manifest symptoms of TB. This finding is concurrent with a report done in southeast Ethiopia [21]. In fact, traditional healers have their own role on providing health services to the community; however, there is longer waiting time to get relief after taking traditional medicines, and most of the healers are neither accredited nor have curable treatment for TB so clients will spend longer time to visit health facilities, and most of them arrive at health facilities with advanced stage of TB.

The types of health facility first consulted by study participants was another variable that showed significantly associated with delay for TB treatment. Study participants who first consulted health post and health center were less likely to delay for TB treatment than those who visited public hospitals initially. However, this finding is in contrast to other study report which was done in Afar region, Ethiopia [22]. This result might be due to the community health network that enhances detection and referral of patients who were suspected to have TB to the appropriate level of diagnosis. On top of this, public hospitals would have high burden of client flow that leads to poor quality of health service and delayed TB diagnosis and initiation of treatment as compared to lower level health facilities; as a result, patients would not prefer to visit hospitals at their first instance of development of TB symptoms.

On the contrary, variables such as age, sex, occupation, type of TB, HIV status, distance to the public health facility, knowledge about TB, and perceived stigma did not show significant association in this study. Similarly, a study conducted in Brazil revealed age and gender had no association with delay in TB treatment [29]; however, studies done in Vietnam [8], south east Ethiopia [11], and Syrian Arab [21] showed a significant association between age and gender.

5. Conclusion and Recommendations

In this study, the proportion of delay in tuberculosis treatment was low as compared to other studies but significant numbers of clients delayed to reach at health facilities get appropriate diagnostic service and receive anti-TB medication. Being a rural residence, lower level of education, low economy, visiting traditional healers during the onset of symptoms, and consulting health post and health center other than public hospital were found to be determinant factors of delay for TB treatment. Though the proportion of delay was low as compared to other studies, still, there is a need to strengthen early detection, diagnosis, and treatment strategies on tuberculosis infection to further minimize complications and spread of the disease. Providing regular health education to the community about TB infection emphasizes the rural community and promotes health professionals mass campaign on TB prevention is mandatory. Strengthening

TABLE 2: The proportion of delays in tuberculosis treatment among DOTS patients at Debremarkos PHF, North West Ethiopia, 2018.

Type of delays	Duration of delays	Gender		Median	IQR	Min	Max
		Male	Female				
Patient delays	<20 days	87	87	20	15-20	12	60
	≥20 days	57	69				
Health system delays	<4 days	99	98	4	3-5	1	9
	≥4 days	45	58				
Total delays	<23 days	76	79	23	19-28	13	64
	≥23 days	68	77				

TABLE 3: The result of logistic regression showing association of variables with total delay for TB treatment at Debremarkos town public health facilities, North West Ethiopia, 2018.

Variables	Categories	Total Rx delay		COR (95% CI)	AOR (95% CI)	*P* value
		Yes	No			
Age	<20 years	10	14	1	1	
	20-39 years	86	101	1.19 (0.5, 2.8)	0.690 (0.2, 2.35)	0.553
	≥40 years	49	40	1.72 (0.69, 4.27)	0.68 (0.16, 2.7)	0.591
Residence	Rural	68	50	1.85 (1.16, 2.96)	1.141 (1.1, 2.61)	0.001*
	Urban	77	105	1	1	
Educational	No education	56	43	1.97 (1.1, 3.7)	2.35 (1.6, 2.6)	0.001**
	Read and write	19	11	2.62 (1.1, 6.4)	1.519 (1.3, 7.4)	0.045*
	Primary school	19	11	2.62 (1.1, 6.4)	2.186 (1.5, 9.1)	0.020*
	2ndry school	24	49	0.74 (0.37, 1.48)	0.71 (0.24, 2.1)	0.52
	College+	27	41	1	1	
Income	≤500	44	44	1.62 (0.87, 3.02)	6.37 (1.73, 23.4)	0.005*
	501-1500	72	64	1.82 (1.03, 3.23)	1.44 (0.58, 3.6)	0.440
	≥1501	29	47	1	1	
First actions taken	Consult HCP	113	132	1	1	
	Self-medication	4	4	1.17 (0.29, 4.77)	1.02 (0.21, 5.06)	0.976
	Visit traditional healers	15	6	2.92 (1.09, 7.77)	4.475 (1.2, 16.6)	0.025*
	Use nonprescribed drugs	13	13	1.167 (0.5, 2.63)	1.08 (0.38, 3.04)	0.88
HF first consulted	Health post	5	9	0.327 (0.10, 1.0)	0.101 (0.02, 0.5)	0.005*
	Health center	66	102	0.381 (0.23, 0.6)	0.31 (0.17, 0.57)	0.001**
	Public hospital	73	43	1	1	

*Significant association (*P* value less than 0.05); **significant at less than 0.01.

health care professional's capacity and technique of early case detection, diagnosis, and treatment; enhancing quality of care in the health facilities; and integrating traditional healers with formal health care system to build a structured referral system of patients are important implications which reduce delays of TB treatment and achieve national TB control program.

6. Limitation of the Study

Since information regarding date of onset of tuberculosis symptoms is based on participants' self-report, recall bias may occur. The study does not address some sensitive issues that need to be touched with qualitative design. This study does not include rural health facilities; as a result, its generalizability is in question.

Authors' Contributions

The authors have contributed in the conception, study design, acquisition of data, analysis, and interpretation of data and drafting of the manuscript.

Acknowledgments

The authors would like to acknowledge the DOTS health facilities in Debremarkos town; all study participants, all data collectors, and all the respective administrators of health institutions; and the University of Gondar for its financial support. The university has covered the cost of data collection, entry, and other related material costs.

References

[1] D. G. Datiko, M. A. Yassin, S. J. Theobald et al., "Health extension workers improve tuberculosis case finding and treatment outcome in Ethiopia: a large-scale implementation study," *BMJ Global Health*, vol. 2, no. 4, article e000390, 2017.

[2] A. H. Kebede, Z. Alebachew, F. Tsegaye et al., "The first population-based national tuberculosis prevalence survey in Ethiopia, 2010-2011," *The International Journal of Tuberculosis and Lung Disease*, vol. 18, no. 6, pp. 635–639, 2014.

[3] D. M. Needham, S. D. Foster, G. Tomlinson, and P. Godfrey-Faussett, "Socio-economic, gender and health services factors affecting diagnostic delay for tuberculosis patients in urban Zambia," *Tropical Medicine & International Health*, vol. 6, no. 4, pp. 256–259, 2001.

[4] S. E. Saqib, M. M. Ahmad, C. Amezcua-Prieto, and M.-R. Virginia, "Treatment delay among pulmonary tuberculosis patients within the Pakistan national tuberculosis control program," *The American Journal of Tropical Medicine and Hygiene*, vol. 99, no. 1, pp. 143–149, 2018.

[5] C. Chang and A. Esterman, "Diagnostic delay among pulmonary tuberculosis patients in Sarawak, Malaysia: a cross-sectional study," *Rural & Remote Health*, vol. 7, no. 2, 2007.

[6] S. Khazaei, M. A. Mansournia, S. Nematollahi et al., "Determinants of delay in tuberculosis diagnosis in Hamadan province, 2006–2014," *Egyptian Journal of Chest Diseases and Tuberculosis*, vol. 65, no. 4, pp. 811–815, 2016.

[7] World Health Organization, Regional Office for the Eastern Mediterranean, *Diagnostic and Treatment Delay in Tuberculosis*, 2006, https://apps.who.int/iris/handle/10665/116501.

[8] N. T. Huong, M. Vree, B. D. Duong et al., "Delays in the diagnosis and treatment of tuberculosis patients in Vietnam: a cross-sectional study," *BMC Public Health*, vol. 7, no. 1, p. 110, 2007.

[9] G. Meintjes, H. Schoeman, C. Morroni, D. Wilson, and G. Maartens, "Patient and provider delay in tuberculosis suspects from communities with a high HIV prevalence in South Africa: a cross-sectional study," *BMC Infectious Diseases*, vol. 8, no. 1, p. 72, 2008.

[10] S. G. Mfinanga, B. K. Mutayoba, A. Kahwa et al., "The magnitude and factors associated with delays in management of smear positive tuberculosis in Dar es Salaam, Tanzania," *BMC Health Services Research*, vol. 8, no. 1, p. 158, 2008.

[11] F. Maamari, "Case-Finding Tuberculosis Patients: Diagnostic and Treatment Delays and Their Determinants," *Eastern Mediterranean Health Journal*, vol. 4, no. 3, pp. 531–545, 2008.

[12] R. Basnet, S. G. Hinderaker, D. Enarson, P. Malla, and O. Mørkve, "Delay in the diagnosis of tuberculosis in Nepal," *BMC Public Health*, vol. 9, no. 1, p. 236, 2009.

[13] E. R. Wandwalo and O. Mørkve, "Delay in tuberculosis case-finding and treatment in Mwanza, Tanzania," *The International Journal of Tuberculosis and Lung Disease*, vol. 4, no. 2, pp. 133–138, 2000.

[14] M. Lambert and P. Van Der Stuyft, *Delays to Tuberculosis Treatment: Shall We Continue to Blame the Victim?*, Blackwell Publishing, 2005.

[15] M. S. Kiwuwa, K. Charles, and M. K. Harriet, "Patient and health service delay in pulmonary tuberculosis patients attending a referral hospital: a cross-sectional study," *BMC Public Health*, vol. 5, no. 1, p. 122, 2005.

[16] E. S. Ngadaya, G. S. Mfinanga, E. R. Wandwalo, and O. Morkve, "Delay in tuberculosis case detection in Pwani region, Tanzania. A cross sectional study," *Bmc Health Services Research*, vol. 9, no. 1, p. 196, 2009.

[17] C. T. Sreeramareddy, Z. Z. Qin, S. Satyanarayana, R. Subbaraman, and M. Pai, "Delays in diagnosis and treatment of pulmonary tuberculosis in India: a systematic review," *The International Journal of Tuberculosis and Lung Disease*, vol. 18, no. 3, pp. 255–266, 2014.

[18] Z. Bursac, C. H. Gauss, D. K. Williams, and D. W. Hosmer, "Purposeful selection of variables in logistic regression," *Source Code for Biology and Medicine*, vol. 3, no. 1, p. 17, 2008.

[19] E. Buregyeya, B. Criel, F. Nuwaha, and R. Colebunders, "Delays in diagnosis and treatment of pulmonary tuberculosis in Wakiso and Mukono districts, Uganda," *Bmc Public Health*, vol. 14, no. 1, p. 586, 2014.

[20] A. Asefa and W. Teshome, "Total delay in treatment among smear positive pulmonary tuberculosis patients in five primary health centers, southern Ethiopia: a cross sectional study," *Plos One*, vol. 9, no. 7, article e102884, 2014.

[21] A. Hussen, S. Biadgilign, F. Tessema, S. Mohammed, K. Deribe, and A. Deribew, "Treatment delay among pulmonary tuberculosis patients in pastoralist communities in Bale Zone, Southeast Ethiopia," *BMC Research Notes*, vol. 5, no. 1, p. 320, 2012.

[22] M. Belay, G. Bjune, G. Ameni, and F. Abebe, "Diagnostic and treatment delay among tuberculosis patients in Afar region, Ethiopia: a cross-sectional study," *BMC Public Health*, vol. 12, no. 1, p. 369, 2012.

[23] L. Makwakwa, M.-l. Sheu, C.-Y. Chiang, S.-L. Lin, and P. W. Chang, "Patient and health system delays in the diagnosis and treatment of new and retreatment pulmonary tuberculosis cases in Malawi," *BMC Infectious Diseases*, vol. 14, no. 1, p. 132, 2014.

[24] K. C. Takarinda, A. D. Harries, B. Nyathi, M. Ngwenya, T. Mutasa-Apollo, and C. Sandy, "Tuberculosis treatment delays and associated factors within the Zimbabwe national tuberculosis programme," *BMC Public Health*, vol. 15, no. 1, p. 29, 2015.

[25] A. Tegegn and M. Yazachew, "Delays in tuberculosis treatment and associated factors in Jimma Zone, Southwest Ethiopia," *Ethiopian Journal of Health Sciences*, vol. 19, no. 1, 2009.

[26] K. N. Ukwaja, I. Alobu, C. O. Nweke, and E. C. Onyenwe, "Healthcare-seeking behavior, treatment delays and its determinants among pulmonary tuberculosis patients in rural Nigeria: a cross-sectional study," *BMC Health Services Research*, vol. 13, no. 1, p. 25, 2013.

[27] D. G. Storla, S. Yimer, and G. A. Bjune, "A systematic review of delay in the diagnosis and treatment of tuberculosis," *BMC Public Health*, vol. 8, no. 1, p. 15, 2008.

[28] S. Bogale, E. Diro, A. M. Shiferaw, and M. K. Yenit, "Factors associated with the length of delay with tuberculosis diagnosis and treatment among adult tuberculosis patients attending at public health facilities in Gondar town, Northwest, Ethiopia," *BMC Infectious Diseases*, vol. 17, no. 1, p. 145, 2017.

[29] M. M. de Loureiro, R. L. Guerra, M. Cailleaux-Cezar, J. E. Golub, and M. B. Conde, "Time from symptom onset to the initiation of treatment of pulmonary tuberculosis in a city with a high incidence of the disease," *Jornal Brasileiro de Pneumologia*, vol. 38, no. 2, pp. 202–209, 2012.

3

Diagnostic Yield of Fluorescence and Ziehl-Neelsen Staining Techniques in the Diagnosis of Pulmonary Tuberculosis: A Comparative Study in a District Health Facility

Eben Godsway Dzodanu,[1] Justice Afrifa,[1,2] Desmond Omane Acheampong,[3] and Isaac Dadzie[1]

[1] *Department of Medical Laboratory Science, University of Cape Coast, Cape Coast, Ghana*
[2] *Scientific Research Center, The Second Affiliated Hospital of Harbin Medical University, Harbin, China*
[3] *Department of Biomedical Sciences, University of Cape Coast, Cape Coast, Ghana*

Correspondence should be addressed to Isaac Dadzie; idadzie@ucc.edu.gh

Academic Editor: Amit Kaushik

Background. Despite the recent advancement in diagnostic methods, the smear microscopy remains the gold standard for the diagnosis of pulmonary tuberculosis in high burden countries like Ghana. Notwithstanding, fluorescence staining technique provides a more efficient option for the detection of *Mycobacterium tuberculosis* positive smears. This study therefore aimed at assessing the diagnostic performance of fluorescence microscopy (FM) and Ziehl-Neelsen (ZN) staining techniques in the diagnosis of pulmonary tuberculosis. *Methods.* A comparative study was carried out on 100 patients who reported at the Out Patients Department (OPD) or the Directly Observed Therapy (DOT) center of the Kade Government Hospital and were suspected of having pulmonary tuberculosis. Two (2) sputum samples each were collected. This included one spot and one morning sample. The smears were prepared and stained with FM and ZN staining techniques. Xpert MTB/RIF assay was also performed. *Results.* Of the 200 samples analyzed, 71 (35.5%), 46 (23.0%), and 84 (42.0%) were positive for pulmonary tuberculosis when FM, ZN, and XPERT MTB/RIF assays were used, respectively. The mean reading time of FM was three times faster than the ZN technique with very good acceptance (1.5min: 4.6min). The sensitivity and specificity of fluorescent staining to that of XPERT MTB/RIF assay were 84.5% and 100%, respectively, while those of ZN staining were 54.8% and 100%, respectively. *Conclusion.* For a routine laboratory test in a resource-limited setting, our study has demonstrated that fluorescence staining technique is a more sensitive test for the diagnosis of pulmonary tuberculosis as compared to the conventional ZN technique.

1. Introduction

Tuberculosis caused by *Mycobacterium tuberculosis* remains a major public health problem with approximately one-third of the world's population affected. In 2017, 10 million people were infected with tuberculosis and 1.6 million died from the disease. Over 95% of tuberculosis deaths occur in low- and middle-income countries.[1].

A faster, simpler, more accurate, and less expensive means of diagnosis of tuberculosis is necessary for the control of people infected with the disease as wells as preventing its spread in the community [2]. Various investigations can be used to help in the diagnosis of tuberculosis, and these include chest radiographs, clinical suspicion, staining for acid-fast bacilli, culture for mycobacteria, and nucleic acid amplification assays. Sputum smear microscopy is the most preferred and rapid test that is widely used for the detection and diagnosis of pulmonary tuberculosis [2, 3]. The bacilli in the sputum can be detected either by ZN or fluorescence staining techniques. Sputum microscopy is helpful to assess the response to treatment and to establish a cure or failure at the end of treatment.

In many developing countries, the diagnosis of tuberculosis is mostly based on the ZN staining technique [4]. The sensitivity of sputum smear microscopy by ZN method, however, is reported to be low and variable, ranging from 20%

to 80%, often depending on the diligence with which specimens are collected, smears are made, and stained smears are examined [4–7]. This procedure leaves a significant number of cases undetected, especially if it becomes the only means of diagnosis. FM was introduced to improve the outcomes of sputum smear microscopy. The sensitivity of conventional FM provides far better yield and detection of positive smears than the ZN and takes less time to perform [8–10]. There is however a lingering doubt about the specificity of FM as there is the possibility of false positives which may be due to the incorporation of fluorochrome dyes by inorganic objects [11, 12]. Additionally, cost constraint is a limitation of the FM [13] especially, in a low to medium income countries such as Ghana.

In Ghana, diagnosis of pulmonary tuberculosis has involved the use of conventional light microscopy to examine ZN stained direct smears. The FM is gradually replacing ZN stained smear microscopy, while the use of molecular techniques for TB diagnosis is mainly limited to the teaching and regional hospitals. There is currently no documented evidence in the country evaluating the application of the techniques for the diagnosis of pulmonary tuberculosis. Hence, this study compares the diagnostic efficacy of these three methods for the detection of pulmonary diagnosis of tuberculosis.

2. Materials and Methods

This prospective study was carried out at Kade Government Hospital in the Eastern Region by trained biomedical scientists. Samples were collected between 08:00 am and 12:00 noon each day. The study population consisted of patients suspected of pulmonary tuberculosis and have reported at the OPD/DOT center of the Kade Government Hospital. A total of 100 patients were recruited for the study.

2.1. Sample Collection and Preparation. The study subjects (hundred patients) were requested to submit two sputum samples each in a clean, sterile, leak-proof, wide-mouth containers. In total, 200 samples were collected. One sample from each patient was taken on the spot and the subjects were provided with a second prelabeled container for a morning sample to be taken at home. Preparation of smear for staining was done as described elsewhere [14]. For each sample, the smears were made in duplicate. Positive and negative control smears were also prepared.

2.2. Ziehl-Neelsen (ZN) Staining Procedure. The smears were arranged in serial order on staining bridge, with smear side up and flooded with filtered 0.1% Carbol Fuchsin. The smears were steamed and allowed to stain for 5 minutes, rinsed with water, and drained. They were decolorized with 25% sulphuric acid for 5 minutes, rinsed with water, and drained. They were then counterstained with 0.1% methylene blue solution for 1 minute and rinsed with water. The smear was allowed to air dry and examined microscopically using the oil immersion (100x) objective.

2.3. Fluorescence Microscopy Staining Procedure. The smears were flooded with filtered 0.1% auramine for at least 20 minutes. They were then rinsed with water and drained. Acid alcohol decolorizing solution (0.5%) was applied on the smear for 30 to 60 seconds, rinsed with water, and drained. They were then flooded with 0.5% potassium permanganate counterstain for a maximum of 1 minute and rinsed with water. The smears were allowed to air dry and examined microscopically using the dry (40x) objective lens of an LED illumination-based fluorescence microscope (Zeiss primo star iLED).

2.4. Xpert MTB/RIF Assay Procedure. Xpert MTB/ RIF assay was performed following the protocol of the manufacturer (Cepheid Inc., Sunnyvale, CA, USA). Samples were collected in containers provided and treated with sample reagent in a proportion of 2:1 and incubated for 15 minutes at room temperature. Two milliliters (2 ml) of the reagent treated sample was pipetted into the sample chamber of the Xpert cartridge. The Xpert cartridge was then placed into the GeneXpert instrument system and run. Results were generated after 90 min.

2.5. Ethical Consideration. Study approval was sought from the authorities of the Kade Government Hospital. Written informed consent was sought from all participants before recruitment. Records were kept strictly confidential.

3. Data Analysis

Data were entered in Microsoft, and the statistical analysis was performed using SPSS software, version 23.0 (IBM Inc.). Data were expressed in percentages for the different variables. Kappa test was used to determine the correlation between diagnostic tests and the receiver operating characteristic curve was used to determine the sensitivity and specificity of tests. P-value <0.05 was considered statistically significant. Xpert MTB/RIF assay was taken as reference when ZN and fluorescence microscopy tests were compared. Samples that were positive and negative by GeneXpert were considered true positive and true negative.

4. Results

A total of 200 samples received from 100 individuals were screened for the presence of acid-fast bacilli (AFB) using the ZN and fluorescence microscopy staining techniques. In the absence of culture, Xpert MTB/RIF, which amplifies and detects specific gene target of *Mycobacterium tuberculosis,* was used as a reference.

Table 1 shows the results of the diagnostic tests used in the study. Of the 200 samples analyzed, 46 (23.0%), 71 (35.5%), and 84 (42.0%) were positive for pulmonary tuberculosis when ZN staining, fluorescence staining, and Xpert MTB/RIF assay were used, respectively. Of the 100 subjects recruited for the study, FM yielded 37 (37%) whereas ZN staining identified 25 (25%) of them to be infected with the AFB.

TABLE 1: Comparison of diagnostic tests used.

	Fluorescent staining			Ziehl-Neelsen staining		Xpert MTB/Rif	
	Spot (N=100)	EM (N=100)	(N=200)	Spot (N=100)	EM (N=100)	(N=200)	(N=200)
Positive	34(34)	37(37)	71 (35.5)	21(21)	25(25)	46 (23.0)	84 (42.0)
Negative	66(66)	63(63)	129 (64.5)	79(79)	75(75)	154 (77.0)	116 (58.0)
				Sputum Grading			
Scanty			12 (6.0)		2 (1.0)		
1+			20 (10.0)		10 (5.0)		
2+			21 (10.5)		24 (12.0)		
3+			18 (9.0)		10 (5.0)		

Data is represented in raw figures and percentages. EM: early morning sample.

TABLE 2: Correlation of fluorescence and ZN staining techniques with Xpert MTB/Rif.

Staining Technique	XPERT MTB/Rif Positive	XPERT MTB/Rif Negative	Kappa	P-value	PPV (%)	NPV (%)
Fluorescence						
Positive	71 (84.5)	0 (0.0)	0.864	p≤0.001	100	92.1
Negative	13 (15.5)	116 (100)				
ZN						
Positive	46 (54.8)	0 (0.0)	0.584	p≤0.001	100	77.3
Negative	38 (45.2)	116 (100)				

Data is represented in raw figures and percentages. P-value is statistically significant if $p < 0.05$ as compared between Xpert MTB/Rif and fluorescence microscopy, Xpert MTB/Rif and ZN.

Table 2 compares the results of ZN and fluorescence staining with the Xpert MTB/RIF test. Of the 84 positive samples, 38 (45.2%) were missed by ZN staining technique and 13 (15.5%) were missed by FM. Both fluorescence and ZN staining techniques showed a positive correlation with Xpert MTB/RIF diagnostic technique; however, fluorescent staining had a stronger correlation compared to ZN staining (kappa=0.864, p≤0.001 versus kappa=0.584, p≤0.001). It could also be observed that all the samples that were negative by Xpert MTB/RIF test were also negative by both ZN and fluorescence staining.

Tables 3 and 4 compare the diagnostic performance of ZN to that of FM. Fluorescence staining showed a positive correlation with ZN staining technique (kappa=0.680, p≤0.001). It could be seen that 25 (35.2%) of the samples that were positive by fluorescence microscopy were missed by ZN staining whereas only 1 (0.8%) sample that was positive by the ZN staining was negative by FM. The two tests had the same specificity (100%); however, the sensitivity of fluorescent staining (84.5%) was higher than that of ZN staining (54.8). The ROC analysis (Figure 1) also proved fluorescent staining (AUC= 0.923) to be a better diagnostic test than ZN staining (AUC= 0.774), when the tests were compared to the reference.

Table 5 shows the comparison of the diagnostic yield of spot and early morning sputum samples as stained by fluorescence and ZN staining techniques. Of the 37 early morning samples that tested positive for AFB, 34 (91.8%) of their corresponding spot samples also tested positive with 3(8.1%) testing negative when fluorescent staining technique was used. There was a strong agreement between early

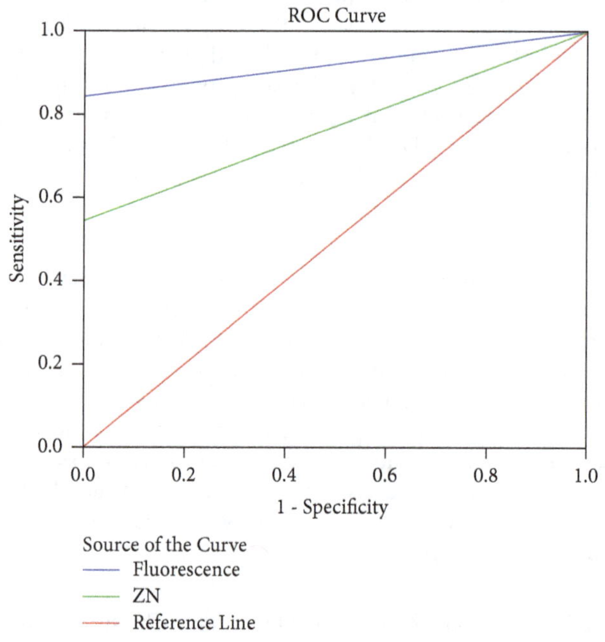

FIGURE 1: Receiver operator characteristic curve.

morning and spot samples as indicated by the Cohens Kappa (0.935); however, the difference was statistically significant ($p<0.05$). Also, of the 25 early morning samples that tested positive for AFB, 21 (84.0%) of their corresponding spot

TABLE 3: Comparison of diagnostic performance of fluorescence staining to ZN staining.

ZN	Fluorescence		Kappa	P-value
	Positive	Negative		
Positive	46 (64.8)	1 (0.8)	0.680	p≤0.001
Negative	25 (35.2)	128 (99.2)		

Data is represented in raw figures and percentages. P-value is statistically significant if $p < 0.05$ as compared between FM and ZN.

TABLE 4: Receiver operator characteristic (ROC) curve parameters.

Technique	Sensitivity	Specificity	AUC	95%CI	P-value
Fluorescence	84.5%	100%	0.923	0.876-0.969	p≤0.001
ZN	54.8%	100%	0.774	0.702-0.846	p≤0.001

Xpert MTB/Rif used as reference diagnostic test; AUC: area under curve. Data is represented in percentages. P-value is statistically significant if $p < 0.05$ as compared between Xpert MTB/Rif and fluorescence microscopy, Xpert MTB/Rif, and Ziehl-Neelsen.

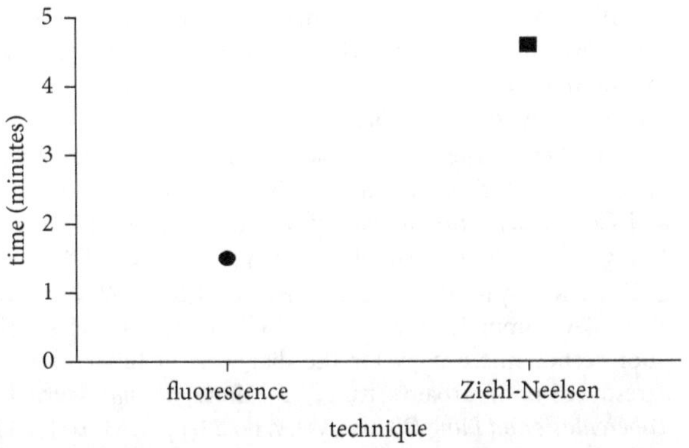

FIGURE 2: Average time taken to observe fluorescence and ZN stained smears.

samples also tested positive with 4 (16.0%) testing negative when ZN staining technique was used.

The mean reading time of fluorescent staining technique was three times faster than the ZN technique with very good acceptance (1.5 min: 4.6 min) (Figure 2)

5. Discussion

Growth detection of AFB in culture considered the most sensitive method for diagnosis of TB is not routinely done in our health facilities mainly due to the slow growth of the bacteria and the lack of equipment required for the test. Prompt diagnosis of TB, therefore, is achieved by AFB smear microscopy, mostly by the ZN technique and recently by the fluorescence microscopy and the Xpert MTB/RIF in few facilities that have them. We compared the results of ZN stain smear and fluorescence staining with Xpert MTB/RIF test for detection of AFB in sputum samples.

Results of this study demonstrated that Xpert MTB/RIF diagnosed approximately 15% more of the 200 samples screened than FM and as high as 45% more than ZN. The superior performance of Xpert MTB/RIF over fluorescence and ZN microscopy in the diagnosis of pulmonary tuberculosis has been established in many studies [15–18]. Also, FM produced a higher diagnostic yield compared to that of ZN staining technique among our study samples. This finding confirms the previously reported superior performance of FM over the conventional ZN technique for AFB detection [19–21]. Comparatively, the fluorescence microscopy generated readings at a rate that is approximately three times faster than ZN technique, thus helping save approximately 2 minutes per slide (66%) which corroborate findings of a study conducted by Marais, Brittle [22]. Therefore, the introduction of LED-FM would be time-saving and allow for quality microscopy.

The study revealed a higher percentage of false negatives from ZN staining technique (45.2%) as compared to FM (15.5%) and this is consistent with a study carried out in Sinamangal, Nepal [19], which showed that the percentage of false negative by FM staining was only 2.78%, and was in sharp contrast to that of ZN (40.27%). FM was also able to detect more paucibacillary cases than ZN. The better case detection rates of FM over ZN were comparable to reports found in several studies [8, 23–25].

A significant benchmark for an alternative diagnostic method is its ability to establish a linear relationship with the gold standard. Interestingly, both FM and ZN techniques correlated positively with Xpert MTB/RIF diagnostic technique. Fluorescent staining, however, showed a stronger linear relationship as compared to ZN staining (kappa=0.864, p≤0.001 versus kappa=0584, p≤0.001). Elsewhere, Stella et al. observed similar findings when both the FM and ZN techniques were compared to the PCR method (kappa FM versus PCR=0.60; ZN versus PCR=0.54) [26].

In an ideal situation, a diagnostic technique should be 100% specific and 100% sensitive. Our results indicated that both the ZN and FM techniques showed similar specificity (100%) when compared to that of Xpert MTB/RIF; however, in relation to Xpert MTB/RIF, FM (84.5%) was more sensitive than ZN staining (54.8%). In general, it has been reported that, in the diagnosis of pulmonary tuberculosis, the fluorescence staining technique provides better sensitivity and specificity when compared to the ZN [27, 28].

This study showed that, in both FM and ZN staining techniques, early morning samples yielded more AFB as compared to spot samples. Interestingly, sputum samples positive for smear collected at the spot were also positive for

TABLE 5: Comparison of diagnostic yield of "spot" and "early morning" sputum samples.

Spot	EM Positive	EM Negative	Kappa	P value
Fluorescence				
Positive	34(91.8)	0(0.0)	0.935	p≤0.001
Negative	3(8.1)	63(100.0)		
ZN				
Positive	21(84.0)	0(0.0)	0.887	p≤0.001
Negative	4(16.0)	75(100.0)		

Data is represented in raw figures and percentages. P-value is statistically significant if p< 0.05 as compared between "spot" and "early morning (EM)" sputum samples. EM: early morning.

samples collected early in the morning. This agrees with a study carried out by Myneedu et al. and which showed that the first sputum sample (spot sample) collected immediately in the vicinity of the laboratory showed a reduced smear positivity as compared to morning samples. Similarly, they also reported that all AFB positive spot samples were also positive for AFB in the early morning smears [29]. To reduce diagnostic defaulting, this result calls for a second look at the standard 2-day protocol of collecting samples on two consecutive days for diagnosis of pulmonary tuberculosis. Early morning samples prove to be ideal when onetime sample collection is to be adopted.

In conclusion, our findings show the FM technique to be of a more diagnostic value compared with the ZN technique. It is more sensitive and can detect accurately paucibacillary cases and this has implication on early treatment of pulmonary tuberculosis.

Disclosure

The authors did not receive funding from any funding body. The research was performed as part of the employment of the authors from the University of Cape Coast.

References

[1] Organization WH, "Global tuberculosis report 2018," Tech. Rep., Geneva, Switzerland, 2018.

[2] Organization WH, "Early detection of tuberculosis: an overview of approaches, guidelines and tools," Tech. Rep., World Health Organization, Geneva, Switzerland, 2011.

[3] P. C. Hopewell, M. Pai, D. Maher, M. Uplekar, and M. C. Raviglione, "International standards for tuberculosis care," *The Lancet Infectious Diseases*, vol. 6, no. 11, pp. 710–725, 2006.

[4] Y. J. Ryu, "Diagnosis of pulmonary tuberculosis: recent advances and diagnostic algorithms," *Tuberculosis and Respiratory Diseases*, vol. 78, no. 2, pp. 64–71, 2015.

[5] K. R. Steingart, A. Ramsay, and M. Pai, "Optimizing sputum smear microscopy for the diagnosis of pulmonary tuberculosis," *Expert Review of Anti-infective Therapy*, vol. 5, no. 3, pp. 327–331, 2007.

[6] R. A. Cohen, S. Muzaffar, D. Schwartz et al., "Diagnosis of pulmonary tuberculosis using PCR assays on sputum collected within 24 hours of hospital admission," *American Journal of Respiratory and Critical Care Medicine*, vol. 157, no. 1, pp. 156–161, 1998.

[7] P. Mathew, Y.-H. Kuo, B. Vazirani, R. H. K. Eng, and M. P. Weinstein, "Are three sputum acid-fast bacillus smears necessary for discontinuing tuberculosis isolation?" *Journal of Clinical Microbiology*, vol. 40, no. 9, pp. 3482–3484, 2002.

[8] T. Hänscheid, "The future looks bright: low-cost fluorescent microscopes for detection of Mycobacterium tuberculosis and Coccidiae," *Transactions of the Royal Society of Tropical Medicine and Hygiene*, vol. 102, no. 6, pp. 520-521, 2008.

[9] L. E. A. Kivihya-Ndugga, M. R. A. Van Cleeff, W. A. Githui et al., "A comprehensive comparison of Ziehi-Neelsen and fluorescence microscopy for the diagnosis of tuberculosis in a resource-poor urban setting," *The International Journal of Tuberculosis and Lung Disease*, vol. 7, no. 12, pp. 1163–1171, 2003.

[10] P. Bell, "Fluorescence microscopy in the laboratory diagnosis and assessment of pulmonary tuberculosis," *Central African Journal of Medicine*, vol. 8, no. 1, pp. 4–9, 1962.

[11] J. C. Boyd and J. J. Marr, "Decreasing reliability of acid fast smear techniques for detection of tuberculosis," *Annals of Internal Medicine*, vol. 82, no. 4, pp. 489–492, 1975.

[12] G. P. Kubica, "Correlation of acid-fast staining methods with culture results for mycobacteria," *Bulletin of the International Union against Tuberculosis*, vol. 55, no. 3-4, pp. 117–124, 1980.

[13] K. R. Steingart, M. Henry, V. Ng et al., "Fluorescence versus conventional sputum smear microscopy for tuberculosis: a systematic review," *The Lancet Infectious Diseases*, vol. 6, no. 9, pp. 570–581, 2006.

[14] D. A. Mitchison, "Standard smears for grading the content of acid-fast bacilli in sputum," *Tuberculosis*, vol. 47, no. 3, pp. 289–291, 1966.

[15] M. K. Munir, S. Rehman, M. Aasim, R. Iqbal, and S. Saeed, "Comparison of Ziehl Neelson microscopy with GeneXpert for detection of Mycobacterium tuberculosis," *IOSR Journal of Dental and Medical Sciences*, vol. 14, no. 11, pp. 56–60, 2015.

[16] R. Bajrami, G. Mulliqi, A. Kurti, G. Lila, and L. Raka, "Comparison of genexpert MTB/RIF and conventional methods for the diagnosis of tuberculosis in Kosovo," *The Journal of Infection in Developing Countries*, vol. 10, no. 4, pp. 418–422, 2016.

[17] G. Alvarez-Uria, J. M. Azcona, M. Midde, P. K. Naik, S. Reddy, and R. Reddy, "Rapid diagnosis of pulmonary and extrapulmonary tuberculosis in HIV-infected patients. comparison of LED fluorescent microscopy and the GeneXpert MTB/RIF assay in a district hospital in India," *Tuberculosis Research and Treatment*, vol. 2012, Article ID 932862, 4 pages, 2012.

[18] A. E. M. Ahmed, N. Yousif, M. ELhassan et al., "Diagnostic perfomance of ziehl-neelsen, flourescent auramine O stains and Genexpert for the detection of mycobacterium tuberculosis," *IOSR Journal of Dental and Medical Sciences*, vol. 17, no. 2, 2018.

[19] S. Laifangbam, H. L. Singh, N. B. Singh, K. M. Devi, and N. T. Singh, "A comparative study of fluorescent microscopy with Ziehl-Neelsen staining and culture for the diagnosis of pulmonary tuberculosis," *Kathmandu University Medical Journal*, vol. 7, no. 27, pp. 226–230, 2009.

[20] A. O. Nazar, A. M. Mustafa, k. H. Mona, and M. T. Mohamed, "Comparative study of auramine-O staining and Ziehl-Neelsen for diagnosis of pulmonary tuberculosis," *Natural Science*, vol. 12, no. 11, pp. 59–63, 2014.

[21] N. Van Hung, D. N. Sy, R. M. Anthony, F. G. Cobelens, and D. van Soolingen, "Fluorescence microscopy for tuberculosis diagnosis," *The Lancet Infectious Diseases*, vol. 7, no. 4, pp. 238-239, 2007.

[22] B. J. Marais, W. Brittle, K. Painczyk et al., "Use of light-emitting diode fluorescence microscopy to detect acid-fast bacilli in sputum," *Clinical Infectious Diseases*, vol. 47, no. 2, pp. 203–207, 2008.

[23] N. P. Singh and S. C. Parija, "The value of fluorescence microscopy of auramine stained sputum smears for the diagnosis of pulmonary tuberculosis," *Southeast Asian Journal of Tropical Medicine and Public Health*, vol. 29, no. 4, pp. 860–863, 1998.

[24] V. Annam, M. Kulkarni, and R. Puranik, "Comparison of the modified fluorescent method and conventional Ziehl-Neelsen method in the detection of acidfast bacilli in lymphnode aspirates," *Cyto Journal*, vol. 6, no. 13, 2009.

[25] K. Prasanthi and A. R. Kumari, "Efficacy of fluorochrome stain in the diagnosis of pulmonary tuberculosis co-infected with HIV," *Indian Journal of Medical Microbiology*, vol. 23, no. 3, pp. 179–181, 2005.

[26] S. S. S. Lima, W. T. Clemente, M. Palaci, R. V. Rosa, C. M. D. F. Antunes, and J. C. Serufo, "Conventional and molecular techniques in the diagnosis of pulmonary tuberculosis: a comparative study," *Jornal Brasileiro de Pneumologia*, vol. 34, no. 12, pp. 1056–1062, 2008.

[27] W. Githui, F. Kitui, E. S. Juma, D. O. Obwana, J. Mwai, and D. Kwamanga, "A comparative study on the reliability of the fluorescence microscopy and Ziehl-Neelsen method in the diagnosis of pulmonary tuberculosis.," *East African Medical Journal*, vol. 70, no. 5, pp. 263–266, 1993.

[28] S. Hooja, N. Pal, B. Malhotra, S. Goyal, V. Kumar, and L. Vyas, "Comparison of Ziehl Neelsen and Auramine O staining methods on direct and concentrated smears in clinical specimens," *Indian Journal of Tuberculosis*, vol. 58, no. 2, pp. 72–76, 2011.

[29] V. P. Myneedu, A. K. Verma, P. P. Sharma, and D. Behera, "A pilot study of same day sputumsmear examination, its feasibility and usefulness in diagnosis of Pulmonary TB," *Indian Journal of Tuberculosis*, vol. 58, no. 4, pp. 160–167, 2011.

4

Pulmonary Tuberculosis among Male Inmates in the Largest Prison of Eastern Nepal

Gambhir Shrestha ,[1] Deepak Kumar Yadav,[2] Rabin Gautam,[3] Rashmi Mulmi,[1] Dharanidhar Baral,[2] and Paras Kumar Pokharel[2]

[1]*Department of Cancer Prevention, Control and Research, B.P. Koirala Memorial Cancer Hospital, Bharatpur, Chitwan, Nepal*
[2]*School of Public Health and Community Medicine, B.P. Koirala Institute of Health Sciences, Dharan, Sunsari, Nepal*
[3]*National Tuberculosis Program, Health Research and Social Development Forum, Thapathali, Kathmandu, Nepal*

Correspondence should be addressed to Gambhir Shrestha; gamvir.stha@gmail.com

Academic Editor: José R. Lapa e Silva

Introduction. The prevalence of Pulmonary Tuberculosis (PTB) is much higher in the prison population than in the general population. This study aims to find out the prevalence of PTB and its associated factors among inmates in eastern Nepal. *Methods.* This cross-sectional study was conducted in Jhumka Regional Prison, the largest male prison of Eastern Nepal from September 2014 to August 2015. Semi-structured questionnaires were used to identify individuals with a cough more than one-week duration among 434 randomly selected inmates. Screening of PTB was done by sputum smear test and/or GeneXpert test. Prevalence of TB was defined as the number of cases detected during the study period divided by the total number of inmates screened during that period. Fisher's exact test was used to find out the association of PTB with related variables. *Results.* A total of 434 inmates were screened for PTB with mean age 35.7 years and body mass index 22.7 kg/m^2. A total of 68 inmates had a productive cough of more than a week and two patients were already on anti-tuberculosis therapy at the time of screening. Sixty sputum samples were considered for sputum smear/GeneXpert test and 6 of them (10%) had positive results. The prevalence of TB in the Prison was 1843/100,000 population. Chest pain and abnormal chest auscultation findings were found to be significantly associated with PTB. *Conclusions.* This study showed that there was a high rate of PTB among inmates in Nepal. The results suggest a need for effective screening of PTB and strategies to improve management including reduction of PTB transmission in the prison.

1. Background

The prevalence of infectious diseases, chronic diseases, blood-borne viruses, and sexually transmitted diseases are much higher in the prison population than in the general population [1–7]. Pulmonary Tuberculosis (PTB) has been reported up to 100 times more in the prison population than the civilian population [8]. First, higher rates of TB in the prison setting has been attributed to prisoners who are from population groups already at high risk of TB infection and disease (addicted to alcohol, drug users, homelessness, living in unfavorable social conditions such as poverty and misery). Second, prisons promote transmission of TB infection through prolonged and repeated exposure due to overcrowding, inadequate ventilation, and late case detection. Third, poor nutritional status and coexisting pathology like HIV in prison predispose them to higher chances of TB transmission [9].

TB is a serious cause of morbidity and mortality in prison among the inmates. The prison system often faces various problems that hinder TB control lack of laboratory facility and other diagnostic tools, interrupted supply and stock out of drugs, inadequate infection control measures, lack of coordination between civilian and prison health services, and low priority for health care to inmates [10].

TB remains a major public health problem in Nepal and is the sixth leading cause of death in the country. With a population of around 30 million, the number of cases registered at National TB Program as of 2015 includes 34121 cases (case notification rate 123/100,000) with approximately

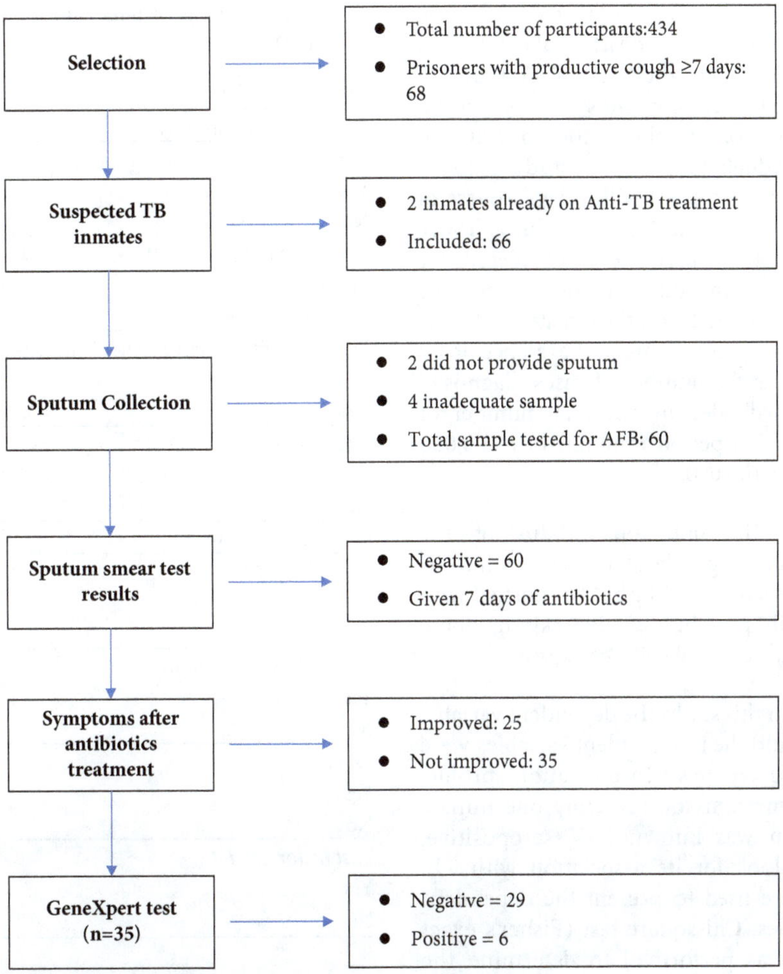

FIGURE 1: Screening of PTB among inmates in the prison.

8000–10,000 cases to be missing every year. As of 2015, the estimated prevalence rate was 211/100,000 population, and with the annual estimated incidence of 158/100000 [11, 12].

Prison is one of the areas where Urban TB control program (DOTS) has been implemented in Nepal; however, there is inadequate human resource along with the absence of a key focal person to look after TB in prisons. Furthermore, there are no surveillance data available regarding tuberculosis in prison setting in Nepal. To our best knowledge, this is the first study of its kind to find out the prevalence and associated factors of PTB in a Nepalese prison.

2. Methods

2.1. Study Setting and Design. Screening of PTB among inmates was conducted in Jhumka Regional Prison, the largest adult male prison in the Eastern Development Region of Nepal from September 2014 to August 2015. The prison capacity is of 1500 prisoners.

2.2. Sampling Technique. This paper is a part of a large study and has followed the methods of Shrestha et al. 2017 [13]. The health needs, risky behaviours, and depression among the inmates of same population have been presented elsewhere [13, 14]. Briefly, out of total 1203 inmates in the prison, 450 were randomly selected, of whom 434 gave consent for the study.

2.3. Ethical Approval. Ethical Review Board approval was obtained from B.P. Koirala Institute of Health Sciences. The Department of Prison Management, Ministry of Home Affairs, Government of Nepal granted permission to conduct study in the prison. Informed written consent from the participants was taken prior to the interview.

2.4. Methods of Data Collection. All eligible participants were interviewed in-person by a community physician, who collected detailed information on socio-demographic characteristics, imprisonment characteristics, substance use disorders, and symptoms of tuberculosis using a semi-structured questionnaire. A detailed clinical examination was also performed.

2.5. Screening for Tuberculosis. Prisoners with a productive cough more than a week were considered TB suspects and two sputum samples (one on-the-spot and second early morning samples) were collected for Ziehl–Neelsen (ZN) sputum smear test. The acid-fast bacilli microscopy was performed by a certified laboratory technician in nearby Baklori Health Post following the guidelines set by the National TB Program (NTP). The NTP guideline recommends use of nonTB antibiotics and restricts use of quinolone group of drugs in chest symptomatic individuals [15]. In this study, patients with negative smear test were treated with 7 days' course of antibiotics (Amoxicillin) as per the NTP guidelines. Those whose symptoms did not improve were considered for GeneXpert test at B.P. Koirala Institute of Health Sciences for suspected sputum smears (Figure 1). All the inmates with PTB were placed on anti-tuberculosis treatment. Prevalence of TB in prison was calculated as the number of cases diagnosed during the study period divided by the total number of inmates screened during that period multiplied by 100,000 and expressed as cases per 100,000.

2.6. Nutritional Status. The nutritional status of the inmates was classified according to body mass index into (i) underweight with BMI less than 18.5 kg/m^2 (ii) normal with range 18.5–24.99 kg/m^2 (iii) pre-obese 25–29.99 kg/m^2, obese class I 30–34.99 kg/m^2 and severe obesity ≥40 kg/m^2.

2.7. Statistical Analysis. In this study, the dependent variable was TB among inmates and the independent variables were sociodemographic characteristics, incarceration profile, substance abuse, and symptoms of TB. Only one inmate in the study population was known HIV seropositive, and hence we did not look for its association with TB. Descriptive statistics were used to present the dependent and independent variables. Chi-square test (Fisher's exact test where applicable) was performed to determine the association of tuberculosis with the independent variables. Statistical Package for Social Sciences (SPSS, version 20) was used for all statistical analyses. A p-value of <0.05 was considered as statistically significant.

Table 1: Symptoms of tuberculosis among inmates in the prison (n = 434).

Symptoms of TB	n (%)
Respiratory symptoms	
Cough	
Yes	172 (39.6)
No	262 (60.4)
Type of cough (n = 172)	
Productive	79 (45.9)
Non-productive	93 (54.1)
Duration of productive cough in days (n = 79)	
<7	11 (13.9)
≥7	68 (86.1)
Chest pain	
Yes	40 (9.2)
No	394 (90.8)
General symptoms	
Loss of appetite	
Yes	181 (42.2)
No	251 (57.8)
Weight loss in 3 months	
Yes	239 (55.1)
No	195 (44.9)
Fever	
Yes	8 (1.8)
No	426 (98.2)
Past history of TB	
Yes	22 (5.1)
No	412 (94.9)

Table 2: Nutritional status of inmates in the prison (n = 434).

Nutritional status (kg/m^2)	n (%)
Underweight (<18.5)	25 (5.8)
Normal (18.5–24.99)	317 (73.0)
Pre-obese (25–29.99)	84 (19.4)
Obese Class I (30–34.99)	8 (1.8)

3. Results

The age of the participants ranged from 18 to 81 years with a mean of 35.73 years (SD 13.25). About 172 (39.6%) of the participating inmates had a cough at the time of interview and 79 (45.9%) of them had the productive type of cough, and among these with productive cough, 68 (86.1%) had a cough of 7 days and more. About 42.2% of the inmates reported recent loss of appetite and more than half (55.1%) reported loss of weight during the last 3 months. Very few (1.8%) had a fever at the time of interview and 9.2% reported of having chest pain. Inmates with a past history of tuberculosis were 5.1% (Table 1).

The mean BMI was found to be 22.76 (SD 2.93) which ranged from 15 to 33 kg/m^2. About three-fourths of the inmates were found to have normal range of BMI while only 6% were underweight, 19% were pre-obese and 2% were Obese class I (Table 2).

A total of 68 inmates had a productive cough ≥7 days of which two were already on anti-tuberculosis therapy and hence 66 inmates were suspected of TB. Two inmates did not provide a sputum sample so 64 inmates were considered for sputum smear/GeneXpert test for tuberculosis. Four samples were rejected due to inadequate sample and hence 60 samples were tested. All the sample were negative for sputum AFB smear test. After 7 days of antibiotics treatment, 25 inmates symptomatically improved. Remaining 35 inmates did not improve and one sample was sent for GeneXpert test. Six samples (10%) had a positive test result for TB in GeneXpert test of which one had rifampicin resistant (Figure 1). Of the 434 inmates evaluated, 6 newly diagnosed and 2 under anti-tubercular treatment i.e., 8 inmates (1.84%) had active tuberculosis in the prison i.e., the prevalence of TB in Jhumka Regional Prison was **1843/100,000** population.

Age, education, duration of stay in prison, previous incarceration, overcrowding, and substance use disorders were not found to statistically significant with the prevalence of tuberculosis (Table 3).

In this study, fever, duration of cough, weight loss, loss of appetite, BMI, and past history of TB were not found to be the significantly associated with tuberculosis. Only chest pain and

TABLE 3: Association of TB among inmates with related variables.

Characteristics	Total suspected TB (n = 68)	TB suspects with sputum test (n = 60)	Inmates with TB (n = 6)	Inmates without TB (n = 54)	p-value
Age (in years)					
18–44	42 (61.8)	38 (63.3)	2 (5.3)	36 (94.7)	0.179
≥45	26 (38.2)	22 (36.7)	4 (18.2)	18 (81.8)	
Education					
Illiterate	28 (41.2)	25 (41.7)	4 (16.0)	21 (84.0)	0.223
Literate	40 (58.8)	35 (58.3)	2 (5.7)	33 (94.3)	
Time held in prison					
<12 months	7 (10.3)	7 (11.7)	1 (14.3)	6 (85.7)	0.541
≥12 months	61 (89.7)	53 (88.3)	5 (9.4)	48 (90.6)	
Previous incarceration					
Yes	13 (19.1)	10 (16.7)	3 (30.0)	7 (70.0)	0.052
No	55 (80.9)	50 (83.3)	3 (6.0)	47 (94.0)	
Inmates per cell					
≤50	36 (52.9)	31 (51.7)	3 (9.7)	28 (90.3)	1.000
>50	32 (47.1)	29 (48.3)	3 (10.3)	26 (89.7)	
Alcohol intake					
Yes	48 (70.6)	43 (71.7)	4 (9.3)	39 (90.7)	1.000
Never	20 (29.4)	17 (28.3)	2 (11.8)	15 (88.2)	
Smoking status					
Current user	36 (52.9)	32 (53.3)	4 (12.5)	28 (87.5)	0.675
Nonuser/Ex-user	32 (47.1)	28 (46.7)	2 (7.1)	26 (92.9)	
Chewing tobacco					
Current user	37 (54.4)	33 (55.0)	4 (12.1)	29 (87.9)	0.681
Nonuser/Ex-user	31 (45.6)	27 (45.0)	2 (7.4)	25 (92.6)	
Illicit drug use					
Yes	15 (22.1)	11 (18.3)	0 (0.0)	11 (100)	0.581
No	53 (77.9)	49 (81.7)	6 (12.2)	43 (87.8)	
Injectable drug use					
Yes	6 (8.8)	3 (5.0)	1 (33.3)	2 (66.7)	0.275
No	62 (91.2)	57 (95.0)	5 (8.8)	52 (91.2)	

abnormal chest finding on auscultation (i.e., wheezes and crackles) were found to be statistically significant with the presence of tuberculosis (p = 0.012 and 0.027, respectively) (Table 4).

4. Discussion

The prevalence of PTB in Nepalese prison was found to be 1843/100000 population, which is 8.7 times higher than the general population. This study reflects important insights into the burden of tuberculosis in the country, particularly in the high-risk prison setting. The detection of 6 new undiagnosed PTB cases shows the vulnerability of the jail inmates for the disease. The prevalence of tuberculosis is similar to other studies [16–18]. However, the rate of tuberculosis in prisoners compared with that in the general population varies depending on the prison location [19]. The high prevalence of PTB in prison settings highlights the importance of implementing systematic tuberculosis screening program in correctional facilities within the country. Such high prevalence could have a potential impact on the overall national TB control program due to potential spread to and through visitors, prison staffs, and discharged inmates themselves [18].

In this study, there was no significant association between the age group with the disease. This finding is in accordance with other studies [18, 20]. It was also observed that more older age group populations (>45 years) have TB compared to the younger people. This is in contrast to the study done in Africa, where the primary age group affected has been the younger age group [17, 21].

In this study, the duration of cough did not have any association with tuberculosis. This is similar to the study done by Moges et al. [18]. Although, fever and cough are cardinal symptoms for diagnosis of tuberculosis and various studies have pointed out an association of these symptoms with TB disease [16, 17, 22]. Our lack of association could be due to the substantial lag time associated between symptoms and diagnosis. However, even in this study, we saw the association of inmates with history of chest pain and tuberculosis similar to other studies [17, 23]. Abnormal chest finding during auscultation was found to be a associated with PTB. Along

TABLE 4: Association of TB among inmates with signs and symptoms.

Signs/Symptoms	Total suspected TB (n = 68)	TB suspects with sputum test (n = 60)	Inmates with TB (n = 6)	Inmates without TB (n = 54)	p-value
Fever					
Yes	6 (8.8)	6 (10.0)	1 (16.7)	5 (83.3)	0.484
No	62 (91.2)	54 (90.0)	5 (9.3)	49 (90.7)	
Duration of cough					
≤4 weeks	47 (69.1)	41 (68.3)	3 (7.3)	38 (92.7)	0.370
>4 weeks	21 (30.9)	19 (19.7)	3 (15.8)	16 (84.2)	
Weight loss in 3 months					
Yes	47 (69.1)	42 (70.0)	5 (11.9)	37 (88.1)	0.658
No	21 (30.9)	18 (30.0)	1 (5.6)	17 (94.4)	
Recent loss of appetite					
Yes	37 (54.4)	30 (50.0)	4 (13.3)	26 (86.7)	0.671
No	31 (45.6)	30 (50.0)	2 (6.7)	28 (93.3)	
Chest pain					
Yes	13 (19.1)	12 (20.0)	4 (33.3)	8 (66.7)	0.012*
No	55 (80.9)	48 (80.0)	2 (4.2)	46 (95.8)	
Chest auscultation#					
Abnormal	8 (88.2)	8 (13.3)	3 (37.5)	5 (62.5)	0.027*
Normal	60 (11.8)	52 (86.7)	3 (5.8)	49 (94.2)	
BMI (kg/m²)					
<18.5	7 (10.3)	5 (8.3)	1 (20)	4 (80)	0.421
≥18.5	61 (89.7)	55 (91.7)	5 (9.1)	50 (90.9)	
Past history of TB					
Yes	6 (8.8)	6 (10.0)	1 (16.7)	5 (83.3)	0.484
No	62 (91.2)	54 (90.0)	5 (9.3)	49 (90.7)	

*Significant/ #only wheezes and crackles were found on auscultation.

with the symptoms, a careful and detailed clinical examination can help in PTB diagnosis. This association has not been tested in other prison studies, hence further research can be done in this regard.

Weight loss, loss of appetite, and malnutrition have been important risk factors associated with tuberculosis in various studies [18, 20, 24]. However, this study does not show this association. Some other studies also do not show this association [16, 17].

The present study also did not find an association between substance use disorder, overcrowding, length of incarceration and previous incarceration. Various studies conducted have similar findings [18, 21, 25, 26]. In contrast to this, a study conducted in Cameroon found a positive association of prison stay of less than 12 months and a history of previous incarceration with PTB [27]. This observation could be explained by the low number of confirmed TB cases detected to confer any association with these factors with tuberculosis.

This study highlights considerable strength and weaknesses. To our best knowledge, this is the first study which shows the high burden of Tuberculosis in a prison setting in Nepal. Prison health is sadly neglected and under-addressed in most parts of the world [28]. Nepal in line with many countries does not have specific prison health policies. Our study findings underline the importance of periodic and timely screening and diagnosis of TB in prisons and timely institution of TB treatment to control the transmission of the infection [29]. Proper screening for tuberculosis symptoms is highly recommended as the first line of defence in prison.

We also acknowledge the limitation of our study where we could do screening among only 434 inmates (small sample size) due to the control prison setting environment. Furthermore, our diagnosis mostly relied on the sputum microscopy examination, where the yield is substantially lower compared to the modern diagnostic methods like GeneXpert. Not all sputum samples could be sent for GeneXpert due to resource constraint of GeneXpert machines in setting like Nepal. Sputum culture, and X-ray screening of suspected inmates were not done, which could have further helped diagnose TB.

Furthermore, the cross-sectional design of this study does not allow us to make definitive inferences about the effect of the risk factors in association with tuberculosis. Lastly, as this study is done only in one male prison, it cannot be generalized to other prisons of the country.

5. Conclusions

This study found a high prevalence of PTB among inmates in Nepal than the general population. Our study highlights the vulnerability of inmates to tuberculosis and stresses the need for effective screening for TB in new and continuing prisoners and appropriate measures to halt the transmission of the disease in the high-risk prison environment. Isolation of active PTB patients and early diagnosis and treatment should be implemented to control the disease and to reduce the incidence of TB in prisons.

Abbreviations

TB: Tuberculosis
PTB: Pulmonary tuberculosis
HIV: Human immunodeficiency virus
BMI: Body mass index
NTP: National tuberculosis program
ZN: Ziehl–Neelsen
ATT: Anti-tubercular treatment.

Authors' Contributions

GS, DKY, and PKP designed the study. GS and DB were responsible for streamlining the research idea and finalizing the questionnaire. GS and RG collected the data. GS, DB, and RM were involved in data cleaning and statistical analysis. All authors contributed to the interpretation of the results. GS, RG, and RM wrote the preliminary drafts. All authors read and approved the final version of the manuscript.

Acknowledgments

We express our gratitude to the Jhumka Regional Prison's authority for giving us permission to conduct this study. We are thankful to all the inmates who helped us and participated in the study. A part of this study was presented at "Third National Summit of Health and Population Scientists in Nepal 2017" conference.

References

[1] "Health in prison," http://www.euro.who.int/__data/assets/pdf_file/0009/99018/E90174.pdf.

[2] A. M. Kazi, S. A. Shah, C. A. Jenkins, B. E. Shepherd, and S. H. Vermund, "Risk factors and prevalence of tuberculosis, human immunodeficiency virus, syphilis, hepatitis B virus, and hepatitis C virus among prisoners in Pakistan," *International Journal of Infectious Diseases*, vol. 14, 3pp. e60–e66, 2010.

[3] O. Simooya, "Infections in prison in low and middle income countries: prevalence and prevention strategies," *The Open Infectious Diseases Journal*, vol. 4, no. 2, pp. 33–37, 2010.

[4] J. Baillargeon, S. A. Black, J. Pulvino, and K. Dunn, "The disease profile of Texas prison inmates," *Annals of epidemiology*, vol. 10, no. 2, pp. 74–80, 2000.

[5] I. A. Binswanger, P. M. Krueger, and J. F. Steiner, "Prevalence of chronic medical conditions among jail and prison inmates in the USA compared with the general population," *Journal of Epidemiology and Community Health*, vol. 63, no. 11, pp. 912–919, 2009.

[6] D. Indig, L. Topp, B. Ross et al., *2009 NSW Inmate Health Survey: Key Findings Report*, Justice Health, Pagewood NSW 2035, 2010.

[7] M. Esposito, "The health of Italian prison inmates today: a critical approach," *Journal of Correctional Health Care*, vol. 16, no. 3, pp. 230–238, 2010.

[8] F. Biadglegne, A. C. Rodloff, and U. Sack, "A first insight into high prevalence of undiagnosed smear-negative pulmonary tuberculosis in northern ethiopian prisons: implications for greater investment and quality control," *PLoS One*, vol. 9, no. 9, Article ID e106869, 2014.

[9] A. Bone, A. Aerts, M. Grzemska et al., "Tuberculosis control in prisons: a manual for programme managers," *Institutional Respository for Information Sharing*, 2000.

[10] M. Dara, C. D. Acosta, N. V. S. V. Melchers et al., "Tuberculosis control in prisons: current situation and research gaps," *International Journal of Infectious Diseases*, vol. 32, pp. 111–117, 2015.

[11] Ministry of Health, GOH, *Annual Report 2015/2016*, Department of Health Services MoH, Government of Nepal, Kathmandu, 2016.

[12] "Annual TB Report 2013," http://www.searo.who.int/entity/tb/annual_tb_report_2013.pdf.

[13] G. Shrestha, D. K. Yadav, N. Sapkota et al., "Depression among inmates in a regional prison of eastern Nepal: a cross-sectional study," *BMC Psychiatry*, vol. 17, no. 1, p. 348, 2017.

[14] G. Shrestha, R. Mulmi, D. K. Yadav et al., "Health needs and risky behaviours among inmates in the largest prison of Eastern Nepal," *International Journal of Prisoner Health*, vol. 14, no. 4, pp. 254–267, 2018.

[15] *National Tuberculosis Control Programme: General Manual*, National Tuberculosis Control Programme, Department of Health Services, Ministry of Health and Population, Nepal, Thimi, Bhaktapur, Nepal, 3rd edition, 2012.

[16] A. C. M. lemos, E. D. Matos, and C. N. Bittencourt, "Prevalence of active and latent TB among inmates in a prison hospital in Bahia, Brazil," *Jornal Brasileiro de Pneumologia*, vol. 35, no. 1, pp. 63–68, 2009.

[17] D. S. Abebe, G. Bjune, G. Ameni, D. Biffa, and F. Abebe, "Prevalence of pulmonary tuberculosis and associated risk factors in Eastern Ethiopian prisons," *International Journal of Tuberculosis and Lung Disease*, vol. 15, no. 5, pp. 668–673, 2011.

[18] B. Moges, B. Amare, F. Asfaw et al., "Prevalence of smear positive pulmonary tuberculosis among prisoners in North Gondar Zone Prison, Northwest Ethiopia," *BMC Infectious Diseases*, vol. 12, no. 1, p. 352, 2012.

[19] R. B. Wallace, *Wallace/Maxcy-Rosenau-Last Public Health and Preventive Medicine*, McGraw Hill Medical, New York, 15th edition, 2007.

[20] S. X. Jittimanee, N. Ngamtrairai, M. C. White, and S. Jittimanee, "A prevalence survey for smear-positive tuberculosis in Thai Prisons," *International Journal of Tuberculosis and Lung Disease*, vol. 11, no. 5, pp. 556–561, 2007.

[21] P. Nyasulu, S. Mogoere, T. Umanah, and G. Setswe, "Determinants of pulmonary tuberculosis among inmates at Mangaung maximum correctional facility in Bloemfontein, South Africa," *Tuberculosis Research and Treatment*, vol. 2015, Article ID 752709, pp. 1–7, 2015.

[22] B. Séri, A. Koffi, C. Danel et al., "Prevalence of pulmonary tuberculosis among prison inmates: a cross-sectional survey at the correctional and detention facility of Abidjan, Côte d'Ivoire," *PLoS One*, vol. 12, no. 7, Article ID e0181995, 2017.

[23] A. Sanchez, G. Gerhardt, S. Natal et al., "Prevalence of pulmonary tuberculosis and comparative evaluation of screening strategies in a Brazilian Prison," *International Journal of Tuberculosis and Lung Disease*, vol. 9, no. 6, pp. 633–639, 2005.

[24] S. Banu, A. Hossain, M. K. M. Uddin et al., "Pulmonary tuberculosis and drug resistance in Dhaka Central Jail, the Largest Prison in Bangladesh," *PLoS One*, vol. 5, no. 5, Article ID e10759, 2010.

[25] L. Telisinghe, K. L. Fielding, J. L. Malden et al., "High tuberculosis prevalence in a South African Prison: the need for routine tuberculosis screening," *PLoS One*, vol. 9, no. 1, Article ID e87262, 2014.

[26] D. E. Winetsky, O. Almukhamedov, D. Pulatov, N. Vezhnina, A. Dooronbekova, and B. Zhussupov, "Prevalence, risk factors and social context of active pulmonary tuberculosis among prison inmates in Tajikistan," *PLoS One*, vol. 9, no. 1, Article ID e86046, 2014.

[27] J. Noeske, C. Kuaban, G. Amougou, A. Piubello, and R. Pouillot, "Pulmonary tuberculosis in the central prison of DoualaCameroon," *East African Medical Journal*, vol. 83, no. 1, pp. 25–30, 2006.

[28] B. M. Prasad, B. Thapa, S. S. Chadha et al., "Status of tuberculosis services in Indian prisons," *International Journal of Infectious Diseases*, vol. 56, pp. 117–121, 2017.

[29] M. Dara and C. D. Acosta, "Tuberculosis prevention and control in prisons: do we know enough?," *International Journal of Tuberculosis and Lung Disease*, vol. 18, no. 7, pp. 758–759, 2014.

5

Predictors of Adverse TB Treatment Outcome among TB/HIV Patients Compared with Non-HIV Patients in the Greater Accra Regional Hospital from 2008 to 2016

Kenneth Mawuta Hayibor,[1,2] Delia Akosua Bandoh,[2] Adwoa Asante-Poku,[1] and Ernest Kenu[2]

[1]Noguchi Memorial Institute for Medical Research, University of Ghana, Ghana
[2]School of Public Health, University of Ghana, Ghana

Correspondence should be addressed to Ernest Kenu; ernest_kenu@yahoo.com

Academic Editor: Vincent Jarlier

Introduction. The convergence of TB and HIV dual epidemics is a major public health challenge in Ghana as well as many developing countries. Treatment outcome monitoring is a vital part of the surveillance needed to successfully eliminate TB. The impact of HIV status and demographic and treatment-related factors on adverse TB treatment outcome has not been studied in the Greater Accra Regional Hospital. This study determined factors associated with TB treatment outcome in patients with TB-HIV coinfection and TB-only infection in the hospital. *Method.* A cross-sectional study was carried out in the Greater Accra Regional Hospital. We reviewed TB treatment cards of patients who received treatment for tuberculosis in the hospital from 2008 to 2016. Data on treatment outcome and sociodemographic and clinical characteristics were extracted on TB-only-infected and TB/HIV-coinfected patients. The chi-squared test and binary and multiple logistic regression models were used to assess factors associated with adverse treatment outcome. *Results.* Out of the 758 patient records analyzed, 174 (22.9%) were TB-HIV-coinfected patients. Overall treatment success for all TB patients was 88.1% (668/758). About 11.9% (90/758) of the patients had an adverse treatment outcome, including treatment failure 0.9% (7/758), defaulting 0.9% (7/758), and death 10.0% (76/758). TB-HIV-coinfected patients' treatment success was 78.1% (136/174). TB-only patients' treatment success was 91.4% (532/582). Independent predictors of adverse treatment outcome were found to be as follows: being HIV positive (aOR: 3.85, 95% CI: 2.19-6.75; $p < 0.01$); aged 65 and above (aOR: 1.76, 95% CI: 1.44-1.54; $p = 0.01$); and previously failed TB treatment (aOR: 5.02, 95% CI: 2.09-28.87; $p < 0.01$). *Conclusion.* Treatment outcome for TB-HIV-coinfected patients is below the WHO target. HIV status, age, and category of patient of the TB patients were associated with adverse treatment outcome. Strengthening the TB/HIV collaborative efforts by stakeholders is required for good treatment outcomes.

1. Introduction

Tuberculosis (TB) and Human Immunodeficiency Virus (HIV) are diseases of global public health concern despite the existing prevention and control strategies [1]. TB is caused mainly by Mycobacterium tuberculosis, and it is curable. However, without early detection and diagnosis, it is difficult to treat. HIV is another infectious disease; however, there is no known cure at the moment. The HIV pandemic poses a great challenge to the control of the TB epidemic by changing the natural progression of latent TB to active TB and also impacting on the epidemiology and clinical outcomes of TB [2]. TB is a leading killer among people living with HIV. At least one in four deaths among people living with HIV can be attributed to TB, and many of these deaths occur in resource-limited settings especially in sub-Saharan Africa [2].

There were 10.4 million incident cases of TB worldwide in 2015, of which about 10% were coinfected with HIV and there were about 1.4 million deaths, of which 400,000 deaths were among people coinfected with HIV [3]. The sub-Saharan African region bears the highest global TB/HIV burden, and over 50% of TB cases are coinfected with HIV [3].

Ghana is one of the high-burdened TB/HIV countries in the world [4]. The prevalence of TB in Ghana in 2015 was estimated to be 356 per 100,000 population, and 22.5% of the TB patients are coinfected with HIV [5]. The impact of HIV on TB, and the implications for TB and HIV control, has been acknowledged as a public health challenge in Ghana.

There was a policy change in Ghana in July 2007 on collaboration of TB and HIV activities. The TB/HIV policy which was in line with the WHO recommendations consists of three linked sets of activities: effective implementation of the Stop TB Strategy for TB control, improved HIV prevention and care, and implementation of a TB and HIV coinfection clinic [2]. This policy was fully implemented in the Greater Accra Regional Hospital (GARH) in December 2007. The GARH has one of the best collaborative TB and HIV activities supported by the National Tuberculosis Control and National HIV/AIDS Control Programs with cross-referral mechanisms with other health facilities. However, since the integration of TB/HIV activities, there are few published reports on TB treatment outcomes among TB/HIV patients compared with non-HIV patients likewise the impact of HIV status and demographic and treatment-related factors on adverse TB treatment outcome in the GARH.

The World Health Organization (WHO) recommends that TB treatment outcomes be monitored, as monitoring is a vital part of the surveillance needed to successfully eliminate TB [6]. Treatment monitoring also serves as a tool to assess the TB treatment quality provided by the health care system [7]. There are six possible TB treatment outcomes: the patient may be cured, completed treatment, treatment failure, default treatment, transferred out to another facility, or died. Treatment success is when a patient is cured or completed treatment. Regardless of the number of reported TB cases in a setting, key treatment outcomes are expected to improve in line with WHO treatment outcome benchmarks. Currently, the international benchmark for assessing countries' performance with respect to cure rates is 85%.

This study reports on the prevalence of HIV and treatment outcome of TB patients who received treatment at a Directly Observed Therapy Short-course (DOTS) center in the GARH from 2008 to 2016. It further reports on the background and clinical characteristics associated with adverse treatment outcome among the TB patients. The GARH was one of the first health facilities in Ghana that integrated TB-HIV activities.

2. Methods

2.1. Study Design and Setting. This was a cross-sectional study of treatment outcomes of all TB cases registered from January 2008 to December 2016 in the GARH. The GARH serves the whole of the Greater Accra Region of Ghana, and it is a major referral center. The hospital has a DOTS center and a dedicated TB laboratory for TB cases' diagnosis, treatment, and monitoring according to NTP guidelines and protocols. All patients diagnosed with TB are made to undergo HIV counseling, testing, and treatment.

2.2. Data Collection and Study Variables. Data for this study was obtained from the TB register and patients' treatment cards at the DOT center of the hospital. The TB register is a standardized document used by all DOTS centers in Ghana. From March to May 2017, data was extracted from the TB register and treatment cards using a specially developed data extraction form. The background characteristics (age, sex, distance of residence to the DOTS center, and treatment supporter availability), clinical characteristics (category of patient, HIV status, diabetes status, TB diagnostic category, and adverse reaction to the anti-TB drug), and treatment outcome (cured, treatment complete, died, defaulted, and treatment failure) were the variables of interest. The WHO definitions of the six-treatment outcome category, type of patient, and TB diagnostic category were used [6].

2.3. Data Handling and Analysis. The abstraction forms were cross-checked for completion. Data were coded, entered, and cleaned using Microsoft Excel 2016 and imported into STATA 14 statistical software for analysis.

Data were summarized using frequencies and percentages to describe background characteristics, clinical characteristics, and treatment outcomes. A chi-squared test of association was used to determine significant differences in characteristics between TB-only and TB/HIV coinfection patients. Bivariate and multiple logistic regression models were used to identify significant predictors of adverse TB treatment outcomes in all TB patients. Statistical significance was set at a p value of 0.05 at 95% confidence level.

2.4. Ethical Approval. Ethical approval was obtained from the Ethical Review Committee of Ghana Health Service, Research and Development Division, Accra (Reference No. GHS/RDD/ERC/Admin/App/17/434). Permission to conduct the study was obtained from the Central Administration and the Deputy Director of Nursing Services of the DOT center at the GARH. To ensure privacy and confidentiality, data abstraction was done in a room provided by the hospital authority. Access to the data obtained from the TB cards was limited to the study investigators. No identifying information such as names was captured from the records. Data collected were solely used for research purpose. Confidentiality and anonymity were maintained from data entry into the data abstraction forms and into the computer before data analysis.

3. Results

A total of 761 TB patients were registered at the Greater Accra Regional Hospital from January 2008 to December 2016. Treatment outcome was not documented for three patients; therefore, only 758 cases were included in the analysis.

3.1. Background Characteristics of TB Patients by HIV Status. Table 1 describes the background characteristics of TB cases

TABLE 1: Background characteristics of TB cases according to HIV status in the Greater Accra Regional Hospital, 2008-2016 ($n = 758$).

Characteristics	TB-HIV n (%)	TB-only n (%)	Total n (%)	p value
Age				<0.001*
<15	27 (15.2)	37 (6.3)	64 (8.4)	
15-24	10 (5.8)	81 (13.9)	91 (12.0)	
25-34	36 (20.7)	134 (23.0)	170 (22.4)	
35-44	57 (32.8)	119 (20.4)	176 (23.2)	
45-54	36 (20.7)	93 (15.9)	129 (17.0)	
55-64	6 (3.5)	65 (11.1)	71 (9.4)	
>64	2 (1.2)	55 (9.4)	57 (7.5)	
Sex				<0.001*
Male	92 (52.9)	434 (74.3)	526 (69.4)	
Female	82 (47.1)	150 (25.7)	232 (30.6)	
Area of residence				0.972
Urban	134 (77.0)	449 (76.9)	583 (76.9)	
Periurban	40 (23.0)	135 (23.1)	175 (23.1)	
Distance to the hospital				0.513
<5 km	133 (76.4)	460 (78.8)	593 (78.2)	
≥5 km	41 (23.6)	124 (21.2)	165 (21.8)	
Treatment supporter available[a]				0.212
Yes	173 (99.4)	570 (97.6)	743 (98.0)	
No	1 (6.7)	14 (2.4)	15 (2.0)	

*Significant at $p < 0.05$. [a]Significance was determined using Fisher's exact test.

in the GARH, 2008-2016. Majority of the patients were in the age group 25-44. There were 526 (69.4%) males, and there were 232 (47.1%) females. With the patients' area of residence, 77% of TB/HIV-coinfected patients and TB-only patients resided in an urban area. Most of the patients live less than 5 km away from the hospital. Almost all the patients in both categories had treatment supporters. There was a statistically significant difference in age ($p < 0.001$) and sex ($p < 0.001$) between TB-HIV patients and TB-only patients. However, there was no evidence of statistical difference between the two categories of patients with respect to distance to the hospital ($p = 0.51$), area of residence ($p = 0.97$), and available treatment supporter ($p = 0.13$).

3.2. Disease Characteristics of TB Patients with or without HIV. Majority of the patients in both categories were mostly newly diagnosed cases. Seventy-nine percent of the TB/HIV patients were new cases likewise 73.5% for the TB-only patients. More than half of the TB-only patients were smear positive (57.7%). Most of patients' (both TB/HIV and TB-only) chest X-rays were suggestive of TB. Sixty-two percent of the patients that experienced adverse drug reactions were TB/HIV-coinfected patients.

There was a statistically significant difference in TB classification ($p < 0.01$) between TB-HIV-coinfected patients and TB-only patients. There was no significant association between TB-HIV-coinfected patients and TB-only patients with type of patient ($p = 0.25$), chest X-ray ($p = 0.09$), duration of treatment ($p = 0.75$), diabetes ($p = 0.27$), and adverse treatment reaction ($p = 0.052$) (Table 2).

3.3. TB Cases by HIV Status. The highest number of TB cases over the period was 120, which was recorded in 2012, and the lowest was in 57 in 2016 (Figure 1). The proportion of TB patients coinfected with HIV over the period was 22.9% (174/758). There was a gradual increase in the number of TB cases from 2008 to 2012 except 2010, and then there was a gradual decrease till 2016, and this was likewise for TB-HIV-coinfected cases.

3.4. Treatment Outcomes of TB Patients with or without HIV. Treatment success for patients coinfected with TB and HIV was 77.0% (134/174) (95% CI: 0.70-0.83). TB-only patients' treatment success was 91.4% (534/584) (95% CI: 0.89-0.94). The overall treatment success was 88.1% (668/758) (95% CI: 0.86-0.90) Twelve percent (90/758) of the patients had an adverse outcome. Thirty-five (20.1%) of the HIV-positive patients and 43 (7.4%) of the HIV negative patients died (Table 3).

3.5. Predictors of Adverse TB Treatment Outcomes. Multiple logistic regression revealed that after adjusting for six other variables, HIV status, age, and category of patient were significantly associated with adverse treatment outcome (Table 4). TB patients coinfected with HIV had 4.5 times higher chance of adverse treatment outcome compared to non-HIV TB patients (aOR: 4.5, 95% CI: 2.6-7.8; $p < 0.01$). Likewise, the odds of experiencing adverse treatment is 4 times as great in patients' aged above 64 years than that of patients below 15 years (aOR: 4.0, 95% CI: 1.44-1.54; $p = 0.01$). Patients who have previously defaulted treatment had

TABLE 2: Disease characteristics of TB cases according to HIV status in the Greater Accra Regional Hospital, 2008-2016.

Characteristics (758)	TB-HIV *n* (%)	TB-only *n* (%)	Total *n* (%)	*p* value
Category of patient[a]				0.149
New	139 (78.9)	429 (73.5)	568 (74.93)	
Relapse	5 (2.9)	13 (2.2)	18 (2.37)	
Defaulter	0	12 (2.1)	12 (1.6)	
Failure	1 (0.6)	3 (0.5)	4 (0.5)	
Undefined	28 (16.1)	125 (21.4)	153 (20.2)	
Transferred in	1 (0.6)	2 (0.3)	3 (0.4)	
TB classification				<0.001*
Smear positive	74 (42.5)	337 (57.7)	411 (54.2)	
Smear negative	65 (37.4)	109 (18.7)	174 (23.0)	
Extrapulmonary	35 (20.1)	138 (23.6)	173 (22.8)	
Chest X-ray				0.085
Suggestive	114 (65.5)	340 (58.2)	454 (59.9)	
Not suggestive	60 (34.5)	244 (41.8)	304 (40.1)	
Duration of treatment				0.750
<6 months	15 (8.6)	55 (9.4)	70 (9.2)	
≥6 months	159 (91.4)	529 (90.6)	688 (90.8)	
Diabetes				0.274
Yes	8 (4.6)	17 (2.9)	25 (3.3)	
No	166 (95.4)	567 (97.1)	733 (96.7)	
Adverse treatment reaction[a]				0.052
Yes	4 (2.3)	3 (0.5)	7 (0.9)	
No	170 (97.7)	581 (99.5)	751 (99.1)	

*Significant at $p < 0.05$. [a]Significance was determined using Fisher's exact test.

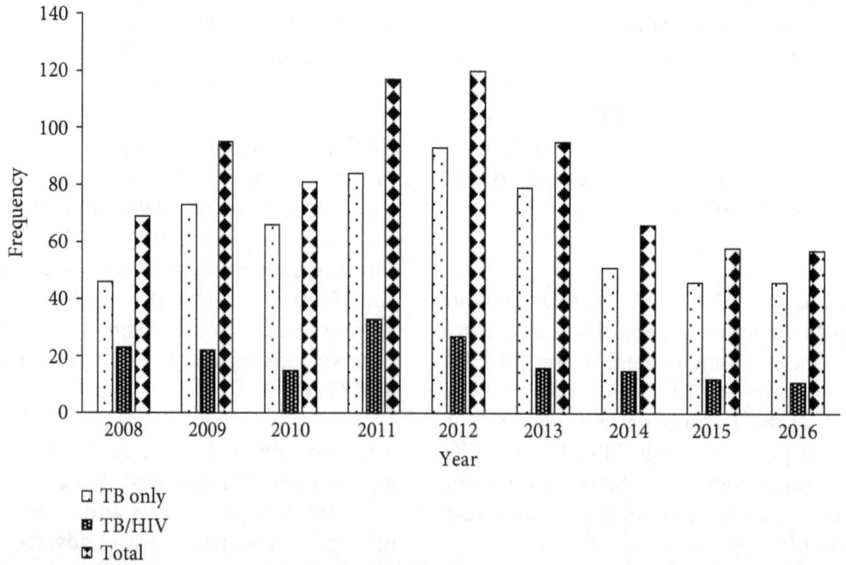

FIGURE 1: TB cases by HIV status registered in the Greater Accra Regional Hospital, 2008-2016.

8.1 times higher odds of having adverse treatment outcome compared to new patients (aOR: 8.12 95% CI: 2.19-30.08; $p = 0.002$). The odds of adverse treatment outcomes was 5.2 times higher among patients that previously failed TB treatment compared to new TB patients, though this was not statistically significant (aOR: 5.2, 95%: CI 0.49-55.36; $p = 0.17$).

TABLE 3: Treatment outcomes of TB cases according to HIV status in the Greater Accra Regional Hospital, 2008-2016.

Variable	TB-HIV	TB-only	Total (%)	*p* value
Treatment outcome				<0.001
Cured	58 (33.8)	288 (49.3)	346 (45.6)	
Treatment completed	76 (43.7)	246 (42.1)	322 (42.5)	
Treatment failure	2 (1.2)	5 (0.9)	7 (0.9)	
Died	34 (19.5)	42 (7.2)	76 (10.0)	
Defaulted	4 (2.3)	3 (0.5)	7 (0.9)	
Overall treatment outcome				<0.001
Treatment success*	134 (77.0)	534 (91.4)	668 (88.1)	
Adverse treatment**	40 (23.0)	50 (8.6)	90 (11.9)	

*Sum of treatment outcomes cured and treatment completed. **Sum of treatment outcomes treatment default, died, and defaulted.

TABLE 4: Logistic regression analysis of predictor variables of adverse treatment outcome among TB patients in the Greater Accra Regional Hospital, 2008-2016.

Variables	Treatment outcome: Trt. success* *N* (%)	Treatment outcome: Adverse trt.** *N* (%)	aOR	95% CI	*p* value
Age					
<15	52 (7.8)	12 (13.33)	Ref		
15-24	85 (12.7)	6 (6.7)	0.61	0.20-1.87	0.39
25-34	150 (22.5)	20 (22.2)	0.92	0.39-2.17	0.85
35-44	157 (23.5)	19 (21.1)	0.75	0.32-1.77	0.51
45-54	119 (17.8)	10 (11.1)	0.51	0.19-1.32	0.16
55-64	64 (9.58)	7 (7.8)	0.96	0.29-2.48	0.95
>64	41 (6.1)	16 (17.8)	4.00	1.54-10.34	0.004
Sex					
Male	469 (70.2)	57 (63.3)	Ref		
Female	199 (29.8)	33 (36.7)	0.94	0.57-1.597	0.81
Category of patient					
New	510 (76.4)	58 (64.4)	Ref		
Relapse	16 (2.4)	2 (2.2)	1.40	0.29-6.74	0.67
Defaulter	8 (1.20)	4 (4.4)	8.12	2.19-30.08	0.002
Undefined	128 (19.2)	25 (27.8)	1.33	0.45-3.89	0.60
Failure	3 (0.5)	1 (1.1)	5.22	0.49-55.36	0.17
Transferred in	3 (0.45)	0	1.00	—	—
TB classification					
Positive	376 (56.3)	35 (38.9)	Ref		
Negative	147 (22.0)	27 (30.0)	1.34	0.74-2.46	0.34
Extrapulmonary	145 (21.7)	28 (31.1)	1.73	0.59-5.08	0.31
Adverse treatment reaction					
Yes	4 (0.6)	3 (3.3)	3.90	0.78-19.48	0.10
No	664 (99.4)	87 (96.7)	Ref		
TB patient coinfected with HIV					
No	534 (79.9)	50 (55.6)	Ref		
Yes	134 (20.1)	40 (44.4)	4.48	2.59-7.77	<0.01

Trt. = treatment. *Sum of treatment outcomes cured and treatment completed. **Sum of treatment outcomes treatment default, died, and defaulted.

4. Discussion

This study was set to determine factors associated with TB treatment outcome in patients with TB-HIV coinfection and TB-only infection in the GARH. The main findings of the study were as follows: 22.9% of all TB patient records reviewed were coinfected with HIV; the overall treatment success for TB patients was 88.1% while that of the patients coinfected with HIV was 77.3%. Adverse treatment outcome was associated with HIV coinfection, previously defaulted treatment, previously failed treatment, and aged above 64 years.

Studies conducted in the African region on TB/HIV coinfection showed varied values ranging between 2.9% and 72.3%, with pooled prevalence of 23.5% [8]. The HIV prevalence recorded in this study is comparable to the Ghana national average of 22% [9] and a study in Ethiopia (25%) [10]. However, it is higher than the current global estimate of 15% and much lower than the African regional estimate of 36% [5]. This finding reveals why Ghana is considered to be one of the high-burdened TB/HIV countries in the world by the WHO [4].

WHO recommends treatment outcome monitoring among TB patients as an essential component for TB control and surveillance. The overall treatment success recorded in this study is higher than most of the studies conducted in the African subregion [11–14]. The high overall treatment success recorded in this study may be attributed to prudent following of the WHO treatment guidelines. An implication of the high treatment success rate recorded is that Ghana is likely to meet the End TB targets if this trend continues.

TB/HIV-coinfected patients in this study had more adverse treatment outcomes than patients with TB only. Globally, TB-associated mortality in coinfected patients is three times higher than mortality among TB-only patients [5]. TB/HIV-coinfected patients in this study had more adverse treatment outcomes than patients with TB only. Moreover, coinfected patients have an increased risk of experiencing adverse treatment outcomes compared to TB-only-infected patients. Adverse treatment outcomes associated with TB/HIV coinfection have been shown by several studies [8, 11, 15–18]. The reasons for the adverse treatment outcome may be due to immunosuppression [19], drug interactions between rifampicin a major anti-TB drug and some antiretroviral agents [20, 21], suboptimal drug concentrations of anti-TB drugs [22], and a malabsorption of the anti-TB drugs [23]. Also, late diagnosis of HIV [24], alternation of the clinical manifestation of TB [22, 25], lack of a rapid and sensitive TB diagnostic test [26, 27], and unavailability/inaccessibility of antiretroviral therapy [28] may be the cause of the adverse treatment outcomes.

Globally, TB/HIV coinfection rates have been falling since 2008 [5]; however, in our study, the rate increased gradually and peaked at the year 2011, before a gradual decrease year after year (Figure 1). This gradual decrease in our study suggests that the current TB and HIV collaborative activities in the hospital must be encouraged to further reduce the coinfection rate. Moreover, a study in five districts in the Volta Region of Ghana revealed a stable TB/HIV coinfection from 2012 to 2015 [11]. TB-associated mortality in coinfected patients globally is three times higher than mortality among TB-only patients [5]. TB/HIV-coinfected patients in this study had more adverse treatment outcomes than patients with TB only. Coinfected patients have an increased risk of experiencing adverse treatment outcomes compared to TB-only-infected patients.

Our findings revealed that males were more susceptible than females, and this is consistent with a study done in Southern Ethiopia [12], but this is in contrast with studies conducted in the Volta Region of Ghana [11], Gondar [13] and Gambella [14]. Our findings might be due to most males spending more time at their workplaces and outside their homes than females, which predisposed them for susceptibility of TB infection. However, another possible explanation could be that females underutilized the DOTS services at the hospital.

Majority of the TB patients were aged between 25 and 45. Persons within this age group are usually sexually active. HIV/TB coinfection is more common in the sexually active age group (18). This finding is consistent with several studies that have also identified TB/HIV coinfection rates to be higher in persons within these age groups [9, 19, 20]. However, it is contrasted by a study where majority of the coinfected patients were below 15 years [11].

This study observed that patients who previously failed treatment and patients who return after previously defaulting treatment have an increased risk of developing adverse treatment outcomes compared to newly registered patients. This shows that more attention needs to be given to this category of patients and the reason for their previous treatment failure needs to be investigated.

It was also observed that TB patients aged above 64 were more likely to experience adverse treatment outcome compared to patients' aged below 15 years. This finding is consistent with studies conducted in Gondar University Teaching Hospital, Northwest Ethiopia, where the elderly were more likely to die than the younger ones [13]. Patients aged 64 and above may have adverse treatment outcome due to their immune systems as they age.

This study is a cross-sectional study and based only on records that were available in the GARH. It should be seen that the study incorporated data of patients with completed information of their treatment outcome at the hospital. We could not collect additional data needed, which could affect treatment outcome such as educational status and occupation, to confirm or refute our findings. In particular, we did not have access to ART history among our group of HIV-coinfected patients, and therefore, we could not assess its effect on our findings. It is likely though that most of them were not receiving ART and care or were diagnosed late in the course of their HIV disease. Despite this limitation, the study provided useful information on the treatment outcomes of TB/HIV-coinfected patients and TB-only-infected patients in the GARH. Findings may be useful to the National TB Control Program, the National AIDS Control Program, and the hospital authorities.

5. Conclusion

Our findings indicate that TB-HIV coinfection among the TB patient records reviewed was very high. Treatment success for TB patients was 88.1% while that of the patients coinfected with HIV was 77%. Significant predictors of adverse treatment outcomes were TB/HIV coinfection, aged 64 years and above, and having previously failed treatment. Factors associated with adverse treatment outcomes in TB/HIV-coinfected patients and patients that have previously failed treatment should be investigated. Strengthening the TB/HIV collaborative efforts is required for good treatment outcomes.

Acknowledgments

We would like to acknowledge the staff of the hospital who facilitated our data collection process. This work was funded by the authors of this study.

References

[1] M. Raviglione and G. Sulis, "Tuberculosis 2015: burden, challenges and strategy for control and elimination," *Infectious Disease Reports*, vol. 8, no. 2, p. 6570, 2016.

[2] H. G. Delphine Sculier and World Health Organization, *WHO policy on collaborative TB/HIV activities : guidelines for national programmes and other stakeholders*, 2004.

[3] WHO, *WHO | Tuberculosis*, WHO, Geneva, 2018, March 2018, http://www.who.int/mediacentre/factsheets/fs104/en/.

[4] World Health Organization, *Use of high burden country lists for TB by WHO in the post-2015 era meeting of WHO's Strategic and Technical Advisory Group for TB (STAG-TB)*, 2015, March 2018, http://www.who.int/tb/publications/global_report/high_tb_burdencountrylists2016-2020.pdf.

[5] World Health Organisation, *Global Tuberculosis Report 2015*, WHO Library Cataloguing-in-Publication Data, Geneva, 2015, March 2018, http://www.who.int/tb/publications/global_report/gtbr15_main_text.pdf.

[6] World Health Organisation, *WHO | Guidelines for treatment of tuberculosis*, WHO, Geneva, 2015.

[7] Stop TB Partnership (World Health Organization), *The global plan to stop TB 2011-2015 : transforming the fight : towards elimination of tuberculosis*, Stop TB Partnership, Geneva, 2010.

[8] J. Gao, P. Zheng, and H. Fu, "Prevalence of TB/HIV co-infection in countries except China: a systematic review and meta-analysis," *PLoS One*, vol. 8, no. 5, article e64915, 2013.

[9] World Health Organization, *Ghana country statistics*, WHO. Accra, Ghana, 2016, https://www.who.int/countries/gha/en/.

[10] F. Biadglegne, B. Anagaw, T. Debebe, and B. Anagaw, "A retrospective study on the outcomes of tuberculosis treatment in Felege Hiwot Referral Hospital, Northwest Ethopia," *International Journal of Medicine and Medical Sciences*, vol. 5, no. -February, pp. 85–91, 2013.

[11] E. Osei, J. Der, R. Owusu, P. Kofie, and W. K. Axame, *The burden of HIV on tuberculosis patients in the Volta region of Ghana from 2012 to 2015 : implication for tuberculosis control*, pp. 1–9, 2017.

[12] B. Getahun, G. Ameni, G. Medhin, and S. Biadgilign, "Treatment outcome of tuberculosis patients under directly observed treatment in Addis Ababa, Ethiopia," *The Brazilian Journal of Infectious Diseases*, vol. 17, no. 5, pp. 521–528, 2013.

[13] B. Tessema, A. Muche, A. Bekele, D. Reissig, F. Emmrich, and U. Sack, "Treatment outcome of tuberculosis patients at Gondar University Teaching Hospital, Northwest Ethiopia. A five - year retrospective study," *BMC Public Health*, vol. 9, no. 1, p. 371, 2009.

[14] S. Sisay, B. Mengistu, W. Erku, and D. Woldeyohannes, "Directly Observed Treatment Short-course (DOTS) for tuberculosis control program in Gambella Regional State, Ethiopia: ten years experience," *BMC Research Notes*, vol. 7, no. 1, p. 44, 2014.

[15] M. J. van der Werf, C. Ködmön, P. Zucs, V. Hollo, A. J. Amato-Gauci, and A. Pharris, "Tuberculosis and HIV coinfection in Europe," *AIDS*, vol. 30, no. 18, pp. 2845–2853, 2016.

[16] M. Sanchez, P. Bartholomay, D. Arakaki-Sanchez et al., "Outcomes of TB treatment by HIV status in National Recording Systems in Brazil, 2003–2008," *PLoS One*, vol. 7, no. 3, article e33129, 2012.

[17] T. N. do Prado, A. E. Miranda, F. M. de Souza et al., "Factors associated with tuberculosis by HIV status in the Brazilian national surveillance system: a cross sectional study," *BMC Infectious Diseases*, vol. 14, no. 1, 2014.

[18] W. J. Burman and B. E. Jones, "Treatment of HIV-related tuberculosis in the era of effective antiretroviral therapy," *American Journal of Respiratory and Critical Care Medicine*, vol. 164, no. 1, pp. 7–12, 2001.

[19] C. J. Waitt and S. B. Squire, "A systematic review of risk factors for death in adults during and after tuberculosis treatment [review article]," *The International Journal of Tuberculosis and Lung Disease*, vol. 15, no. 7, pp. 871–885, 2011.

[20] D. P. Holland, C. D. Hamilton, A. C. Weintrob et al., "Therapeutic drug monitoring of antimycobacterial drugs in patients with both tuberculosis and advanced human immunodeficiency virus infection," *Pharmacotherapy*, vol. 29, no. 5, pp. 503–510, 2009.

[21] S. Vijay, P. Kumar, L. S. Chauhan, S. V. Narayan Rao, and P. Vaidyanathan, "Treatment outcome and mortality at one and half year follow-up of HIV infected TB patients under TB control programme in a district of South India," *PLoS One*, vol. 6, no. 7, article e21008, 2011.

[22] T. R. Sterling, P. A. Pham, and R. E. Chaisson, "HIV infection–related tuberculosis: clinical manifestations and treatment," *Clinical Infectious Diseases*, vol. 50, no. s3, pp. S223–S230, 2010.

[23] B. Karo, G. Krause, V. Hollo et al., "Impact of HIV infection on treatment outcome of tuberculosis in Europe," *AIDS*, vol. 30, no. 7, pp. 1089–1098, 2016.

[24] N. A. Ifebunandu, K. N. Ukwaja, and S. N. Obi, "Treatment outcome of HIV-associated tuberculosis in a resource-poor setting," *Tropical Doctor*, vol. 42, no. 2, pp. 74–76, 2012.

[25] A. Pawlowski, M. Jansson, M. Sköld, M. E. Rottenberg, and G. Källenius, "Tuberculosis and HIV co-infection," *PLoS Pathogens*, vol. 8, no. 2, article e1002464, 2012.

[26] B. Sawadogo, K. S. Tint, M. Tshimanga, L. Kuonza, and L. Ouedraogo, "Risk factors for tuberculosis treatment failure among pulmonary tuberculosis patients in four health regions of Burkina Faso, 2009: case control study," *The Pan African Medical Journal*, vol. 21, p. 152, 2015.

[27] E. Osei, P. Akweongo, and F. Binka, "Factors associated with DELAY in diagnosis among tuberculosis patients in Hohoe

Municipality, Ghana," *BMC Public Health*, vol. 15, no. 1, p. 721, 2015.

[28] L. King, S. S. Munsiff, and S. D. Ahuja, "Achieving international targets for tuberculosis treatment success among HIV-positive patients in New York City SUMMARY," *The Lancet Infectious Diseases*, vol. 14, no. December 2004, pp. 1613–1620, 2010.

6

Mycobacterial Lineages Associated with Drug Resistance in Patients with Extrapulmonary Tuberculosis in Addis Ababa, Ethiopia

Getu Diriba,[1,2] Abebaw Kebede,[1,3] Habteyes Hailu Tola,[1] Ayinalem Alemu,[1] Bazezew Yenew,[1] Shewki Moga,[1] Desalegn Addise,[1] Zemedu Mohammed,[1] Muluwork Getahun,[1] Mengistu Fantahun,[4] Mengistu Tadesse,[1] Biniyam Dagne,[1] Misikir Amare,[1] Gebeyehu Assefa,[5] Dessie Abera,[2] and Kassu Desta[2]

[1]*Ethiopian Public Health Institute, Addis Ababa, Ethiopia*
[2]*Department of Medical Laboratory Sciences, College of Health Sciences, Addis Ababa University, Addis Ababa, Ethiopia*
[3]*Department of Microbial, Cellular and Molecular Biology, College of Natural and Computational Sciences, Addis Ababa University, Addis Ababa, Ethiopia*
[4]*St. Paul's Hospital Millennium Medical College, Addis Ababa, Ethiopia*
[5]*Armauer Hansen Research Institute, Addis Ababa, Ethiopia*

Correspondence should be addressed to Getu Diriba; getud2020@gmail.com

Academic Editor: Adwoa Asante-Poku

Background. In Ethiopia, tuberculosis (TB) is one of the most common causes of illness and death. However, there is limited information available on lineages associated with drug resistance among extrapulmonary tuberculosis patients in Ethiopia. In this study, researchers looked into *Mycobacterium tuberculosis* lineages linked to drug resistance in patients with extrapulmonary tuberculosis in Addis Ababa, Ethiopia. *Methods.* On 151 *Mycobacterium tuberculosis* isolates, a cross-sectional analysis was performed. Spoligotyping was used to characterize mycobacterial lineages, while a phenotypic drug susceptibility test was performed to determine the drug resistance pattern. Data were analyzed using SPSS version 23. *Results.* Among 151 *Mycobacterium tuberculosis* complex (MTBC) genotyped isolates, four lineages (L1–L4), and *Mycobacterium bovis* were identified. The predominantly identified lineage was Euro-American (73.5%) followed by East-African-Indian (19.2%). Any drug resistance (RR) and multidrug-resistant (MDR) tuberculosis was identified among 16.2% and 7.2% of the Euro-American lineage, respectively, while it was 30.8% and 15.4% among the East-African-Indian lineages. Among all three preextensively drug-resistance (pre-XDR) cases identified, two isolates belong to T3-ETH, and the other one strain was not defined by the database. There was no statistically significant association between any type of drug resistance and either lineage or sublineages of *Mycobacterium tuberculosis. Conclusion.* A higher proportion of any type of drug resistance and MDR was detected among the East-African-Indian lineage compared to others. However, there was no statistically significant association between any type of drug resistance and either lineages or sublineages. Thus, the authors recommend a large-scale study.

1. Introduction

Currently, tuberculosis (TB) is the first and the 10th global cause of death among infectious diseases and all diseases [1]. It is a global public health issue that affects approximately one-fourth of the world's population [1]. Based on the 2020 Global TB report, it is estimated that about 10 million people develop TB. Across the globe, there were 1.2 million TB deaths among HIV-negative people and 208, 000 deaths among HIV-positive people [1, 2]. The Mycobacterium tuberculosis complex (MTBC), the causative agent of TB, spreads from one person to the other through sneezing, coughing, and talking. Tuberculosis is mainly a disease of the lung (pulmonary TB), but it also affects other body parts (extrapulmonary TB) [1, 3].

Nowadays, TB control programs are challenged due to the emergence of drug-resistant TB and in particular multidrug-resistant (MDR) and extensively drug-resistance TB (XDR-TB) [4]. Globally, the burden of multidrug- or rifampicin-resistant TB (MDR/RR-TB) as a share of the number of TB cases remains stable. In 2019, an estimated 3.3% of new TB cases and 18% of previously treated cases had MDR/RRTB. In absolute numbers, there were an estimated 465, 000 incident cases of RR-TB burden [1, 5, 6]. Additionally, XDR-TB accounts for 7.4% of MDR-TB worldwide [5].

Ethiopia is among the 14 high TB, MDR-TB, and TB-HIV burden countries in the world. Based on the 2020 global TB report, the prevalence of MDR-TB among new and retreatment cases was reported to be 0.71% and 16%, respectively [1, 7]. Besides, the pre-XDR-TB and XDR-TB isolates accounted for 5.7% and 0.6%, respectively [8].

These nine MTBC genetic lineages are categories into modern lineages, intermediate lineage, and ancestral lineages. The "modern" clades of tuberculosis lineage are East Asian, East-African-Indian, and Euro-American lineages (lineages 2 and 3 and 4 and 7) and lineages 7 [9–12], whereas Indo-Oceanic (lineage 1), *Mycobacterium bovis*, and *Mycobacterium africanum* West African 1 and West African 2 (lineages 5 and 6) are ancestral lineages. The newly identified lineages 8 and 9 are an intermediate lineage [11, 12]. The East Asian and Euro-American lineages are the most common worldwide, and they are likely more virulent than other MTBC lineages [13]. The Latin American Mediterranean family and Euro-American (lineage 4) are the most common in Ethiopia [14]. A new lineage (lineage 7) has recently been identified, which is primarily found in Ethiopia and the Horn of Africa [15, 16].

A previous study conducted in the USA reported that the Euro-American, East Asian, Indo-Oceanic, and East African-Indian bacterial lineages were the predominantly identified bacterial lineages found in exclusively extrapulmonary tuberculosis patients (EPTB). Likewise, in exclusively PTB cases, the predominantly identified lineages were Euro-American, East Asian, Indo-Oceanic, and East African-Indian bacterial lineages [17]. In a given situation, characterization of those lineages in EPTB may provide better insights on strain pathogenicity and further will help to document global TB epidemiology [18]. Even though some published studies characterized the drug resistance pattern of MTBC in EPTB patients in Ethiopia [19], there is limited information on the association between specific mycobacterial lineages and sublineages with drug resistance in EPTB patients. Thus, the aim of this study was to identify the Mycobacterial lineages linked to drug resistance in extrapulmonary tuberculosis patients in Addis Ababa, Ethiopia.

2. Materials and Methods

2.1. Study Setting. In this study, we characterized about 151 MTBC isolates identified from 151 patients with extrapulmonary tuberculosis. The isolates were based on samples (abscess, ascetic fluid, CSF, lymph node aspirate, pleural fluid, peritoneal fluid, pericardium fluid, pus) collected from EPTB patients in the selected eight public hospitals located in Addis Ababa from 2016 to 2017. Drug-susceptibility testing and spoligotyping of Mycobacterial isolates are performed at the Ethiopian Public Health Institute. The laboratory provides TB research services, TB diagnosis, and drug susceptibility tests by well-experienced professionals using advanced technologies.

2.2. Study Design and Period. Primary data were collected in a period between December 2016 and August 2017, while the current laboratory-based cross-sectional study was conducted from November 2019 to April 2020 using the stored MTB isolates identified from extrapulmonary cases in Addis Ababa, Ethiopia.

2.3. Laboratory Tests

2.3.1. Drug-Susceptibility Testing. All isolates were subjected to drug susceptibility testing (DST) with first-line anti-TB drugs streptomycin (STM; 1 g/ml), isoniazid (INH; 0.1 g/ml), rifampicin (RIF; 40 g/ml), ethambutol (EMB; 5 g/ml), and pyrazinamide (PZA; 100/ml) using the MGIT 960 [20]. Second-line DST was performed on multidrug-resistant isolates using second-line anti-TB drugs such as amikacin (AMK; 1.0 g/ml), capreomycin (CAP; 1.25 g/ml), ethionamide (ETH; 2.5 g/ml), kanamycin (KAN; 2.5 g/ml), moxifloxacin (MOX; 2.5 g/ml), and ofloxacin (OFX; 2.0 g/m [21]). Reference strain MTB H37Rv was used for quality control.

2.3.2. Spoligotyping. Genomic DNA was extracted from grown subcultured isolates by transferring 500 μl growth *Mycobacterium tuberculosis* isolate into 1.5 cryovial tubes, followed by heat inactivation for 20 minutes at 95°C and release the mycobacterial DNA. Recovered DNA was either immediately used for PCR amplification or stored at -20°C until use [22]. Spoligotyping was carried out according to the standard protocol developed by Kamerbeek et al. [23]. We run both positive and negative controls for each run. For the positive control, we used characterized strains of H37Rv and BCG strains. While for the negative control, molecular grade water is used. Hybridized PCR products were incubated with streptavidin peroxidase conjugate, and the membrane was exposed to a chemiluminescence system, followed by exposure to X-ray film. The film was then developed using standard photochemical procedures (Amersham International, Buckinghamshire, United Kingdom) [23]. Spoligotype international type (SIT) and the family assignment were performed using the MIRU-VNTR*plus* database.

2.3.3. Data Analysis. The spoligotype data analysis was conducted using the MIRU-VNTRplus database software for strain identification [24]. The database is used to assign the spoligotype international type (SIT) and family assignment. All data that were collected are entered into a Microsoft Excel sheet and analyzed using SPSS version 23. Frequencies and proportions were determined to characterize the type of lineages, sublineages, and the DST pattern. Odds ratio along with the 95% CI was used to assess the association between the drug resistance pattern and the type of mycobacterial lineages and sublineages. A P value < 0.05 was considered as a statistically significant difference.

3. Results

3.1. Mycobacterial Lineages Identified. Among the 151 isolates, we identified four main lineages with nine sublineages. Euro-American strain (L4) was the most frequent lineage (111 isolates, 73.5%), followed by the East-African-India (L3) (26 isolates, 17.2%). At the sublineage level, the most prevalent sublineages identified were T family (47 isolates, 31.1%), followed by T3-ETH (33 isolates, 21.9%), Central Asia Strain (26 isolates, 17.2%), Haarlem (15 isolates, 9.9%), and unknown (nine isolates, 6.0%) (Table 1).

3.2. Mycobacterium tuberculosis Lineages and their Drug Resistance Patterns. The spoligotype patterns and their associated drug resistance were analyzed for the 151 mycobacterial isolates analyzed in this study. Out of 151 isolates tested, 122 were sensitive to all first-line anti-TB drugs and belong to different lineages like Euro-American (L4, 61.6%), East-African-Indian (L3, 11.9%), East-Asian (L2, 0.7%), Bovis (1.3%), and unknown strain (5.4%). Among all 151 isolates, we observed 29 drug-resistant isolates. Among the Euro-American lineages (L4), the resistance pattern to first-line anti-TB drugs was as follows: STM (5, 4.5%), INH (14, 12.6%), RIF (8, 7.2%), EMB (2, 1.3%), PZA (14, 12.9%), and MDR-TB (8, 7.2%). Of the East-African-Indian lineages (L3), 3 (11.5%), 5 (19.2%), 4 (15.4%), 6 (23.1%), and 4 (15.4%) lineages became resistant to STR, INH, RIF, PZA, and MDR-TB, respectively. In the current study, only one isolate was identified as Indo-Oceanic (L1), and the isolate was resistant to STR, INH, and RIF. However, a single East-Asian (L2) Beijing isolate becomes susceptible to all drugs. Among the three *Mycobacterium bovis* identified, one strain becomes resistant to INH and PZA. MDR-TB was identified in 6.3% [7], 0.9% [1], 15.4% [4], 100% [1], and 11.1% [1] of T3-ETH, Haarlem, CAS, EAI5, and undefined mycobacterial sublineages, respectively (Table 2).

Of the 14 MDR-TB isolates that had also been submitted to DST for second-line DST (AMK, CAP, ETH, KAN, MOX, and OFX), only three pre-XDR cases were identified. Of these three isolates, two isolates that belong to T3-ETH became resistant to MOX and OFX. The other one strain, which is not defined strain in the database, becomes resistant to CAP and ETH (Table 3).

Any type of drug resistance was identified in 16.2% [18], 30.8% [8], and 11.1% [1] among the Euro-American lineage, East-African-Indian lineage, and unknown strains, respectively. However, in this study, a statistically significant association was not observed for Euro-American lineage (COR; 0.51, 95% CI, 0.216-1.204), East-African-Indian lineage (COR; 2.201, 95% CI, 0.846-5.724), other lineages (COR; 2.938, 95% CI, 0.468-18452), and the strain with undefined lineage (COR; 0.509, 95% CI, 0.61-4.238) with any type of drug resistance. Similarly, in subgroup analysis, there was no statistically significant association between the type of sublineage and any type of drug resistance (Table 4).

Table 1: Distribution of *Mycobacterium tuberculosis* complex (MTBC) lineages and families among extrapulmonary TB isolates ($n = 151$).

Lineages (L)	Sublineages	Frequency	Percent
Euro-American (L4)		111	73.5%
	T	47	31.1%
	T3-ETH	33	21.9%
	Haarlem	15	9.9%
	X1	1	0.7%
	LAM	6	4.0%
	Ural	6	4.0%
East-African-Indian (L3)	CAS	26	17.2%
Indo-Oceanic (L1)	EAI5	1	0.7%
East-Asian (L2)	Beijing	1	0.7%
Bovis	BOV	3	2.0%
Unknown strain	Not defined	9	5.3%

EAI: East-African-Indian; IO: Indo-Oceanic; EAI: East-African-Indian; CAS: Central Asian Strain; H: Harlem; BOV: Bovis; LAM: Latin American Mediterranean; ETH: Ethiopia; L: lineages.

4. Discussion

The present study describes the circulating MTBC lineages and the associated drug-resistance pattern among MTBC isolates collected from EPTB patients. In Ethiopia, few studies have been performed using extrapulmonary samples, and the MTBC lineages associated with drug resistance are poorly described in the country. According to the results of the current analysis, the Euro-American lineage (L 4) was the most prevalent (73.5%), followed by the East-African-Indian (L3) lineage (19.2%). Additionally, we showed that the T family strain predominates (31.1%), followed by T3-ETH (21.9%), Central Asia Strain (17.2%), Haarlem (9.9%), and *Mycobacterium bovis* (2%). A higher proportion of drug resistance was identified among the East-African-Indian lineage (30.8%), followed by the Euro-American lineage (16.2%). However, this study revealed that there was no statistically significant association between any type of drug resistance and either the type of mycobacterial lineage or sublineage.

In the present study, Indo-Oceanic lineage, East-African-Indian lineage, East-Asian lineage, and the Euro-American lineage were identified. Lineage 4 (Euro-American lineage) was the most prevalent among the lineages listed. The dominant prevalence of lineage 4 (Euro-American) and lineage 3 (East-African-Indian) has already been shown in previous studies in Ethiopia [14, 25, 26]. The Euro-American lineage was found to be the most prevalent lineage in Ethiopia and the United States, confirming our results [15, 17, 27–29]. Likewise, a previously conducted study revealed that the T family that is categorized under Euro-American was predominant [30]. In Sudan, MTBC lineage 4 (the Euro-American lineage) was also the most common

Table 2: Distribution of first-line drug-resistance with *Mycobacterium tuberculosis* complex lineages and families among extrapulmonary TB ($N = 151$).

Lineages (Ls) (*n*)	Sublineages	Resistance *N* (%)					
		STR	INH	RIF	EMB	PZA	MDR-TB
Euro-American (L4) (111)		5 (4.5)	14 (12.6)	8 (7.2)	2 (1.8)	14 (12.6)	8 (7.2)
	T	1 (0.9)	2 (1.8)	0	1 (0.9)	2 (1.8)	0
	T3-ETH	3 (2.7)	10 (9.0)	7 (6.3)	1 (0.9)	0	7 (6.3)
	Haarlem	1 (0.9)	1 (0.9)	1 (0.9)	0	3 (2.7)	1 (0.9)
	X1	0	0	0	0	0	0
	LAM	0	1 (0.9)	0	0	2 (1.8)	0
	Ural	0	0	0	0	1 (0.9)	0
East-African-Indian (L3) [26]	CAS	3 (11.5)	5 (19.2)	4 (15.4)	0	6 (23.1)	4 (15.4)
Indo-Oceanic (L1) [1]	EAI5	1 (100)	1 (100)	1 (100)	0	0	1 (100)
East-Asian (L2) [1]	Beijing	0	0	0	0	0	0
Bovis [3]	BOV	0	1 (33.3)	0	0	1 (33.3)	0
Unknown strain [9]	Not defined	0	1 (11.1)	1 (11.1)	1 (11.0)	1 (11.1)	1 (11.1)

EA: Euro-American; EAI: East-African-Indian; IO: Indo-Oceanic; EAI: East-African-Indian; CAS: Central Asian Strain; H: Harlem; BOV: Bovis; LAM: Latin American Mediterranean; ETH: Ethiopia; L: lineages; STM: streptomycin; INH: isoniazid; RIF: rifampicin; EMB: ethambutol; PZA: pyrazinamide; MDR: multidrug resistance.

Table 3: Distribution of second-line anti-TB drug-resistance with lineages and families among MDR isolates among EPTB cases ($N = 14$).

Lineages (Ls) (*n*)	Sublineages	Resistance *N* (%)					
		AMK	CAP	ETH	KAN	MOX	OFX	Pre-XDR-TB
Euro-American (L4) [8]								
	T3-ETH	0	0	0	0	2 (25.0)	2 (25.0)	2 (25.0)
Unknown strain [1]	Not defined	0	1 (100)	1 (100)	0	0	0	1 (100)

ETH: ethinomidine; L: lineages; OFX: ofloxacin; CAP: capreomycin; AMK: amikacin; KAN: kanamycin; MOX: moxifloxacin; ETH: ethionamide.

Table 4: Association between any drug resistance and lineages and sublineage genotype of *Mycobacterium tuberculosis* among extrapulmonary TB isolates ($n = 151$).

Characteristic	Variable	Any drug resistance		Total	COR (95% CI)	*P*
		Sensitive	Resistant			
Lineages (L)	Euro-American	93	18	111	0.51 (0.216-1.204)	0.124
	East-African-Indian	18	8	26	2.201 (0.846-5.724)	0.106
	Unknown strain	8	1	9	0.509 (0.61-4.238)	0.532
	Others lineages	3	2	5	2.938 (0.468-18452)	0.250
Sublineages	T	43	4	47	0.294 (0.096-0.900)	0.032
	T3-ETH	24	9	33	1.837 (0.744-4.540)	0.187
	Haarlem	13	2	15	0.621 (0.132-2.918)	0.546
	LAM	4	2	6	2.185 (0.380-12.551)	0.381
	Ural	5	1	6	0.949 (0.102-8.824)	0.963
	CAS	21	5	26	1.943 (0.755-4.998)	0.168
	Unknown strain	8	1	9	0.509 (0.61-4.238)	0.532
	Other sublineages	4	2	6	1.965 (0.236-16.363)	0.532

EAI: East-African-Indian; CAS: Central Asian Strain; H: Harlem; LAM: Latin American-Mediterranean; ETH: Ethiopia; L: lineages; CI: confidence interval; COR: crude odds ratio; other lineages: Indo-Oceanic, East-Asian, and Bovis; other sublineages: EAI5, Beijing, and Bovis.

(71.6%) [29]. Previously conducted studies in India also identified 76.05%, 67.5, and 59.3% of Euro-American strains [31–33]. The Euro-American lineage's widespread distribution may be due to its virulence and population movement between areas, which promotes its transmission.

Drug resistance to each first-line anti-TB drug, including STM, INH, RMP, EMB, and PZA, was observed to be more prevalent in the EAI lineage and the Euro-American among MTBC genotypes in this study, although not statistically significant. Previous studies in Ethiopia have linked MTBC of the Euro-American lineage with resistance to first-line anti-TB drugs [34, 35]. In our study, East-African-Indian lineage in CAS sublineage was found to be driving the massive spread of drug resistance TB to compare the other than strains.

In the present study, a higher prevalence of MDR was found among the CAS-Delhi/East-African-Indian (lineage 3) followed by the T3-ETH/Euro-American lineage (lineage 4). Likewise, previous studies conducted in Ethiopia reported a higher prevalence of MDR among T3-ETH and CAS-Delhi/East-African-Indian MTBC strains that were isolated from lymph node aspirates [36] .

Resistance to INH was the most frequent in the Euro-American (L4) lineage with predominantly the T3-ETH sublineage. Likewise, the INH mono-resistance was predominantly identified in the T3-ETH sublineage. Previous studies from Ethiopia conducted using direct spoligotyping have also reported similar detection rates of INH mono-resistant isolates belonged to diverse families within Euro-American (L4) [37]. As a consequence, it is necessary to develop a closer surveillance system in the country, with a particular emphasis on isolates where resistance to isoniazid is observed, and to reduce the evolution of DR to MDR and subsequent dispersion within the population.

In the current study, XDR-TB was not identified, despite the fact that 25% of MDR-TB patients of the Euro-American (L4) had pre-XDR-TB cases. In addition, the most frequent resistance proportion was observed in the T3-ETH sublineage. However, we were unable to compare our data to that of other studies in the country because there was no data on pre-XDR/XDR Mycobacterium tuberculosis resistance isolates in combination with EPTB genotypes. However, the finding is in agreement with a previous investigation in Mexico where the Euro-American lineage was predominantly identified among the pre-XDR/XDR *Mycobacterium tuberculosis* isolates [38]. More importantly, the higher prevalence rate of MDR-TB strains with additional resistance to the second-line anti-TB drugs in this study warrants the urgent need for reinforcement of the TB control program [28]. Finally, this study has some limitations. First, the sample size was relatively small. Secondly, the study was based on the mycobacterial isolates collected from EPTB patients residing in a single city, Addis Ababa, which might not represent the whole country.

5. Conclusions

In conclusion, MTBC strains showed considerable genetic diversity in Addis Ababa, Ethiopia. Euro-American (L4) with T3-ETH sublineage strain family and the East-African-Indian (L3) in CAS sublineages were the dominant lineages in both the total MTBC and drug-resistance MTBC strains. No statistically significant association was observed between any type of drug resistance with MTBC lineage or sublineages. Thus, a study on a larger number of MTBC isolates and comparing from both PTB and EPTB is needed to clearly describe the epidemiology of MTBC lineages associated with drug resistance in extrapulmonary tuberculosis patients.

Abbreviations

AMK: Amikacin
BOV: Bovis
CAP: Capreomycin
CAS: Central Asian Strain
CI: Confidence interval
COR: Crude odds ratio
EA: Euro-American
EAI: East-African-Indian
IO: Indo-Oceanic
EAI: East-African-Indian
EMB: Ethambutol
ETH: Ethiopia
H: Harlem
INH: Isoniazid
KAN: Kanamycin
L: Lineages
LAM: Latin American Mediterranean
MDR: Multidrug resistance
MOX: Moxifloxacin
MTBC: Mycobacterium tuberculosis complex
OFX: Ofloxacin
PZA: Pyrazinamide
RIF: Rifampicin
STM: Streptomycin
TB: Tuberculosis
XDR: Extensively drug-resistance.

Consent

No consent was necessary.

Authors' Contributions

GD, AK, HHT, KD, AA, and DA have conceived the study protocol and prepared the assay system. MF, BY, AA, BD, MA, SM, DA, MT, and GA have made substantial contributions to the acquisition of clinical data. GD, BY, MG, BD, MA, and AA performed laboratory tests and analyzed data. ZM has made contributions to combine clinical and laboratory data. GD, AK, HHT, KD, AA, ZM, and DA analyzed the results, drafted the manuscript, and revised it. All authors discussed the results and approved the final manuscript.

Acknowledgments

The authors would like to acknowledge the Ethiopian Public Health Institute and Addis Ababa University for providing materials and facilities during this study. The authors are also grateful for the study participants whose specimens and data were used in this study.

References

[1] *World Health Organization Global Tubeclosis Report*, 2020.

[2] L. M. Muyaya, E. M. Musanda, and J. L. Tamuzi, "Human immunodeficiency virus-associated tuberculosis care in Botswana: evidence from a real-world setting," *BMC Infectious Diseases*, vol. 19, no. 1, p. 767, 2019.

[3] E. O. Babafemi, B. P. Cherian, B. Ouma, and G. Mogoko, "Paediatric tuberculosis diagnosis using Mycobacterium tuberculosis real-time polymerase chain reaction assay: protocol for systematic review and meta-analysis," *Systematic Reviews*, vol. 8, no. 1, p. 225, 2019.

[4] K. J. Seung, S. Keshavjee, and M. L. Rich, "Multidrug-resistant tuberculosis and extensively drug-resistant tuberculosis," *Cold Spring Harbor Perspectives in Medicine*, vol. 5, no. 9, 2015.

[5] M. Park, G. Satta, and O. M. Kon, "An update on multidrug-resistant tuberculosis," *Clinical Medicine*, vol. 19, no. 2, pp. 135–139, 2019.

[6] R. Matambo, K. C. Takarinda, P. Thekkur et al., "Treatment outcomes of multi drug resistant and rifampicin resistant tuberculosis in Zimbabwe: a cohort analysis of patients initiated on treatment during 2010 to 2015," *PLoS One*, vol. 15, no. 4, p. e0230848, 2020.

[7] A. Alemu, Z. W. Bitew, and T. Worku, "Poor treatment outcome and its predictors among drug-resistant tuberculosis patients in Ethiopia: a systematic review and meta-analysis," *International Journal of Infectious Diseases*, vol. 98, pp. 420–439, 2020.

[8] A. Shibabaw, B. Gelaw, W. Gebreyes, R. Robinson, S. H. Wang, and B. Tessema, "The burden of pre-extensively and extensively drug-resistant tuberculosis among MDR-TB patients in the Amhara region, Ethiopia," *Ethiopia. PLoS One.*, vol. 15, no. 2, article e0229040, 2020.

[9] S. Gagneux, K. DeRiemer, T. Van et al., "Variable host-pathogen compatibility in Mycobacterium tuberculosis," *Proceedings of the National Academy of Sciences of the United States of America*, vol. 103, no. 8, pp. 2869–2873, 2006.

[10] M. Senghore, B. Diarra, F. Gehre et al., "Evolution of _Mycobacterium tuberculosis_ complex lineages and their role in an emerging threat of multidrug resistant tuberculosis in Bamako, Mali," *Scientific Reports*, vol. 10, no. 1, p. 327, 2020.

[11] C. N. Sanoussi, D. Affolabi, L. Rigouts, S. Anagonou, and B. de Jong, "Genotypic characterization directly applied to sputum improves the detection of Mycobacterium africanum West African 1, under-represented in positive cultures," *PLoS Neglected Tropical Diseases*, vol. 11, no. 9, article e0005900, 2017.

[12] F. Menardo, L. K. Rutaihwa, M. Zwyer et al., "Local adaptation in populations of Mycobacterium tuberculosis endemic to the Indian Ocean Rim," *F1000Research*, vol. 10, p. 60, 2021.

[13] M. Coscolla and S. Gagneux, "Consequences of genomic diversity in _Mycobacterium tuberculosis_," *Seminars in Immunology*, vol. 26, no. 6, pp. 431–444, 2014.

[14] B. Tulu and G. Ameni, "Spoligotyping based genetic diversity of Mycobacterium tuberculosis in Ethiopia: a systematic review," *BMC Infectious Diseases*, vol. 18, no. 1, p. 140, 2018.

[15] R. Firdessa, S. Berg, E. Hailu et al., "Mycobacterial lineages causing pulmonary and extrapulmonary Tuberculosis, Ethiopia," *Emerging Infectious Diseases*, vol. 19, no. 3, pp. 460–463, 2013.

[16] Y. Blouin, Y. Hauck, C. Soler et al., "Significance of the identification in the Horn of Africa of an exceptionally deep branching Mycobacterium tuberculosis clade," *PLoS One*, vol. 7, no. 12, article e52841, 2012.

[17] X. Qian, D. T. Nguyen, J. Lyu, A. E. Albers, X. Bi, and E. A. Graviss, "Risk factors for extrapulmonary dissemination of tuberculosis and associated mortality during treatment for extrapulmonary tuberculosis," *Emerging Microbes & Infections*, vol. 7, no. 1, pp. 1–14, 2018.

[18] M. R. Farhat, R. Sultana, O. Iartchouk et al., "Genetic determinants of drug resistance in Mycobacterium tuberculosis and their diagnostic value," *American Journal of Respiratory and Critical Care Medicine*, vol. 194, no. 5, pp. 621–630, 2016.

[19] F. Biadglegne, B. Tessema, A. C. Rodloff, and U. Sack, "Magnitude of gene mutations conferring drug resistance in Mycobacterium tuberculosis isolates from lymph node aspirates in Ethiopia," *International Journal of Medical Sciences*, vol. 10, no. 11, pp. 1589–1594, 2013.

[20] P. Zhao, X. J. Li, S. F. Zhang, X. S. Wang, and C. Y. Liu, "Social behaviour risk factors for drug resistant tuberculosis in mainland China: a meta-analysis," *The Journal of International Medical Research*, vol. 40, no. 2, pp. 436–445, 2012.

[21] O. Ignatyeva, I. Kontsevaya, A. Kovalyov et al., "Detection of resistance to second-line antituberculosis drugs by use of the genotype MTBDRsl assay: a multicenter evaluation and feasibility study," *Journal of Clinical Microbiology*, vol. 50, no. 5, pp. 1593–1597, 2012.

[22] P. B. Melchior and H. B. Drugeo, "Inactivation of Mycobacterium tuberculosis for DNA typing analysis inactivation of Mycobacterium tuberculosis for DNA typing analysis," *Journal of Clinical Microbiology*, vol. 37, no. 7, 1999.

[23] J. Kamerbeek, L. Schouls, A. Kolk et al., "Simultaneous detection and strain differentiation of Mycobacterium tuberculosis for diagnosis and epidemiology," *Journal of Clinical Microbiology*, vol. 35, no. 4, pp. 907–914, 1997.

[24] C. Allix-Beguec, D. Harmsen, T. Weniger, P. Supply, and S. Niemann, "Evaluation and strategy for use of MIRU-VNTRplus, a multifunctional database for online analysis of genotyping data and phylogenetic identification of Mycobacterium tuberculosis complex isolates," *Journal of Clinical Microbiology*, vol. 46, no. 8, pp. 2692–2699, 2008.

[25] D. Mekonnen, A. Derbie, A. Chanie, A. Shumet, F. Biadglegne, and Y. Kassahun, "Molecular epidemiology of _M. tuberculosis_ in Ethiopia: A systematic review and meta-analysis," *Tuberculosis (Edinb)*, vol. 118, p. 101858, 2019.

[26] A. Mihret, Y. Bekele, M. Aytenew et al., "Modern lineages of Mycobacterium tuberculosis in Addis Ababa, Ethiopia: implications for the tuberculosis control programe," *African Health Sciences*, vol. 12, no. 3, pp. 339–344, 2012.

[27] I. Comas, E. Hailu, T. Kiros et al., "Population Genomics of _Mycobacterium tuberculosis_ in Ethiopia Contradicts the Virgin Soil Hypothesis for Human Tuberculosis in Sub-Saharan Africa," *Current Biology*, vol. 25, no. 24, pp. 3260–3266, 2015.

[28] D. Damena, S. Tolosa, M. Hailemariam et al., "Genetic diversity and drug susceptibility profiles of Mycobacterium tuberculosis obtained from Saint Peter's TB specialized hospital, Ethiopia," *PLoS One*, vol. 14, no. 6, article e0218545, 2019.

[29] F. A. Khalid, N. Gasmelseed, E. Hailu et al., "Molecular identification of Mycobacterium tuberculosis causing pulmonary tuberculosis in Sudan," *European Academic Research*, vol. 4, no. 9, pp. 7842–7855, 2016.

[30] W. Korma, A. Mihret, J. Hussien, R. Anthony, M. Lakew, and A. Aseffa, "Clinical, molecular and drug sensitivity pattern of mycobacterial isolates from extra-pulmonary tuberculosis cases in Addis Ababa, Ethiopia," *BMC Infectious Diseases*, vol. 15, no. 1, 2015.

[31] S. Sivakumar, Y. Chandramohan, G. R. Kathamuthu et al., "The recent trend in mycobacterial strain diversity among extra pulmonary lymph node tuberculosis and their association with drug resistance and the host immunological response in South India," *BMC Infectious Diseases*, vol. 20, no. 1, p. 894, 2020.

[32] S. Shanmugam, N. Selvakumar, and S. Narayanan, "Drug resistance among different genotypes of _Mycobacterium tuberculosis_ isolated from patients from Tiruvallur, South India," *Infection, Genetics and Evolution*, vol. 11, no. 5, pp. 980–986, 2011.

[33] U. B. Singh, J. Arora, N. Suresh et al., "Genetic biodiversity of _Mycobacterium tuberculosis_ isolates from patients with pulmonary tuberculosis in India," *Infection, Genetics and Evolution*, vol. 7, no. 4, pp. 441–448, 2007.

[34] Z. Bedewi, Y. Mekonnen, A. Worku et al., "_Mycobacterium tuberculosis_ in central Ethiopia: drug sensitivity patterns and association with genotype," *New Microbes and New Infections*, vol. 17, pp. 69–74, 2017.

[35] A. Alelign, A. Zewude, T. Mohammed, S. Tolosa, G. Ameni, and B. Petros, "Molecular detection of Mycobacterium tuberculosis sensitivity to rifampicin and isoniazid in South Gondar Zone, Northwest Ethiopia," *BMC Infectious Diseases*, vol. 19, no. 1, p. 343, 2019.

[36] S. Ayalew, T. Wegayehu, H. Taye et al., "Drug resistance conferring mutation and genetic diversity of Mycobacterium tuberculosis isolates in tuberculosis lymphadenitis Patients; Ethiopia," *Infection and Drug Resistance*, vol. Volume 14, pp. 575–584, 2021.

[37] M. Ejo, G. Torrea, C. Uwizeye et al., "Genetic diversity of the _Mycobacterium tuberculosis_ complex strains from newly diagnosed tuberculosis patients in Northwest Ethiopia reveals a predominance of East-African-Indian and Euro-American lineages," *International Journal of Infectious Diseases*, vol. 103, pp. 72–80, 2021.

[38] A. C. Jiménez-Ruano, C. F. Madrazo-Moya, I. Cancino-Muñoz et al., "Whole genomic sequencing based genotyping reveals a specific X3 sublineage restricted to Mexico and related with multidrug resistance," *Scientific Reports*, vol. 11, no. 1, p. 1870, 2021.

7

Diversity of *Mycobacterium tuberculosis* Complex Lineages Associated with Pulmonary Tuberculosis in Southwestern, Uganda

Lisa Nkatha Micheni,[1,2] Kennedy Kassaza,[1] Hellen Kinyi,[3] Ibrahim Ntulume,[2] and Joel Bazira[1]

[1]*Department of Microbiology, Mbarara University of Science and Technology, P.O. Box 1410 Mbarara, Uganda*
[2]*Department of Microbiology and Immunology, Kampala International University Western Campus, P.O. Box 71, Bushenyi, Uganda*
[3]*Department of Biochemistry, School of Medicine, Kabale University, P.O. Box 317, Kabale, Uganda*

Correspondence should be addressed to Joel Bazira; jbazira@gmail.com

Academic Editor: Adwoa Asante-Poku

Uganda is among the 22 countries in the world with a high burden of tuberculosis. The southwestern region of the country has consistently registered a high TB/HIV incidence rate. This study is aimed at characterizing the *Mycobacterium tuberculosis* complex (MTBC) genotypic diversity in southwestern Uganda. A total of 283 sputum samples from patients with pulmonary tuberculosis were genotyped using specific single nucleotide polymorphism markers for lineages 3 and 4. Most of the patients were males with a mean age of 34. The lineage 4 Ugandan family was found to be the most dominant strains accounting for 59.7% of all cases followed by lineage 3 at 15.2%. The lineage 4 non-Ugandan family accounted for 14.5% of all cases while 4.2% showed amplification for both lineage 4 and lineage 3. Eighteen samples (6.4%) of the strains remained unclassified since they could not be matched to any lineage based on the genotyping technique used. This study demonstrates that a wide diversity of strains is causing pulmonary tuberculosis in this region with those belonging to the lineage 4 Ugandan family being more predominant. However, to confirm this, further studies using more discriminative genotyping methods are necessary.

1. Introduction

Tuberculosis (TB) is an ancient communicable disease that has been in existence over the past millennia and up to date remains a major global public health problem. It is caused by closely related acid-fast bacteria known as *Mycobacterium tuberculosis* complex (MTBC) with seven human-adopted MTBC lineages (designated lineage 1 through lineage 7) and two lineages adapted to various wild and domestic animal species but capable of causing human infection being implicated [1–4]. Epidemiological studies reveal that there is a strong phylogeographical structuring of this organism [5–7] and well adapted to sympatric human populations [8, 9]. This makes these lineages more predominant in specific human populations of certain geographical locations [1, 7, 10]. For instance, lineage 2 (L2) is most predominant in East Asia and is more associated with virulence and drug-resistant than other lineages [11, 12]. L1 (moderately virulent) and L3 mainly occur in areas around the Indian Ocean whereas L5 and L6 are highly restricted to West Africa [13, 14]. L4 is commonly found in Africa, Central America, Europe, and South America [15], while L7 is highly and exclusively restricted in Ethiopia [16]. This adoption could be a result of coevolution [17, 18]. Studies have also shown that human migration greatly contributes to the spread of TB and causes an increase in the genetic diversity of MTBC [9, 19–23].

Uganda is listed among the world's 22 countries with the highest TB burden countries [24] and the third-largest refugee host country in the world after Turkey and Pakistan with over 1.36 million refugees [25–27]. The refugees come from countries such as the Democratic Republic of the Congo (DRC), Burundi, Ethiopia, Eritrea, Rwanda, Somalia, and

South Sudan. Over the past five years, there has been a mass refugee influx from DRC and South Sudan into the country with the southwestern region of the country accommodating most of these refugees. Ninety-two percent (92%) of these refugees live alongside the local communities where accommodation and farming land are given to them [27]. Earlier studies conducted in central Uganda indicate that majority of the TB cases are due to MTBC lineage 4 sublineage Ugandan family (L4-U) [28–30], Euro-American lineage. This sublineage is defined by a deletion in 724 region of difference (RD) and (SNP) typing 33–36, 40 and 43 spoligotype fingerprint spacers missing, and several single nucleotide polymorphisms (SNPs). Similarly, a 2010 study in southwestern Uganda done by Bazira and colleagues using spoligotyping indicated that the majority of TB strains in the region belong to the Uganda genotype [31]. However, the fact that there has been an influx of immigrants in a region that consistently registers high TB incidence rates calls for a greater understanding of the molecular epidemiology and genetic variability of MTBC in the region to enable better control of this causative agent of TB.

2. Methods

2.1. Study Setting. This study was conducted between May 2018 and April 2019 in the southwestern region of Uganda, a region with fifteen administrative districts and borders Tanzania, Rwanda, and the Democratic Republic of Congo (Supplementary File 1: Figure 1). The region is heavily affected by the TB/HIV epidemic and constantly registers high TB incidence rates [32–34]. There were four patient recruitment centers which included two regional referral hospitals (Kabale and Mbarara regional referral hospitals) and two health centers within the refugee camps in the region (Oruchinga and Nakivale health center IV).

2.2. Patient Recruitment and Sample Collection. The patient's clinical information including age, sex, HIV status, previous history of TB, and economic status was recorded. Sputum samples were collected from patients aged ≥18 years. Cases of pulmonary tuberculosis (PTB) were diagnosed at the sample collection centers by either GeneXpert Cepheid test for samples analyzed at the regional referral hospitals or sputum smear microscopy for samples analyzed in the health centers. Those samples diagnosed positive for PTB were then transported (not more than 72 hours after collection time) in a cold box to Mbarara University of Science and Technology Genomics and Translational Laboratory for processing and molecular analysis.

2.3. DNA Extraction and Confirmation of MTB in Sputum Samples. The genomic DNA from each patient sample was processed by standardized protocols [35, 36]. All the samples were then screened and confirmed as MTB by detection of a 123 bp fragment of the IS*6110* gene which is common among the members of the MTBC.

2.4. Single Nucleotide Polymorphism (SNP) Typing. SNP typing to determine the MTB lineages was performed by RT-PCR (Bio-Rad CFX96 Touch™). Lineage-specific primers were as follows: Rv004C for MTB L4-U, Rv2962C for MTB L4-NU, and Rv0129C for MTB L3 based on a previous study of Wampande et al. [37] and their accompanying hybridization probes (Supplementary File 2: Table 1). The MTBC lineages were identified based on differences in melting temperature (T_m). Briefly, the assays were performed in 20 μl reaction mixture containing 3.75 μl of PCR water, 1.25 μl (0.5 μM final concentration) of each primer, 0.625 μl (0.25 μM final concentration) of each probe, 9.5 μl of 2X Lunar® Universal genotyping master mix, and 3 μl (5–50 ng) of extracted genomic DNA. The Bio-Rad CFX96 Touch™ Real-Time PCR Detection System was programmed for PCR amplification and a melting curve stage. For each of the three uniplex assays, the amplification stage consisted of a pre-PCR stage performed at 95°C for 10 min, an amplification stage with denaturation at 95°C for 30 s, primer annealing (50°C for Rv004C or 52°C for Rv0129C or 51°C for Rv2962C) for 30 s, and extension at 60°C for 30 s for 45 cycles. The melting curve analysis consisted of denaturation of the amplicons at 95°C for 10 s to produce single-stranded DNA, probe annealing temperature at 65°C for 05 s with a continuous acquisition mode to allow capture of the fluorescence, and probe melting temperature ranging from 40 to 80°C. In all the assays, kc32969 (L4-U), H37Rv (L4-NU), and delicus (L3) genomic DNA (courtesy of Makerere Molecular Labs) were used as positive control while nontemplate mix as a negative control. The Bio-Rad CFX96 Touch™ software was used to determine the MTB lineages through the analysis of amplicon melting temperature (T_m) (Supplementary File 3: Figure 2).

2.5. Statistical Analysis. Patient demographic data were converted into Excel tables and then exported to SPSS version 25 (IBM, Chicago, USA) for analysis. Bivariate analysis was performed using the chi-square test to determine the relationship between categorical variables (independent variables) and dependent variables. Multinomial logistic regression models were fitted to evaluate the relationship between MTB lineage (dependent variable) and patients' country of origin/ethnicity (primary independent variable). Patients' characteristics of age, gender, and economic status were treated as covariates when fitting the final model. Statistical significance was considered at $p \leq 0.05$. Chi-square and Fisher's exact tests were computed, and a p value of ≤0.05 was considered evidence of a significant difference.

3. Results

A total of 283 samples were genotyped. Majority of the samples (246, 86.9%) were obtained from Ugandan patients. The mean age of the patients was 34 years, and most (73.1%) were males. One hundred and twenty-nine (45.6%) of the patients had unknown serostatus at the time of the study and did not consent to test while 26.9% were HIV seropositive. Among the 283 samples analyzed, 59.7% (169) belonged to lineage 4 Ugandan family (L4-U), 14.5% (41) were other lineage 4 non-Ugandan (L4-NU), and 15.2% (43) lineage 3 (L3) while 4.2% (12) had amplification for both lineage 4 and lineage 3. The remaining 18 (6.4%) strains could not be matched to any

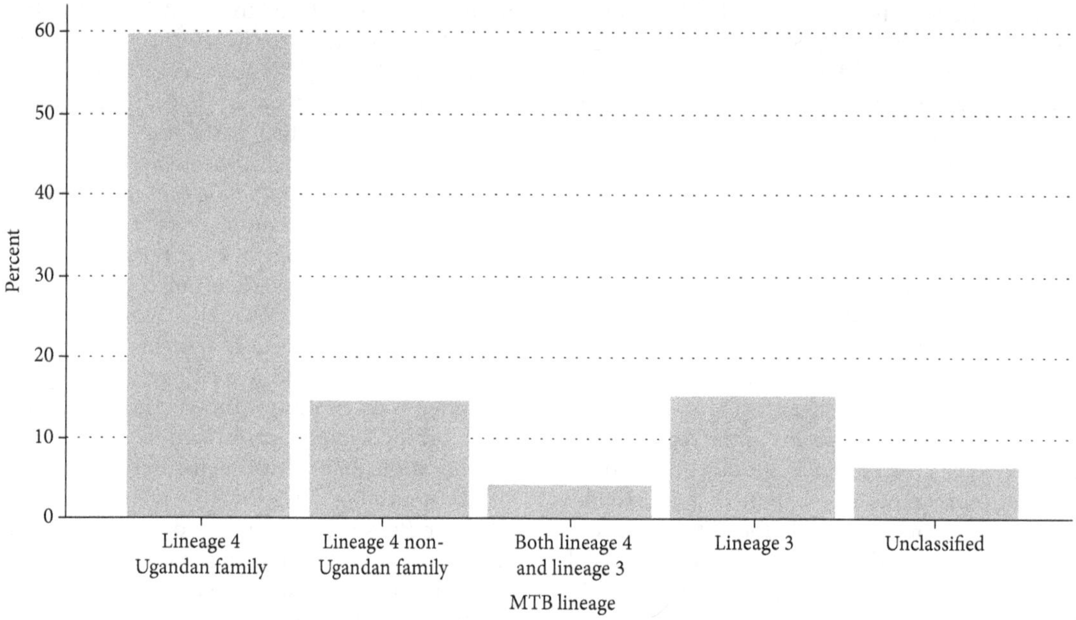

FIGURE 1: Overall prevalence of MTBC lineages causing PTB in southwestern Uganda.

lineage based on the genotyping techniques used (Figure 1). Of the 37 samples from the refugees, 8.1% belonged to L4-U family while 1.1%, 3.2%, and 0.4% were L4-NU, L3, and unclassified strains, respectively. In those samples from the Ugandan patients, 51.6% belonged to L4-U family while 13.4%, 12%, and 6% were L4-NU, L3, and unclassified strains, respectively (Table 1).

Bivariate analysis taking lineage as the outcome showed that the proportions of patients infected with each MTBC lineage did not differ according to age, sex, HIV status, level of income, or history of TB in the past. Despite the fact that the Ugandan genotype was found in a higher proportion of those confirmed by GeneXpert or microscopy, the proportion was not statistically significant ($p = 0.074$) (Table 1). A multinomial logistic regression analysis was further performed to determine the relationship between the independent variable "patients' nationality" and the MTB lineages circulating in southwestern Uganda (Table 2). It was revealed that the Ugandan patients were significantly likely to have L4-U strains (OR: 0.501; 95% CI: 0.143-1.758; p value: 0.281) than the refugee patients when other factors were held constant. Furthermore, the model projected those Ugandan patients were less likely to have strains of lineage 3 (OR = 0.298), both lineages 3 and 4 (OR = 0.868) than the non-Ugandan patients compared to having lineage 4 non-Ugandan family (reference category); however, this was not statistically significant ($p > 0.05$). Conversely, the study showed that Ugandan patients were 1.342 times more likely to have the unclassified strains (95% CI: 0.130-13.54) than the refugee patients when other factors were held constant, but this was not statistically significant ($p > 0.05$).

4. Discussion

To gain insight into the MTBC population structure causing PTB in southwestern Uganda, a region where TB infection is widespread, we utilized SNP typing to analyze 283 sputum samples from Ugandan and non-Ugandan patients diagnosed with PTB. SNP typing was chosen since it was optimized and found to be discriminative by Wampande and colleagues [37]. Our findings revealed heterogeneity of MTBC causing PTB in this area, with L4 being the most predominant lineage, with L4-U family and L4-NU accounting for 59.7% and 14.5% of all cases, respectively. The L4-U family was represented by 51.6% of Ugandan and 8.1% of non-Ugandan patients while L4-NU was represented by 13.4% and 1.1%, respectively. Our results of L4 being the most prevalent in this study are in keeping with reports that indicate TB epidemic in Africa is primarily caused by L4 strains [15]. L4 is phylogenetically complex, with at least ten distinct sublineages that differ in geographical distribution, with local genotypes accounting for a larger proportion of circulating strains in certain regions [15]. For instance, the L4-Cameroon family is almost exclusively found in West Africa [14] while the Latin American-Mediterranean (LAM) family is most predominant in Zambia [38, 39]. Similarly, the L4-U family is more predominant in Uganda as opposed to anywhere else [4, 28, 31, 40]. This is supported by our findings which show that L4-U is most common among the Ugandan patients, as opposed to the refugees and comparable with the 63% recorded in central Uganda [28] and 59.2% reported in an earlier study conducted in Mbarara, southwestern Uganda [31]. Studies indicate that in neighboring countries, the L4-U family is less common. Tanzania, for example, reported 21.8% [40] of L4-U, while Kenya reported 11% [41]. It is thus tempting to speculate that local strains are more likely to transmit in a given local setting compared to others.

Another lineage observed in this study at a relatively high proportion was L3, with a prevalence of 15.2%. The Ugandan patients accounted for 12% of this percentage while non-Ugandans accounted for 3.2%. This finding is comparable to the results of a study conducted in central Uganda, which

TABLE 1: Distribution of patient variables across the MTB lineages in southwestern Uganda.

Variable	Category	Patient's characteristics n (%)	L4-U (n = 169)	L4-NU (n = 41)	MTB lineage Both L4 and L3 (n = 12)	L3 (n = 43)	Unclassified (n = 18)	p value*
Gender	Male	207 (73.1)	120 (42.4)	34 (12)	9 (3.2)	32 (11.3)	12 (4.2)	0.586
	Female	76 (26.9)	49 (17.3)	7 (2.5)	3 (1.1)	11 (3.9)	6 (2.1)	
Age	18-45 years	209 (73.9)	125 (44.2)	29 (10.2)	9 (3.2)	33 (11.7)	13 (4.6)	0.944
	46-65 years	53 (18.7)	29 (10.2)	9 (3.2)	3 (1.1)	8 (2.8)	4 (1.4)	
	≥66 years	21 (7.4)	15 (5.3)	3 (1.1)	0 (0)	2 (0.8)	1 (0.4)	
HIV status	Positive	76 (26.9)	42 (14.8)	12 (4.2)	4 (1.4)	14 (4.9)	4 (1.4)	0.813
	Negative	78 (27.6)	51 (18.0)	9 (3.2)	2 (0.7)	9 (3.2)	7 (2.5)	
	Unknown	129 (45.6)	76 (26.9)	20 (7.1)	6 (2.1)	20 (7.1)	7 (2.5)	
Nationality	Ugandan	246 (86.9)	146 (51.5)	38 (13.4)	11 (3.9)	34 (12.0)	17 (6.0)	0.319
	Non-Ugandan	37 (13.1)	23 (8.1)	3 (1.1)	1 (0.4)	9 (3.2)	1 (0.4)	
Income status	High	23 (8.1)	13 (4.6)	4 (1.4)	1 (0.4)	4 (1.4)	1 (0.4)	0.980
	Low	260 (91.9)	156 (55.1)	37 (13.1)	11 (3.9)	39 (13.8)	17 (6.0)	
TB in the past	No	266 (94)	156 (55.1)	39 (13.8)	12 (4.2)	41 (14.5)	18 (6.4)	0.503
	Yes	17 (6)	13 (4.6)	2 (0.7)	0 (0)	2 (0.7)	0 (0)	
PTB diagnostic results	High/>5AFB/field	148 (52.3)	82 (29)	19 (6.7)	7 (2.5)	31 (11)	9 (3.2)	0.074
	Low/≤5AFB/field	135 (47.7)	87 (30.7)	22 (7.8)	5 (1.8)	12 (4.2)	9 (3.2)	

*p value obtained by chi-square statistic.

TABLE 2: Multinomial analysis of patient's nationality for MTB lineages in southwestern Uganda.

MTB lineage[a]	Predictors	B coefficients	p value*	Odds ratio®	95% CI
Lineage 4 Ugandan family	Intercept	2.037	0.001		
	Ugandan	-0.691	0.281	0.501	0.143–1.758
	Non-Ugandan	0	—	—	
Both lineage 4 and lineage 3	Intercept	-1.099	0.341	—	
	Ugandan	-0.141	0.907	0.868	0.082–9.203
	Non-Ugandan	0	—	—	
Lineage 3	Intercept	1.099	0.099	—	
	Ugandan	-1.210	0.087	0.298	0.075–1.193
	Non-Ugandan	0	—	—	
Unclassified	Intercept	-1.099	0.341	—	
	Ugandan	0.294	0.805	1.342	0.130–13.54
	Non-Ugandan	0	—	—	

[a]Reference category is lineage 4 non-Ugandan family; *p value obtained by logistic regression analysis; ®adjusted OR = odds ratio.

found L3 to be at 11% [28]. Studies conducted in Uganda's neighboring countries such as Tanzania, Sudan, Kenya, and Rwanda have also revealed that L3 (particularly the Central Asian (CAS) family) is a widely implicated lineage in PTB [40]. The MTBC is known to remain stable even in broad cosmopolitan areas such as San Francisco or London where some level of intermingling between locals and immigrants is expected [42]. This is supported by several studies that have shown that MTBC preferably transmits in sympatric host populations [7, 9, 11, 43]. Due to these observations, it is thus easy to speculate that different MTBC lineages could have adapted to different human populations, possibly as a result of MTBC's long coevolutionary history and its human host [6, 8, 17, 18] and that local strains are more likely to transmit in a given local setting compared to others. Our observation that L4-U is predominant in this region is consistent with this hypothesis. However, further work is needed to validate this theory, including studies exploring the interaction between MTBC genetic variation and humans. In our study, 6.4% of the samples were not placed in either of the three lineages screened and may warrant their further characterization to better understand them and to add our knowledge to the molecular epidemiology of TB in this area of Uganda.

5. Limitations of the Study

The use of three unique SNP markers in this study may have restricted our ability to detect other MTBC lineages causing PTB in this region. Nonetheless, our research used SNP markers validated by a local study and took into account the common lineages in circulation in east and central Africa, where the patient population is from.

6. Conclusion

There is heterogeneity of MTBC causing PTB in southwestern Uganda with lineage 4 Ugandan family strains being the most predominant. However, this diversity needs to be ascertained further with more discriminative techniques such as Mycobacterial Interspersed Repeat Units-Variable Number of Tandem Repeat (MIRU-VNTR) typing or whole genome sequencing.

Abbreviations

CAS: Central Asian family
DNA: Deoxyribonucleic acid
EAI: East-African-Indian
L3: *Mycobacterium tuberculosis* lineage 3
L4: *Mycobacterium tuberculosis* lineage 4
L4-NU: *Mycobacterium tuberculosis* lineage 4 other than Ugandan family
L4-U: *Mycobacterium tuberculosis* Ugandan family
LAM: Latin American-Mediterranean
MTB: *Mycobacterium tuberculosis*
MTBC: *Mycobacterium tuberculosis* complex
PTB: Pulmonary tuberculosis
RT-PCR: Real-time polymerase chain reaction
SNP: Single nucleotide polymorphism
TB: Tuberculosis.

Acknowledgments

We thank the colleagues from the molecular biology laboratory at Makerere University Medical School and the staff of TB Laboratory of Mbarara University of Science and Technology for the technical assistance.

References

[1] R. Firdessa, S. Berg, E. Hailu et al., "Mycobacterial lineages causing pulmonary and extrapulmonary tuberculosis, Ethiopia," *Emerging Infectious Diseases*, vol. 19, no. 3, pp. 460–463, 2013.

[2] S. Gagneux, "Genetic diversity in *Mycobacterium tuberculosis*," in *Current Topics in Microbiology and Immunology*, pp. 1–25, Springer, 2013.

[3] S. Gagneux, "Ecology and evolution of *Mycobacterium tuberculosis*," *Nature Reviews Microbiology*, vol. 16, no. 4, pp. 202–213, 2018.

[4] E. M. Wampande, P. Naniima, E. Mupere et al., "Genetic variability and consequence of *Mycobacterium tuberculosis* lineage 3 in Kampala-Uganda," *PLoS One*, vol. 14, no. 9, article e0221644, 2019.

[5] S. Gagneux and P. M. Small, "Global phylogeography of *Mycobacterium tuberculosis* and implications for tuberculosis product development," *The Lancet Infectious Diseases*, vol. 7, no. May, pp. 328–337, 2007.

[6] M. Achtman, "Evolution, population structure, and phylogeography of genetically monomorphic bacterial pathogens," *Annual Review of Microbiology*, vol. 62, no. 1, pp. 53–70, 2008.

[7] I. Mokrousov, "*Mycobacterium tuberculosis* phylogeography in the context of human migration and pathogen's pathobiology: Insights from Beijing and Ural families," *Tuberculosis*, vol. 95, pp. S167–S176, 2015.

[8] S. Gagneux, "Host-pathogen coevolution in human tuberculosis," *Philosophical Transactions of the Royal Society B: Biological Sciences*, vol. 367, no. 1590, pp. 850–859, 2012.

[9] S. Gagneux, K. DeRiemer, T. van et al., "Variable host-pathogen compatibility in *Mycobacterium tuberculosis*," *Proceedings of the National Academy of Sciences of the United States of America*, vol. 103, no. 8, pp. 2869–2873, 2006.

[10] I. Filliol, J. R. Driscoll, D. van Soolingen et al., "Global distribution of *Mycobacterium tuberculosis* spoligotypes," *Emerging Infectious Diseases*, vol. 8, no. 11, pp. 1347–1349, 2002.

[11] Z. Rahim, K. Zaman, A. G. M. van der Zanden et al., "Assessment of population structure and major circulating phylogeographical clades of *Mycobacterium tuberculosis* complex in Bangladesh suggests a high prevalence of a specific subclade of ancient M. tuberculosis genotypes," *Journal of Clinical Microbiology*, vol. 45, no. 11, pp. 3791–3794, 2007.

[12] S. Zamani, M. J. Nasiri, M. Haeili et al., "Determination of circulating *Mycobacterium tuberculosis* strains and transmission patterns among TB patients in Iran, using 15 loci MIRU-VNTR," *International Journal of Mycobacteriology*, vol. 4, p. 119, 2015.

[13] F. Gehre, M. Antonio, F. Faïhun et al., "The first phylogeographic population structure and analysis of transmission dynamics of M. africanum West African 1- combining molecular data from Benin, Nigeria and Sierra Leone," *PLoS One*, vol. 8, no. 10, pp. e77000–e77013, 2013.

[14] S. N. Niobe-Eyangoh, C. Kuaban, P. Sorlin et al., "Genetic biodiversity of *Mycobacterium tuberculosis* complex strains from patients with pulmonary tuberculosis in Cameroon," *Infection, Genetics and Evolution*, vol. 41, no. 6, pp. 2547–2553, 2003.

[15] D. Stucki, D. Brites, L. Jeljeli et al., "*Mycobacterium tuberculosis* lineage 4 comprises globally distributed and geographically

restricted sublineages," *Nature Genetics*, vol. 48, no. 12, pp. 1535–1543, 2016.

[16] H. Nebenzahl-Guimaraes, S. A. Yimer, C. Holm-Hansen, J. de Beer, R. Brosch, and D. van Soolingen, "Genomic characterization of Mycobacterium tuberculosis lineage 7 and a proposed name: 'Aethiops vetus'," *Microbial Genomics*, vol. 2, no. 6, article e000063, 2016.

[17] T. Realpe, N. Correa, J. C. Rozo et al., "Population structure among *Mycobacterium tuberculosis* isolates from pulmonary tuberculosis patients in Colombia," *PLoS One*, vol. 9, no. 4, p. e93848, 2014.

[18] A. L. Banuls, A. Sanou, N. T. Van Anh, and S. Godreuil, "*Mycobacterium tuberculosis*: ecology and evolution of a human bacterium," *Journal of Medical Microbiology*, vol. 64, no. 11, pp. 1261–1269, 2015.

[19] A. Matteelli, K. Lönnroth, D. Mosca et al., "Cameroon's multidrug-resistant tuberculosis treatment programme jeopardised by cross-border migration," *European Respiratory Journal*, vol. 47, no. 2, pp. 686–688, 2016.

[20] I. Mokrousov, H. M. Ly, T. Otten et al., "Origin and primary dispersal of the *Mycobacterium tuberculosis* Beijing genotype: clues from human phylogeography," *Genome Research*, vol. 15, no. 10, pp. 1357–1364, 2005.

[21] I. Comas, E. Hailu, T. Kiros et al., "Population genomics of *Mycobacterium tuberculosis* in Ethiopia contradicts the virgin soil hypothesis for human tuberculosis in sub-Saharan Africa," *Current Biology*, vol. 25, no. 24, pp. 3260–3266, 2015.

[22] E. Alirol, L. Getaz, B. Stoll, F. Chappuis, and L. Loutan, "Urbanisation and infectious diseases in a globalised world," *The Lancet Infectious Diseases*, vol. 11, no. 2, pp. 131–141, 2011.

[23] S. F. Huang, W. J. Su, H. Y. Dou et al., "Association of *Mycobacterium tuberculosis* genotypes and clinical and epidemiological features - A multi-center study in Taiwan," *Infection, Genetics and Evolution*, vol. 12, no. 1, pp. 28–37, 2012.

[24] WHO, *Global Tuberculosis Report*, World Health Organization, 2013.

[25] Norwegian Refugee Council, *Global Report on Internal Displacement*, Norwegian Refugee Council, 2020.

[26] A. Edwards, *Global forced displacement hits record high*, The UN Refugee Agency, 2017.

[27] UNHCR, *Uganda Country Refugee Response Plan*, 2019.

[28] E. M. Wampande, E. Mupere, S. M. Debanne et al., "Long-term dominance of *Mycobacterium* tuberculosisUganda family in peri-urban Kampala-Uganda is not associated with cavitary disease," *BMC Infectious Diseases*, vol. 13, no. 1, 2013.

[29] W. Ssengooba, F. G. Cobelens, L. Nakiyingi et al., "High genotypic discordance of concurrent *Mycobacterium tuberculosis* isolates from sputum and blood of HIV-infected individuals," *PLoS One*, vol. 10, no. 7, article e0132581, 2015.

[30] L. Nabyonga, D. P. Kateete, F. A. Katabazi et al., "Determination of circulating *Mycobacterium tuberculosis* strains and transmission patterns among pulmonary TB patients in Kawempe municipality, Uganda, using MIRU-VNTR," *BMC Research Notes*, vol. 4, no. 1, pp. 4–9, 2011.

[31] J. Bazira, M. Matte, B. B. Asiimwe, and L. M. Joloba, "Genetic diversity of *Mycobacterium tuberculosis* in Mbarara, south western Uganda," *African Health Sciences*, vol. 10, no. 4, pp. 306–311, 2010.

[32] *Uganda Tuberculosis profile*, 2017, https://www.cdc.gov/globalhivtb/where-we-work/Uganda.

[33] M. O. Nwang, J. Kawuma, and M. G. Nabukenya, *Ministry of Health Manual of the National Tuberculosis and Leprosy*, Ministry of Health, Republic of Uganda, 2nd edition, 2010, https://www.who.int/hiv/pub/guidelines/uganda_tb.

[34] Elizabeth Glaser Foundation, *Strengthening the tuberculosis and HIV/AIDS response in the southwest region of Uganda (STAR-SW) project*, 2015.

[35] B. Miljković-Selimović, B. Kocić, T. Babić, and L. Ristić, "Bacterial typing methods," *Acta Fac Medicae Naissensis*, vol. 26, no. 4, pp. 225–233, 2009.

[36] B. A. Forbes, N. Banaiee, K. G. Beavis et al., "Laboratory detection and identification of mycobacteria; approved standard," *Clinical Lab Stand Institute (CLSI)*, vol. 28, no. 17, pp. 14-15, 2008.

[37] E. M. Wampande, S. K. Hatzios, B. Achan et al., "A single-nucleotide-polymorphism real-time PCR assay for genotyping of *Mycobacterium tuberculosis* complex in peri-urban Kampala," *BMC Infectious Diseases*, vol. 15, no. 1, 2015.

[38] C. Mulenga, I. C. Shamputa, D. Mwakazanga, N. Kapata, F. Portaels, and L. Rigouts, "Diversity of *Mycobacterium tuberculosis* genotypes circulating in Ndola, Zambia," *BMC Infectious Diseases*, vol. 10, no. 1, 2010.

[39] E. S. Solo, Y. Suzuki, T. Kaile et al., "Characterization of *Mycobacterium tuberculosis* genotypes and their correlation to multidrug resistance in Lusaka, Zambia," *International Journal of Infectious Diseases*, vol. 102, pp. 489–496, 2021.

[40] E. V. Mbugi, B. Z. Katale, E. M. Streicher et al., "Mapping of *Mycobacterium tuberculosis* complex genetic diversity profiles in Tanzania and other African countries," *PLoS One*, vol. 11, no. 5, p. e0154571, 2016.

[41] W. A. Githui, A. M. Jordaan, E. S. Juma et al., "Identification of MDR-TB Beijing/W and other *Mycobacterium tuberculosis* genotypes in Nairobi, Kenya," *The International Journal of Tuberculosis and Lung Disease*, vol. 8, no. 3, pp. 352–360, 2004.

[42] E. L. Hamblion, A. le Menach, L. F. Anderson et al., "Recent TB transmission, clustering and predictors of large clusters in London, 2010-2012: results from first 3 years of universal MIRU-VNTR strain typing," *Thorax*, vol. 71, no. 8, pp. 749–756, 2016.

[43] R. Stavrum, M. Mphahlele, K. Øvreås et al., "High diversity of *Mycobacterium tuberculosis* genotypes in South Africa and preponderance of mixed infections among ST53 isolates," *Journal of Clinical Microbiology*, vol. 47, no. 6, pp. 1848–1856, 2009.

8

Factors Influencing Adherence to Tuberculosis Treatment in the Ketu North District of the Volta Region, Ghana

Eyram Dogah,[1] Mark Aviisah,[2] Da-Ama Mawulom Kuatewo,[3] Godsway Edem Kpene,[4] Sylvester Yao Lokpo,[4] and Florence Shine Edziah[4]

[1]*Disease Control Unit, Ketu North Municipal Health Directorate, Ghana Health Service, Dzodze, Volta Region, Ghana*
[2]*Department of Health Policy, Planning and Management, School of Public Health, University of Health and Allied Sciences, Hohoe, Ghana*
[3]*Hohoe Municipal Health Directorate, Ghana Health Service, Hohoe, Volta Region, Ghana*
[4]*Department of Medical Laboratory Sciences, School of Allied Health Sciences, University of Health and Allied Sciences, Ho, Ghana*

Correspondence should be addressed to Godsway Edem Kpene; kpene96@gmail.com

Academic Editor: Karl Drlica

Annually, ten million cases of tuberculosis (TB) and about 1.8 million mortalities are recorded. Adherence to TB treatment not only reduces death outcomes but prevents prolonged sickness, transmission to others, and the development of multidrug-resistant TB. This study is aimed at determining the rate of treatment adherence, knowledge of TB infection, and the possible factors influencing adherence to TB treatment in the Ketu North District in the Volta Region of Ghana. A cross-sectional study design was employed. A semistructured questionnaire was used to obtain data from respondents. Adherence to TB treatment and knowledge level about TB infection were assessed. A Chi-square test analysis was used to determine the variables that were associated with treatment adherence. Logistic regression analysis was used to determine potential factors that contribute to treatment adherence. A total of 125 TB registrants were enrolled in the study. The majority (102 (81.6%)) adhered to the TB treatment regimen. However, the level of knowledge about night sweat being a symptom of TB infection was relatively low (78 (62.4%)). Logistic regression analysis revealed that the male gender was about three times more likely (OR = 2.978, 95%CI = 1.173-7.561; $p = 0.022$) to be associated with adherence to TB treatment. However, food availability (OR = 2.208, 95% CI (0.848-5.753); $p = 0.10$) and household size (OR = 0.538, 95% CI (0.195-1.483); $p = 0.23$) were not significantly associated with treatment adherence. In this study, adherence to TB treatment and the knowledge level of TB infection were high. However, the knowledge level of night sweat being a symptom of TB infection was relatively low. Being a male was significantly associated with treatment adherence. An intensified health education on the symptoms of TB infection is therefore recommended.

1. Background

Tuberculosis (TB) is an infectious yet preventable and curable disease caused by *Mycobacterium tuberculosis* [1]. TB affects the lung (pulmonary TB), but it can also affect other parts of the body (extrapulmonary TB). Global reports indicate that about 10 million people were infected with TB in 2019, with some African countries among the leading nations that contributed to the newest TB cases [2]. TB treatment is aimed at ensuring cure for the individual, minimizing the risk of death and disability, and reducing transmission of *M. tuberculosis* [3]. In view of this, the WHO introduced the Directly Observed Treatment (DOT) short-course strategy in 1998 [4] for the purposes of case detection, management, and monitoring [5]. The DOT strategy was also to help improve adherence and enhance treatment outcomes and thus prevent the development of drug resistance [6]. A more recent global target adopted in the United Nations Sustainable Development Goals (SDGs) is to end the TB epidemic by 2030 [7]. Although there appears to be a decline in the annual incident rate, current records show that an estimated 206,030 people worldwide have developed multidrug- or rifampicin-resistant TB (MDR/RR-TB), underscoring the fact that TB infection and control remain a major global public health concern [7].

The WHO defines adherence as the degree to which the person's behavior corresponds with the agreed recommendations from a health care provider [8]. For patients to be successful in TB treatment, they must take the anti-TB drugs for at least six months uninterrupted [3]. However, about half of all TB patients worldwide fail to complete the treatment regimen suggesting the other half to be nonadherent to TB treatment [9]. Some factors proposed to contribute to nonadherence to TB treatment include a false sense of recovery before completing treatment, side effects of the drugs, and ignorance, as well as depression, forgetfulness, and failure to procure medicines from the health facility [5]. Preference for traditional medicine, economic, and geographical difficulties are other suggested factors influencing nonadherence [10].

In West Africa, like most countries in the subregion, Ghana continues to record high TB infection rates as 13,978 new cases were reported in 2018, constituting an incident rate of 32% [11, 12]. The attempt to halt the high prevalence led the country's health ministry to implement a five-year strategic plan (2015-2020) aimed at improving treatment success rate through improved quality clinical care and community TB care [13]. Despite this initiative, records available in the Volta Region show that TB cases remain high, with about 60 and 58.2 TB cases per 100,000 population estimated in 2016 and 2017, respectively [11]. Moreover, there is a dearth of literature on the adherence rate, knowledge level of TB infection, and factors influencing adherence to TB treatment in Ghana, although a previous study in the Eastern Region of Ghana reported a prevalence of 22% noncompliance to treatment among TB patients [14]. Hence, in this study, we aimed to provide information on the rate of treatment adherence and identify factors influencing treatment adherence in the Ketu North District of the Volta Region.

2. Materials and Methods

2.1. Study Design. A cross-sectional study design was employed in this study.

2.2. Study Site Description. Dzodze is the capital of Ketu North District in the Volta Region. Ketu North District shares a boundary with Keta Municipality to the southwest, Akatsi North District to the north, and the Republic of Togo to the east and is bounded by Akatsi South to the east. Ewe is the widely spoken language. Ketu North District has a population of 99,913 with a total number of 26,437 households. The district has an average household of 3.7 persons per household according to the Ghana Statistical Service [15]. There are two hospitals, two clinics, seven health centers, four subdistricts, and thirty-seven CHPS zones. Skilled agriculture, forestry, and fishing constitute the most extensive (47.1%) occupational group, followed by those in craft and related trades (19.8%), and services and sales workers (16.7%). The methods of diagnosing TB in the district include the Acid-Fast Bacilli (AFB) smear microscopy and culture. When a patient is diagnosed with TB, the treatment takes a minimum of six months. The district employs a DOT strategy where a family member or caretaker or a health professional supervises patients to take their medications.

2.3. Study Population. The study population included patients whose records were found in the TB register between November 2014 and August 2016. A health care provider at the facility helped to identify those in the TB register that met the criteria for participation in the study. These patients were informed on the rationale of the study, referred for participation, and contact information was given to ease tracing.

2.4. Inclusion and Exclusion Criteria. The study subjects included registered patients with pulmonary and or extrapulmonary TB, traceable, and consented to be part of the study. However, patients that were drug abusers, were terminally ill, did not give informed consent, and were not traceable were excluded from the study.

2.5. Sample Size Determination. A minimum sample size of 123 was calculated employing the Raosoft online sample size calculator (http://www.raosoft.com/samplesize.html). This was obtained from a total of 180 TB-registered clients, at a 95% confidence interval, 50% response rate, and 5% margin of error.

2.6. Sampling Technique. A convenient and purposive sampling technique was employed. A qualified health worker at the facility helped to identify the 125 respondents who met the inclusion criteria and were reachable.

2.7. Data Collection Procedures. Patients were well informed about the rationale of the study and the consent provided. A structured questionnaire was used to capture data on demographic characteristics and socioeconomic parameters and to assess participants' knowledge about TB, TB treatment, and factors that influence adherence. For confidentiality and anonymity, the names of the respondents were not included in the questionnaire.

2.8. Data Analysis. Data were entered into Microsoft Excel version 13, cleaned, and exported to Social Package for Social Sciences (SPSS) version 23.00 (SPSS Inc., Chicago, USA (http://www.spss.com)) for analysis. Chi-square test and logistic regression analyses were performed to determine the association between variables and adherence and potential factors that could influence adherence to TB treatment, respectively. Variable with p values less than or close to 0.05 after a Chi-square test analysis were included in the logistic regression analysis. At a 95% level of confidence, a p value of less than 0.05 was considered statistically significant.

2.9. Assessment of Knowledge Levels and Definition of Adherence to TB Treatment. The knowledge level of respondents was assessed on TB symptoms, mode of transmission, and treatment duration. The symptoms include coughing, chest pain, weight loss, and night sweats. A right response was regarded as good knowledge (score = 1) while a wrong response was regarded as poor knowledge (score = 0). The total score for an individual below the index score of 4 was regarded as inadequate knowledge while scores above the index score of 4 were regarded as adequate knowledge. Adherence was defined as self-report of having completed TB treatment plus documented evidence from the TB register of having completed treatment regimen as prescribed by the clinician.

2.10. Ethical Consideration. The study was approved by the Ethical Review Committee of Ghana Health Service, Research, and Development Division. Written approval was obtained from Ketu North Health Directorate and St. Anthony Catholic Hospital. Informed consent was obtained from respondents before the interview.

3. Results

The majority of the study participants were males (76 (60.80%)) and Christians (99 (79.2%)), and 42 (33.6%) were between 30 and 39 years. At the time of this study, the majority of the study participants were married (74 (59.2%)) and 116 (92.8%) were employed while 54 (42.2%) attained primary education whereas most respondents were of the Ewe ethnicity 113 (90.40%) (Table 1).

From Table 2, it was observed that all respondents exhibited good knowledge regarding coughing as a symptom. The majority of study respondents demonstrated good knowledge on the mode of TB transmission 100 (80%), duration of treatment (124 (99.2%)), chest pain (117 (93.6)), and weight loss (102 (81.6)) as well as night sweats (78 (62.4)) and coughing 125 (100%) as symptoms of TB infection. When participants were asked when it was appropriate to stop treatment, 121 (96.8) indicated that one needed to continue treatment even when they feel well while 124 (99.2) said it should only be halted when a health worker asks you to stop.

The Chi-square test analysis showed that gender was a significant factor associated with treatment adherence. However, educational level, having treatment supporter, staff attitude, self-perceived wellness, food availability, being on other medication, and household size were not significantly associated with treatment adherence (Table 3).

Males were about thrice as likely to adhere to TB treatment compared to females (OR = 2.978, 95%CI = 1.173-7.561; $p = 0.022$). However, food availability (OR = 2.208, 95% CI (0.848-5.753); $p = 0.10$) and household size (OR = 0.538, 95% CI (0.195-1.483); $p = 0.23$) did not significantly influence adherence to TB treatment (Table 4).

Table 1: Demographic characteristics of the study respondents.

Parameter	Frequency	Percentage
Age (years)	40.23 ± 8.79*	
Age category (years)		
20–29	18	14.4
30–39	42	33.6
40–49	41	32.8
50–59	24	19.2
Gender		
Female	49	39.2
Male	76	60.8
Educational status		
None	20	16.0
Primary	54	42.2
Secondary	43	34.4
Tertiary	8	6.4
Religion		
Christianity	99	79.2
Islam	5	4
Traditional	16	12.8
Others	5	4
Marital status		
Single	16	12.8
Cohabiting	15	12
Married	74	59.2
Separated	11	8.8
Widowed	9	7.2
Ethnicity		
Akan	2	1.6
Ewe	113	90.4
Others	10	8
Employment status		
Employed	116	92.8
Unemployed	9	7.2

Data are presented as figures and percentages. * is expressed as mean ± standard deviation.

4. Discussion

Adherence to TB treatment decreases the risk of drug resistance, prolonged infection, or even death [16]. In the current study, we provide empirical data to the literature on adherence of TB patients to treatment in the Ketu North District in the Volta Region of Ghana, which hitherto was lacking. The adherence rate (81.6%) in this study (Table 3) was higher than that recorded in Suhum in the Eastern Region of Ghana (63%) [14] but lower than rates reported in Tanzania (95.7%) [17] and Ethiopia (90.0%) [18]. Compared to the earlier reports in Suhum, the plausible explanations to the higher adherence rate in our study include increased awareness of TB infection via effective health education in the district and the relatively greater proportion of volunteered treatment supporters (84.80%). Moreover, differences in methodology including study design, type of sampling technique, sample size, and definition of adherence could account for the dissimilarities in the adherence rates between our study and those recorded in Tanzania and Ethiopia.

It is suggested that patients' knowledge about a disease influences treatment adherence and outcome [19]. A previous study in the Sekondi-Takoradi Metropolis observed that failure to recognize symptoms due to TB and stigma negatively affect patients' adherence to treatment [20]. In our study, the overall knowledge level of TB infection was high (119 (95.2%)) (Table 3). Moreover, a greater proportion of

TABLE 2: Respondent's knowledge of TB symptoms, transmission, and treatment duration.

Parameter	Knowledge level Poor	Good
Mode of transmission of TB	25 (20.0)	100 (80.0)
Duration of treatment	1 (0.8)	124 (99.2)
Symptoms of tuberculosis		
Coughing	0 (0.0)	125 (100.0)
Chest pain	8 (6.4)	117 (93.6)
Weight loss	23 (18.4)	102 (81.6)
Night sweat	47 (37.6)	78 (62.4)
When to halt treatment		
When the individual feels well	4 (3.2)	121 (96.8)
When a health worker asks you to stop	1 (0.8)	124 (99.2)
	Inadequate	*Adequate*
Overall knowledge level on TB infection	6 (4.8)	119 (95.2)

Data is presented frequencies and percentages in parentheses.

TABLE 3: Chi-square test analysis of factors associated with treatment adherence.

Parameter	Treatment adherence Total (125 (100))[a]	No (23 (18.4))[b]	Yes (102 (81.6))[b]	p value
Gender				
Female	49 (39.20)	14 (28.57)	35 (71.43)	0.02
Male	76 (60.80)	9 (11.84)	67 (88.16)	
Age category (years)				
<40	60 (48.00)	13 (21.66)	47 (78.34)	0.49
≥40	65 (52.00)	10 (15.38)	55 (84.52)	
Educational level				
Up to primary	74 (59.20)	14 (18.92)	60 (81.08)	0.86
Above primary	51 (40.80)	9 (17.65)	42 (82.35)	
Treatment supporter				
No	19 (15.20)	4 (21.05)	15 (78.95)	0.75
Yes	106 (84.80)	19 (17.92)	87 (82.08)	
Staff attitude				
Friendly	99 (79.20)	18 (18.18)	81 (81.82)	0.90
Nonfriendly	26 (20.80)	5 (19.23)	21 (80.77)	
Self-perceived wellness after initiating treatment				
<2 months	23 (18.40)	6 (26.09)	17 (73.91)	0.29
2-4 months	102 (81.60)	17 (16.67)	85 (83.33)	
On other medications				
No	94 (75.20)	15 (15.96)	79 (84.04)	0.22
Yes	31 (24.80)	8 (25.81)	23 (74.19)	
Food availability				
Available	93 (74.40)	14 (15.05)	79 (84.95)	0.10
Not available	32 (25.60)	9 (28.13)	23 (71.88)	
Household size				
1–2	10 (8.00)	4 (40.00)	6 (60.00)	0.09
3–4	35 (28.00)	8 (22.86)	27 (77.14)	
>4	80 (64.00)	11 (13.75)	69 (86.25)	

Data is presented as figure and percentages in parentheses. p value significant at <0.05. [a]Percentages are calculated columnwise. [b]Percentages are calculated rowwise.

the study respondents demonstrated good knowledge about the mode of transmission (100 (80.0%)), duration of treatment (124 (99.2%)), and symptoms of TB including coughing (125 (100.0%)), chest pain (117 (93.6%)), and weight loss (102 (81.6%)) (Table 2). Indeed, having adequate knowledge about a disease could translate into improved adherence because the patient is less likely to halt treatment during the treatment period [19]. This appears to be the case in this study where the high knowledge level exhibited by the study respondents could account for the high adherence rate recorded. However, the level of knowledge about night sweat being a symptom of TB infection in this study seems to be relatively low (78 (62.4%)) ((Table 2), indicating that more should be done to intensify education on the symptoms of TB infection in the district. This finding is consistent with a prior study in Morocco where only 17.2% of respondents had displayed good knowledge about the causative agent of TB [21] and Equatorial Guinea where 16.84% knew about the mode of transmission [22].

An earlier report in Ghana suggested that patients' compliance with medication was not influenced by their background characteristics [14]. In our study, however, we observed gender to be significantly associated with treatment adherence where the male respondents were about three times more likely to adhere to TB treatment (OR = 2.978, 95%CI = 1.173-7.561; $p = 0.022$) compared to their female counterparts (Table 4). No specific reason can be adduced from the current study. However, further studies are required to confirm this finding and to unravel the possible factors that could contribute to male preponderance to TB treatment adherence in the district. In contrast, females were twice more likely to adhere to TB treatment compared to their male peers in the Tanzanian study [17].

Salifu and Eliason [23] in their study to understand patients' perspectives of barriers and enablers to TB treatment observed that food availability and medication-related side effects impacted negatively on treatment adherence. In contrast, we did not find a significant association between food availability and treatment adherence (OR =2.208, 95% CI (0.848-5.753); $p = 0.10$) (Table 4), although the adherence rates were higher among those who had food available compared to those who did not (Table 3). The feeling of uneasiness after taking medication on an empty stomach or with inadequate food has been reported previously in individuals who had defaulted in TB treatment [23]. Indeed, having a large family size is believed to impact negatively on household food security [24]. Therefore, this impact could also be felt by individuals undergoing TB treatment in such large households. In our study, however, no significant association was observed between household size and treatment adherence (OR = 0.538, 95% CI (0.195-1.483); $p = 0.23$) (Table 4).

The present study is limited by the relatively small sample size; hence, a larger sample size should be used in future studies in the district. Due to the cross-sectional study design employed in this study, cause and effect relationships cannot

TABLE 4: Logistic regression analysis of factors influencing treatment adherence.

Parameter	OR	95% CI	*p* value
Gender			
Female	Ref		
Male	2.978	1.173–7.561	0.02
Food availability			
Available	Ref		
Not available	2.208	0.848–5.753	0.10
Household size			
1–2	Ref		
3–4	0.239	0.058–0.986	0.05
>4	0.538	0.195–1.483	0.23

Data are presented as odds ratio (OR) and 95% confidence interval (CI). p value significant at <0.05.

be established. Notwithstanding, the findings of this study address an important gap in the literature regarding the adherence rate, knowledge level, and possible factors that could contribute to adherence to TB treatment in the Ketu North District in the Volta Region of Ghana.

5. Conclusion

In this study, adherence to TB treatment and the knowledge level of TB infection were high. However, the level of knowledge about night sweat being a symptom of TB infection was relatively low. Being a male was significantly associated with treatment adherence while food availability and household size were not significantly associated with treatment adherence. We recommend an intensified health education on the symptoms of TB infection in the district.

Acknowledgments

We wish to thank the management of the TB unit at the Ketu North District Health Directorate for their assistance in collecting data for this study.

References

[1] WHO, *Global Tuberculosis Report*, World Health Organization, 20th edition, 2015, https://apps.who.int/iris/handle/10665/191102.

[2] WHO, *Tuberculosis Secondary Tuberculosis*, 2019, https://www.who.int/news-room/fact-sheets/detail/tuberculosis.

[3] CDC, *Tuberculosis (TB) Fact Sheet Secondary Tuberculosis (TB) Fact Sheet*, 2011, https://www.cdc.gov/tb/publications/factsheets/general/tb.htm.

[4] C. F. Ubajaka, E. C. Azuike, J. O. Ugoji et al., "Adherence to drug medications amongst tuberculosis patients in a tertiary health institution in south east Nigeria," *International Journal of Clinical Medicine*, vol. 6, no. 6, pp. 399–406, 2015.

[5] F. A. D. Kaona, M. Tuba, S. Siziya, and L. Sikaona, "An assessment of factors contributing to treatment adherence and knowledge of TB transmission among patients on TB treatment," *BMC Public Health*, vol. 4, no. 1, 2004.

[6] S. Yao, W.-H. Huang, S. van den Hof et al., "Treatment adherence among sputum smear-positive pulmonary tuberculosis patients in mountainous areas in China," *BMC Health Services Research*, vol. 11, no. 1, 2011.

[7] WHO, *Global Tuberculosis Report 2018*, 2019.

[8] F. Dobbels, R. Van Damme-Lombaert, J. Vanhaecke, and S. De Geest, "Growing pains: non-adherence with the immunosuppressive regimen in adolescent transplant recipients," *Pediatric transplantation*, vol. 9, no. 3, pp. 381–390, 2005.

[9] S. A. Munro, S. A. Lewin, H. J. Smith, M. E. Engel, A. Fretheim, and J. Volmink, "Patient adherence to tuberculosis treatment: a systematic review of qualitative research," *PLoS Medicine*, vol. 4, no. 7, p. e238, 2007.

[10] A. Rondags, A. B. Himawan, J. F. Metsemakers, and T. N. Kristina, "Factors influencing non-adherence to tuberculosis treatment in Jepara, Central Java, Indonesia," *The Southeast Asian Journal of Tropical Medicine and Public Health*, vol. 45, no. 4, pp. 859–868, 2014.

[11] G. Report, *The Health Sector in Ghana Facts and Figures*, 2018, https://ghanahealthservice.org/download/Facts+Figures_2018.pdf.

[12] Team DHM, *Annual Year Rewiew of Ketu North District Health Directorate*, 2015, In press.

[13] Ministry of Health G, *The National Tuberculosis Health Sector Strategic Plan for Ghana*, 2015, https://www.ccmghana.net/images/PRs/NTP/TB-health-sectorplan-2015-2020.compressed.pdf.

[14] E. Danso, I. Y. Addo, and I. G. Ampomah, "Patients' compliance with tuberculosis medication in Ghana: evidence from a periurban community," *Advances in Public Health*, vol. 2015, Article ID 948487, 6 pages, 2015.

[15] GSS, *Ghana Statistical Services*, 2010, https://statsghana.gov.gh/gssmain/fileUpload/pressrelease/2010_PHC_National_Analytical_Report.pdf.

[16] G. Tesfahuneygn, G. Medhin, and M. Legesse, "Adherence to anti-tuberculosis treatment and treatment outcomes among tuberculosis patients in Alamata District, northeast Ethiopia," *BMC Research Notes*, vol. 8, no. 1, 2015.

[17] A. Mkopi, N. Range, F. Lwilla et al., "Adherence to tuberculosis therapy among patients receiving home-based directly observed treatment: evidence from the United Republic of Tanzania," *PloS one*, vol. 7, no. 12, p. e51828, 2012.

[18] H. H. Tola, K. Holakouie-Naieni, E. Tesfaye, M. A. Mansournia, and M. Yaseri, "Prevalence of tuberculosis treatment non-adherence in Ethiopia: a systematic review and meta-analysis," *The International Journal of Tuberculosis and Lung Disease*, vol. 23, no. 6, pp. 741–749, 2019.

[19] K. Chani, *Factors Affecting Compliance to Tuberculosis Treatment in Andara Kavango Region Namibia*, UNIVERSITY OF SOUTH AFRICA, 2010.

[20] E. A. Dodor, "The feelings and experiences of patients with tuberculosis in the Sekondi-Takoradi Metropolitan district: implications for TB control efforts," *Ghana Medical Journal*, vol. 46, no. 4, pp. 211–218, 2012.

[21] N. Tachfouti, K. Slama, M. Berraho, and C. Nejjari, "The impact of knowledge and attitudes on adherence to tuberculosis treatment: a case-control study in a Moroccan region," *The Pan African Medical Journal*, vol. 12, pp. 52–52, 2012.

[22] G. Fagundez, H. Perez-Freixo, J. Eyene et al., "Treatment

adherence of tuberculosis patients attending two reference units in Equatorial Guinea," *PloS one*, vol. 11, no. 9, p. e0161995, 2016.

[23] Y. Salifu and C. Eliason, "Tuberculosis treatment adherence in Ghana: patients' perspectives of barriers and enablers to treatment," *NUMID HORIZON: An International Journal of Nursing and Midwifery*, vol. 7, pp. 6–23, 2017.

[24] A. O. Olayemi, "Effects of family size on household food security in Osun state, Nigeria," *Asian Journal of Agriculture and Rural Development*, vol. 2, no. 2, pp. 136–141, 2012.

9

Prevalence and Associated Factors of Tuberculosis among Adult Household Contacts of Smear Positive Pulmonary Tuberculosis Patients Treated in Public Health Facilities of Haramaya District, Oromia Region, Eastern Ethiopia

Abinet Adane,[1] Melake Damena,[2] Fitsum Weldegebreal ,[3] and Hussein Mohammed[2]

[1]*East Hararghe Zone, East Hararghe Zonal Health Office, Harar, Ethiopia*
[2]*School of Public Health, College of Health and Medical Sciences, Haramaya University, P.O. Box: 235, Harar, Ethiopia*
[3]*Department of Medical Laboratory Sciences, College of Health and Medical Sciences, Haramaya University, Harar, Ethiopia*

Correspondence should be addressed to Fitsum Weldegebreal; fwmlab2000@gmail.com

Academic Editor: Vincent Jarlier

Background. Tuberculosis is an infectious airborne disease caused by *Mycobacterium tuberculosis.* It still remains a major public health problem which affects all age groups. Risk of exposure is higher in household contact than members of the general population. *Objective.* The aim of this study was to assess the prevalence and associated factors of tuberculosis among adult household contacts of smear positive pulmonary tuberculosis in Haramaya district, Oromia Region, Eastern Ethiopia from February to March, 2019. *Method.* A community based cross-sectional study design was conducted. A total of 454 study participants were selected using systematic sampling method from all adult household contacts of smear positive pulmonary tuberculosis patients treated from July 2017 to December 2018. Data were collected using a pretested and structured questionnaire; and laboratory examination was processed using fluorescent smear microscope. Logistic regression analysis was used to identify the factors associated with the infection of pulmonary tuberculosis and a statistically significant association was declared at P-value < 0.05. *Result.* The overall prevalence of pulmonary tuberculosis among adult household contacts was 7.8% (95% CI: 5.8–10.0). The risk factors for tuberculosis infection among household contacts were eating meals less than three times per day (AOR = 4.31; 95% CI: 1.61, 11.55), drinking raw milk (AOR = 4.12; 95% CI: 1.43, 11.90), having family history of tuberculosis with more than one index case (AOR = 2.7; 95% CI: 1.02, 6.92), living in poor ventilated houses (AOR = 4.02; 95% CI: 1.38, 11.76), and living in inadequate size of living room (AOR = 3.4; 95% CI: 1.30, 8.86). *Conclusion.* In this study, the prevalence of tuberculosis among adult household contacts of smear positive pulmonary tuberculosis is high. Eating meals less than three times per day, drinking raw milk, living in poor ventilated houses, and inadequate sizes of the rooms were identified as contributing factors. Therefore, we recommend that the transmission of tuberculosis can potentially be reduced by a better contact tracing and treatment strategies along with appropriate health education.

1. Introduction

Pulmonary tuberculosis (PTB) is an infectious airborne disease caused mainly by *Mycobacterium tuberculosis.* The main source of infection is untreated smear-positive PTB patients. It typically affects the lungs (PTB) but can also affect other sites as well (extra PTB) [1]. The chance of developing TB is much higher among people with low immune status [2, 3]. Tuberculosis (TB) disease remains a major public health problem which affects all age groups globally [1]. It is one of the top 10 causes of death and the leading cause from a single infectious agent and millions of people continue to fall sick with TB each year [2].

The global TB report showed that there were an estimated 10 million incident cases and 12 million prevalent cases of TB globally. Overall 90% of the infection occurred in adults; of this 9% were people living with HIV (72% in Africa). About 26% of incident TB cases occurred in Africa and 23% of the world's population are estimated to have a latent TB infection, and are thus at risk of developing active TB during their lifetime [2]. Currently, Ethiopia is ranked eighth among the 22 high TB burden countries in the world and at rank three, in Africa. The incidence rate of all forms of TB is estimated at 164 per 100,000 population, leading to an annual mortality rate of 27.5 per 100,000 population [1, 2].

Tuberculosis is exclusively transmitted based on environmental and personal risk factors, especially in a social mixing setting (together with overcrowding) and conditions which prolong the length of exposure to an infectious patient like health system-related factor including delay in diagnosis can increase TB transmission [4, 5]. In addition, the risk of infection following TB exposure is primarily governed by exogenous factors and intrinsic combination of the infectiousness of the source case, proximity to contact and social and behavioral risk factors including smoking, alcohol, and indoor air pollution [4].

Patients with asymptomatic pulmonary tuberculosis transmit the bacilli to risky groups through inhalation. Identify and investigating infected individual among contacts of patients with infectious tuberculosis is the best method of preventing the later development of the disease in populations. In addition to this, contact tracing is very important to establish the primary source of the TB disease and to detect those who are secondarily infected by proper diagnosis and prompt treatment [6–8]. Furthermore, the likelihood of progression from latent TB infection (LTBI) to TB in household contacts is usually higher than in the general population. Household contacts of PTB patients are considered a high-priority population for contact investigation [9–11].

Pulmonary tuberculosis contact investigations are rarely and inconsistently carried out in resource-limited settings of low- and middle-income countries like Ethiopia [12, 13]. Studies conducted in Ethiopia on the prevalence and associated factors of PTB among household contacts were very limited. So, it is necessary to identify the factors which contribute to TB infection and overall status of PTB among household contacts of smears positive TB in the district.

2. Methods and Materials

2.1. Study Area and Period. The study was conducted in Haramaya district, Oromia region, eastern Ethiopia from February to March, 2019. Haramaya is one of 24 districts in east Hararghe zone which is located at 520 km from Addis Ababa; capital city of Ethiopia, and 20 km from the historical city, Harar, with a total land area of 525.64 sq km. It is bordered by Kurfachelle district in north, Dire-Dawa administration in south, Kersa and Kombolcha districts in west and east, respectively. According to population projection set in 2018, the total population of the district is 304,276 among which 152,442 (50.1%) were males and 151,834 (49.9%) were females. Administratively, the district has 2 urban and 31 rural kebeles, with one district hospital, eight health centers, 12 private clinics, and 33 healthposts. All governmental health facilities are providing diagnostic and treatment services for tuberculosis [14].

2.2. Study Design and Population. A community based cross-sectional study design was employed. Adults who had close household contact with PTB infected patients who were on treatment from July 2017 to December 2018 were included while critically sick and mentally ill were excluded from the study.

2.3. Sample Size Determination and Sampling Procedure. The sample size was computed using a single population proportion formula by considering 4.3% proportion of TB cases among household contacts of smear-positive PTB (1), 95% confidence interval, and 2% margin of error. Accordingly, the final sample size with a 5% non-response rate was 454. All public health facilities (one hospital and eight health centers), providing TB diagnosis and treatment services in the district were considered for the study. According to the information retrieved from these health facilities, a total of 240 TB patients were registered and treated from July 2017 to December 2018. First, the total adult household contacts of smear-positive PTB patients ($n = 1152$) were obtained from the district's Community Health Information System registries available at health post. Then the sample size was proportionally allocated to each health facility according to the number of adult household contacts of smear positive PTB patient. Finally, 454 study participants were randomly selected from households.

2.4. Data Collection Tools and Methods. Data were collected using a structured questionnaire developed from previous literature [15–17] and it was pretested on 5% of the study participants in a nearby district (i.e., Aweday district). Data collectors and supervisors were trained on data collection tools and how to observe measure, collect, and transport samples to health facility that helped minimize bias, and maintain the quality of data. Moreover, the supervisors and principal investigator have been supervising field works and they checked the quality of collected data on a daily basis.

The data were collected through face to face interview, observing the house condition, measuring area of house, and collecting data from adult household contacts. Interview and observation were conducted prior to sputum sample collection after informing; getting consents and screen household contacts by using symptoms based algorithm. Household contacts were traced by home to home visits. Sputum microscopy was used to determine tuberculosis among adult household contacts. Household contacts were requested to submit two sputum specimens. Sputum collected at household level was transported to health facility using triple packaging by maintaining cold chain within 5 days. Participants were advised to submit sputum not containing food particle and minimize amount of saliva. Sputum microscopy was done in Haramaya district hospital laboratory using fluorochrome staining technique. In this study Presumptive TB cases were diagnosed if an individual had one or more of the clinical manifestations consistent with TB (i.e. persistent cough of 2 weeks or more, fever for more than 2 weeks, night sweats, and unexplained weight loss) and TB patients were diagnosed if participants had at least one sputum smear positive (1).

2.5. Data Quality Control. Data collectors and supervisors were trained for two days on the data collection tools. The collected data were checked manually on daily basis to check for its completeness and consistency. Double data entry were done by two separate individuals to crosscheck the data entered. The recommended procedure for specimen collection, proper labeling, and storage was followed strictly. The sample was rejected if it contained food particles. Internal and external quality control was also ensured for AFB smear microscopy.

2.6. Data Processing and Analysis. The data were coded and double entered to Epi data version 3.1 and then exported to Statistical Package for Social Sciences (SPSS) version 21 for analysis. Data cleaning was performed by running frequencies and cross tabulation to check accuracy, outliers, consistencies, and missing values. Descriptive statistics (i.e. frequency distribution, proportion, mean, and standard deviation) was used to summarize the variables. Bivariate analysis was performed to assess the potential associations between categorical variables and the outcome. Variables with a p-value of less than 0.25 in the bivariate analysis were entered into the final multivariable logistic regression model to identify the predictors of the outcome. A variable with a P -value less than 0.05 at 95% confidence level was considered statistically significant. The absence of multi-co-linearity was checked by using VIF/tolerance. The model of fitness was checked by Hosmer and Lemeshow, which provided evidence of fitness with a predictor test level of $p = 0.82$.

3. Results

3.1. Socio-Demographic Characteristics. A total of 240 index cases registered in selected public health facilities in the district were included in the study. More than half of the index cases 122 (50.8%) were male and most of them (80%) were from rural areas. From a total of 454 planned household contacts, 451 were included in the study, with a response rate of 99.3%. The mean (±SD) age of the household contacts patients was 31.0 (±11.7) years, range from 18 to 75 years. More than half, 228 (50.6%), of the household contacts were female, majority (73.8%) were from rural areas, and 60.1% were married. One hundred seventy six (39%) of household contacts' relationships with index cases were siblings followed by husband (24.8%) and wife (23.3%). Three hundred thirty eight (74.9%) of the household contacts were farmer in occupation (Table 1).

Table 1: Socio-demographic characteristics of adult household contacts of smear positive PTB patients in Haramaya district, Eastern Ethiopia, 2019 ($n = 451$).

Variables		Frequency	
		Number	Percent (%)
Age (year)	18–27	212	47.0
	28–37	116	25.7
	≥38	123	27.3
Gender	Male	223	49.4
	Female	228	50.6
Marital status	Single	156	34.6
	Married	271	60.1
	Divorced	16	3.5
	Widowed	8	1.8
Ethnicity	Oromo	435	96.5
	Amhara	11	2.4
	Others	5	1.1
Religion	Muslim	441	97.8
	Orthodox	10	2.2
Residence	Urban	118	26.2
	Rural	333	73.8
Educational level	Not read and write	258	57.2
	Read and write	73	16.2
	Primary (1–8)	83	18.4
	Secondary (9–12)	25	5.5
	Collage and above	12	2.7
Occupation	Farmer	338	74.9
	Government employ	5	1.1
	House wife	37	8.2
	Merchant	14	3.1
	Daily labor	15	3.3
	Student	42	9.3
Relationship to the index case	Husband	112	24.8
	Wife	105	23.3
	Sibling	176	39.0
	Others	58	12.9
Monthly income of the family	<1000	273	60.5
	1000–1500	67	14.9
	>1500	111	24.6

3.2. Housing Condition of the Participants. Four hundred sixteen (92.7%) of houses of the study participants were made from mud and wood. Majority 305 (67.6%) of the household contact houses had good ventilation and 314 (69.6%) of the houses had good lighting status. Three hundred sixty sixes (81.2%) of the respondents had separate kitchen room and 408 (90.5%) of household contacts used wood for cooking food (Table 2).

One hundred nine (24.2%), 206 (45.7%), 104 (23.1%), and 12 (2.7%) of household contacts had habit of cigarette smoking, khat chewing, raw milk consuming and alcohol drinking, respectively. Majority (86.3%) of the household contacts had a habit of eating meals ≥3 times per day. Two third (67.6%) of study participants had no family history of TB (Table 3). 362 (80.3%) of household contacts had adequate knowledge about TB.

3.3. Prevalence of Pulmonary Tuberculosis. The overall prevalence of tuberculosis among adult household contacts was 35 (7.8%) (95% CI: 5.8–10). Among household contacts, 206 (45.6%) were symptomatic (had cough > 2 week), and of these 91 (44%) had chest pain, night sweating, and fever. The proportion of tuberculosis among presumptive TB cases was 35 (16.9%). Among detected tuberculosis cases, a relatively higher proportion was observed among age group of 28–37 years (48.6%), male (57.1%), married (71.4%), farmer (85.7%), having monthly average income of <1000 Birr (82.9%), and illiterate (74.3%) adult household contacts (Table 4).

3.4. Associated Factors. In bivariable analyses, age of the adult household contacts, income, ventilation status of houses, lighting status of houses, overcrowdings, presence of separate kitchen, the size of living room, proximity to index

TABLE 2: Housing condition of adult household contacts of smear positive PTB patients in Haramaya district, Eastern Ethiopia, 2019 (n = 451).

Variables		Frequency	
		Number	Percent (%)
Composition of house floor	Mud	418	92.7
	Cement & other	33	7.3
House ventilation status	Good	305	67.6
	Poor	146	32.4
Lighting status	Good	314	69.6
	Poor	137	30.4
Overcrowded	Yes	167	37.0
	No	284	63.0
Cooking energy	Electric	20	4.4
	Wood	408	90.5
	Others	23	5.1
Separated kitchen room	Yes	366	81.2
	No	85	18.8
Duration of index cases registered for treatment	≤6 month	125	27.7
	>6 month	326	72.3
Proximity to TB index case	Sleep on the same bed	217	48.1
	Sleep on different bed	234	51.9
Size of living room	Inadequate	148	32.8
	Adequate	303	67.2

TABLE 3: Behavioral related characteristics of adult household contacts of smear positive PTB patients in Haramaya district, Eastern Ethiopia, 2019 (n = 451).

Host (behavioral) related variables		Frequency (%)	
		Number	Percent (%)
Drinking alcohol	Yes	12	2.7
	No	439	97.3
Cigarette smoking	Yes	109	24.2
	No	342	75.8
Chewing khat	Yes	206	45.7
	No	245	54.3
Drinking raw milk	Yes	104	23.1
	No	347	76.9
Frequency of meals per day	≥3 meals per day	389	86.3
	<3 meals per day	62	13.7
Previously treated for TB	Yes	53	11.8
	No	398	88.2
Family history of TB other than index case	Yes	146	32.4
	No	305	67.6

case, treatment duration of TB index case, family history of TB, smoking cigarette, chewing khat, drinking raw milk, and frequency of meals per day on TB were found to be associated with PTB at p-values less than 0.25.

In multivariable analysis frequency of meals per day, house ventilation status, living room size, drinking raw milk, and family history of TB other than index case remained statistically significant at p-value less than 0.05. Study participants eating meals less than three times per day were 4 times more likely to acquire TB (AOR=4.31; 95% CI: 1.617, 11.545) as compared to those eating meals more than three times per day. Study participants who had history of drinking raw milk were about 4 times more likely to develop tuberculosis (AOR=4.12; 95% CI: 1.43, 11.90) than their counterparts. The odds of getting TB was about 3 times higher among household contacts who had history of TB within family other than index case (AOR=2.7; 95% CI: 1.02, 6.92) compared to those who were not.

The study participants living in the houses with poor ventilation were at risk of getting TB 4.0 times more than likely to develop tuberculosis (AOR=4.02; 95% CI: 1.38, 11.76) compared to their counterparts. Similarly, the likelihood of having TB was about 3 times higher among the contacts dwelling in inadequate room size (less than 4×4 m per person) (AOR=3.4; 95% CI: 1.30, 8.867) when compared to those who were living in an adequately sized room (Table 4).

4. Discussion

The prevalence of TB among adult household contacts of PTB patients was 7.8% (95% CI: 5.8–10.0). Frequency of meals per day, ventilation status of houses, sizes of living rooms, drinking raw milk, and family history of TB other than the index case, were identified as the factors significantly associated with tuberculosis.

The finding is comparable with the other studies in sub-Saharan Africa (7.8%) [18], Peshawar (0.1–14%) [19], and Tanzania (6.4%) [20], but, higher than that reported from Nepal (1.6%) [21], India (1.15%) [7], Pondicherry of India (4.3%) [22], South Africa (3.9%) [23], and Ethiopia (1%) [24]. The variation might be related to differences in the study population, living situation, and overcrowding which are important risks for respiratory diseases, including tuberculosis [25]. Differently, it is lower than the finding reported in a few of the previous studies conducted in Peru (34%) [26], Philippines (12.8%) [27], and Pakistan (15.6%) [28]. This difference could be associated with sample size of the study and diagnostic methods [1].

This study revealed that the likelihood of TB among household contacts eating meals less than three times per day was 4 times higher than that of individuals who eat meals three times or more per day. This is in line with the studies conducted in Tanzania [20] and Pakistan [29]. This might be due to undernutrition or nutritional deficiency that impairs cell-mediated immunity which can lead to progression of latent infection to active TB disease. The differences in the socioeconomic status, lifestyle, and feeding patterns of the household contacts might also explain these differences [30, 31].

Our study showed that household contacts who drink raw milk were 4 times more likely to develop TB compared to their counterparts. This is comparable with the studies conducted in Tanzania [32] and Gojam district of Ethiopia [15]. This might be due to intake of infected milk with the bacteria and which could disseminate from the initial location in the abdomen to other parts of the body via the blood

TABLE 4: Factors associated with Tuberculosis disease among adult household contacts of smear positive PTB patients in Haramaya district, Eastern Ethiopia, 2019 (n = 451).

Variables	Category	Tuberculosis Yes	Tuberculosis No	COR (95% CI)	p-value	AOR (95% CI)	p-value
Age (year)	18–27	13 (6%)	199 (94%)	1		1	
	28–37	15 (13%)	99 (87%)	2.3 (1.06–5.06)	0.04	1.9 (0.55–6.87)	0.31
	≥38	7 (6%)	118 (94%)	0.9 (0.35–2.34)	0.84	0.3 (0.07–1.22)	0.09
Monthly income of the family	<1000	29 (11%)	244 (89%)	13.1 (1.76–97.20)	0.01	6.5 (0.63–68.38)	0.12
	1000–1500	5 (7%)	62 (93%)	8.9 (1.01–77.65)	0.05	15.1 (1.06–217.09)	0.06
	>1500	1 (1%)	110 (99%)	1		1	
House ventilation status**	Poor	29 (19%)	122 (81%)	11.7 (4.71–28.77)	0.01	4.0 (1.382–11.76)	0.01
	Good	6 (2%)	294 (98%)	1		1	
Lighting status	Poor	22 (16%)	115 (84%)	4.4 (2.16–9.09)	0.01	0.78 (0.20–3.09)	0.72
	Good	13 (4%)	301 (96%)	1		1	
Overcrowded	Yes	23 (14%)	144 (86%)	3.6 (1.75–7.49)	0.01	1.3 (0.47–3.44)	0.63
	No	12 (4%)	272 (96%)	1		1	
Separated kitchen	Yes	18 (5%)	348 (95%)	1		1	0.53
	No	17 (20%)	68 (80%)	4.8 (2.37–9.85)	0.01	1.4 (0.47–4.40)	
Size of living room*	Inadequate	24 (16%)	124 (84%)	5.1 (2.44–10.81)	0.01	3.4 (1.30–8.86)	0.01
	Adequate	11 (4%)	292 (96%)	1		1	
Proximity to index case	Sleep on the same bed	19 (9%)	198 (91%)	8.5 (4.12–17.59)	0.01	1.9 (0.61–6.32)	0.26
	Sleep on the different bed	16 (7%)	218 (93%)	1		1	
Treatment duration of index case	≤6 month	15 (12%)	110 (88%)	2.1 (1.03-4.22)	0.04	1.3 (0.46–3.41)	0.66
	>6 month	20 (6%)	306 (94%)	1		1	
Family Hx of TB other than index case*	Yes	22 (15%)	124 (85%)	4.0 (1.95–8.16)	0.01	2.7 (1.02–6.92)	0.047
	No	13 (4%)	292 (96%)	1		1	
Smoking cigarette	Yes	18 (17%)	91 (83%)	3.9 (1.87–7.63)	0.01	1.4 (0.50–3.86)	0.54
	No	17 (5%)	325 (95%)	1		1	
Chewing khat	Yes	28 (14%)	178 (86%)	5.4 (2.28–12.52)	0.01	2.7 (0.91–7.74)	0.07
	No	7 (3%)	238 (97%)	1		1	
Drinking raw milk**	Yes	27 (26%)	77 (74%)	14.9 (6.50–33.97)	0.01	4.1 (1.43–11.90)	0.01
	No	8 (2%)	339 (98%)	1		1	
Frequency of meals per day**	<3 meals per day	21 (34%)	41 (66%)	13.7 (6.49–29.02)	0.01	4.3 (1.61–11.55)	0.004
	≥3 meals per day	14 (4%)	375 (96%)	1		1	
Overall knowledge scored on TB case	Inadequate	21 (24%)	68 (77%)	7.7 (3.72–15.84)	0.01	2.0 (0.72–5.54)	0.18
	Adequate	14 (4%)	348 (96%)	1		1	

*Shows association having p value below 0.05 and **association having p value below 0.01. OR = odd ratio, COR = crude odd ratio, AOR = adjusted odd ratio, CI = confidence interval.

stream, the lymphatic system, or by direct extension to other organs, which can be explained by the high prevalence of Bovine TB in the country [33, 34], and particularly in the study areas.

The likelihood of TB among household contacts with family history of TB other than index case were 8 times higher than that of individuals who did not have family history of TB (AOR=2.78 CI: 1.01–6.92). This is in line with the studies done in India [10], Metema and Gojam in Ethiopia [15]. It is also in support of the WHO report which stated that there was greater occurrence of TB when the contact lived with more than one TB case [9]. It might be due to increased expelled bacilli that maximize the exposure within households.

The study finding showed that contacts dwelling in the house with poor ventilation were 4.0 times more likely at risk of getting TB than those dwelling in the house with good ventilation. This is consistent with the findings of other studies done in Pakistan [34], India [29], meta-analysis in sub-Saharan Africa [35], Addis Ababa, Ethiopia [36], Metema district, Ethiopia [16], and Gojam, Ethiopia [15]. This might be due to poor house ventilation that could increase the likelihood of exposure to tuberculosis by increasing the concentration of TB bacteria within households. However, good ventilation reduces the concentration of TB bacteria so it will decrease the transmission of the TB [37].

Household contacts living in inadequate sizes of rooms were 3 times more likely to get TB than those living in adequate sizes of rooms. This is in agreement with other studies done in sub-Saharan Africa [35], Pakistan [29], and Metema district of Ethiopia [16].This might be related with enclosed spaces and poor air circulation that can accelerate the transmission of TB [37].

Majority of socio-demographic factors assessed in this study did not show a statically significant association with the presence of TB in household contacts. However, community-based study done in high burden settings in Ethiopia [15] and Philippines [27] showed significant association of older age groups with the presence of TB. Similarly, occupational status of the household contacts were not significantly associated with the occurrence of TB in this study which is inconsistent with the study conducted in West Ethiopia [17]. This might be due to difference with study participants, lifestyle, and socioeconomic factors.

This study was not performed without limitations. Causal inferences (temporal relationship) cannot be drawn out since the study is a cross-sectional study. Smear negative cases were not verified using gold standard technique. During observation, there might be intra-observer variations. However, proper training was given to data collectors to minimize these biases. Therefore, this study could provide insights about the prevalence and associated factors of with TB disease among adult household contacts of PTB patients.

5. Conclusion

The overall prevalence of tuberculosis among adult household contacts of pulmonary tuberculosis patients is high. Eating meals less than three times per day, drinking raw milk, having family history of TB other than index case, living in poorly ventilated houses, and inadequate sizes in the living rooms were the independent predictors of the outcome. Appropriate health intervention should be given to the community by health extension workers on TB disease transmission, adequate and balanced diet, and safe dealing with diseased family member. Health facilities should screen all contacts of PTB patients as early as possible to reduce the number of active TB cases, and appropriate prompt treatment should be given to minimize the transmission. Health care providers should strengthen the information given to index cases that their close contacts and perform screening especially to those having the symptoms of TB (coughing, weight loss, and fever) and treat if required.

Authors' Contributions

All authors contributed toward design of the study, writing the proposal, developing tools, data analysis, drafting, and revising the paper and agree to be accountable for all aspects of the work.

Acknowledgments

We would like to thank Haramaya University for financial support. We are also very grateful to the study participants for their participation in the study, and valuable information.

References

[1] FMOH, *Guidelines for Clinical and Programatic Managment TB, TB/HIV and Leprosy in Ethiopia*, Federal Ministry of Health, Addsi Ababa, Ethiopia, 6th edition, 2016.

[2] WHO, *Global Tuberculosis Report*, World Health Organization, Geneva, Switzerland, 2018.

[3] USAID, "Committed to ending TB: Tuberculosis Report to Congress," 2016.

[4] J. Singh, M. M. Sankar, S. Kumar et al., "Incidence and prevalence of tuberculosis among household contacts of pulmonary tuberculosis patients in a peri-urban population of South Delhi, India," *PLoS One*, vol. 8, no. 7, p. e69730, 2013.

[5] KFF, "The U.S. Government and Global Tuberculosis Efforts, Key Facts," 2018, Fact Sheet.

[6] B. I. Omotowo, O. C. Ekwueme, and M. N. Aghaji, "Tuberculosis control mechanisms and contact tracing: knowledge and practice among TB patients at dots centers in southeast Nigeria," *Journal of Biometrics & Biostatistics*, vol. 1, no. 9, 2012.

[7] M. Gupta, A. A. Saibannavar, and V. Kumar, "Household symptomatic contact screening of newly diagnosed sputum smears positive tuberculosis patients - an effective case detection tool," *Lung India*, vol. 33, no. 2, pp. 159–162, 2016.

[8] A. C. Lemos, E. D. Matos, D. B. Sampaio, and E. M. Netto, "Risk of tuberculosis among household contacts in Salvador, Bahia," *Brazilian Journal of Infectious Diseases*, vol. 8, no. 6, pp. 424–430, 2004.

[9] WHO, *Recommendations for Investigating Contacts of Persons with Infectious Tuberculosis in Low- and Middle-Income Countries*, World Health Organization, Geneva, 2012.

[10] D. Nair, N. Rajshekhar, J. S. Klinton et al., "Household contact screening and yield of tuberculosis cases—a clinic based study in Chennai, South India," *PLoS One*, vol. 11, no. 9, p. e0162090, 2016.

[11] FMOH, *Pocket Guide on Clinical Management of TBL and TB/HIV for General Health Workers*, Federal Ministry of Health, Addis Ababa, Ethiopia, 2013.

[12] Word Vision, *Technical Guideline for Tuberculosis (TB) and TB-HIV Program Implementation*, World Vision, Uxbridge, UK, 2017.

[13] EHZHO, *East Hararghe Zonal Annual TB Program Performance Report*, East Hararghe Zone Tuberculosis Control, Harar, Ethiopia, 2018.

[14] Haramaya Woreda Administrative Office, *Annual Administrative Report*, East Hararghe, Oromia, Ethiopia, 2018.

[15] M. Meseret, M. Shibabaw, and G. Tsegaye, "Determinants of tuberculosis among adults in Jabi Tehnan district, West Gojjam zone, Northwest Ethiopia: a case control study," *International Journal of Public Health & Safety*, vol. 2, no. 3, Article ID 1000128, 2017.

[16] C. Tesema, T. Tadesse, M. Gebrehiwot, A. Tsegaw, and F. Weldegebreal, "Environmental and host-related determinants of tuberculosis in Metema district, north-west Ethiopia," *Drug, Healthcare and Patient Safety*, pp. 87–95, 2015.

[17] T. Ephrem, B. Mengiste, F. Mesfin, and W. Godana, "Determinants of active pulmonary tuberculosis in Ambo Hospital, West Ethiopia," *African Journal of Primary Health Care & Family Medicine*, vol. 7, no. 1, p. 8, 2015.

[18] N. S. Shah, C. M. Yuen, M. Heo, A. W. Tolman, and M. C. Becerra, "Yield of contact investigations in households of patients with drug-resistant tuberculosis: systematic review and meta-analysis," *Clinical Infectious Diseases*, vol. 58, pp. 381–391, 2014.

[19] A. Javaid, A. M. Khan, M. A. Khan et al., "Screening outcomes of household contacts of multidrug-resistant tuberculosis patients in Peshawar, Pakistan," *Asian Pacific Journal of Tropical Medicine*, vol. 9, no. 9, pp. 909–912, 2016.

[20] M. Beyanga, B. R. Kidenya, L. G. Adima, E. Ochodo, S. E. Mshana, and C. H. Kasang, "Investigation of household contacts of pulmonary tuberculosis patients increases case detection in Mwanza City, Tanzania," *BMC Infectious Diseases*, vol. 18, p. 110, 2018.

[21] N. Gyawali, R. Gurung, N. Poudyal et al., " Prevalence of tuberculosis in household contacts of sputum smears positive cases and associated demographic risk factors," *Journal of College of Medical Sciences-Nepal*, vol. 14, no. 4, pp. 303–307, 2012.

[22] V. A. Kumar, G. Kalaiselvan, and A. R. Dongre, "Prevalence of tuberculosis among household contacts in Pondicherry: active case finding among new smear positive cases," *Online Journal of Health and Allied Sciences*, vol. 15, no. 1, p. 4, 2016.

[23] K. M. Little, R. Msandiwa, N. Martinson, J. Golub, R. Chaisson, and D. Dowdy, "Yield of household contact tracing for tuberculosis in rural South Africa," *BMC Infectious Diseases*, vol. 18, p. 299, 2018.

[24] Z. Gashu, D. Jerene, M. Ensermu et al., "The yield of community-based "retrospective" tuberculosis contact investigation in a high burden setting in Ethiopia," *PLoS One*, vol. 11, no. 8, p. e0160514, 2016.

[25] T. Kompala, S. Shenoi, and G. Friedland, "Transmission of tuberculosis in resource-limited settings," *Current HIV/AIDS Reports*, vol. 10, no. 3, pp. 264–272, 2013.

[26] L. Otero, L. Shah, K. Verdonck et al., "A prospective longitudinal study of tuberculosis among household contacts of smear-positive tuberculosis cases in Lima, Peru," *BMC Infectious Diseases*, vol. 16, no. 1, 2016.

[27] I. G. Sia, B. R. Orillaza, J. L. Sauver et al., "Tuberculosis attributed to household contacts in the Philippines," *International Journal of Tuberculosis and Lung Disease*, vol. 14, no. 1, pp. 122–125, 2010.

[28] R. Iqbal, K. Munir, S. Bashir et al., "Screening for tuberculosis among household contacts of index patients," *Pakistan Journal of Medical Research*, vol. 52, no. 4, p. 96, 2013.

[29] A. Khaliq, I. H. Khan, M. W. Akhtar, and M. N. Chaudhry, "Environmental risk factors and social determinants of pulmonary tuberculosis in Pakistan," *Epidemiology (Sunnyvale)*, vol. 2015, no. 5, p. 3, 2015.

[30] WHO, *Guideline: Nutritional Care and Support for Patients with Tuberculosis*, World Health Organization, Geneva, 2013.

[31] P. Chandrasekaran, N. Saravanan, R. Bethunaickan, and S. Tripathy, "Malnutrition: modulator of immune responses in tuberculosis," *Frontiers in Immunology*, vol. 8, p. 1316, 2017.

[32] S. G. Finanga, O. Mørkve, R. R. Kazwala, S. Cleaveland, J. M. Sharp, and G. Shirima, "The role of livestock keeping in tuberculosis trends in Arusha, Tanzania," *International Journal of Tuberculosis and Lung Disease*, vol. 7, pp. 695–704, 2008.

[33] A. Girmay, S. Weldegbriel, and B. Afera, "Assessment of bovine tuberculosis in dairy farms and its public health importance in and around Adigrat district," 2015.

[34] K. Srivastava, S. Kant, and A. Verma, "Role of environmental factors in transmission of tuberculosis," *Dynamics of Human Health*, vol. 2, no. 4, p. 12, 2015.

[35] I. S. Saidu, Z. Nasir, and B. W. Goni, "Social determinants of tuberculosis in sub-Saharan Africa: a systematic review," *Global Journal of Medicen and Public Health*, vol. 3, no. 4, p. 14, 2014.2277-9604

[36] E. Shimeles, F. Enquselassie, A. Aseffa, M. Tilahun, A. Mekonen, and G. Wondimagegn, "Risk factors for tuberculosis: a case–control study in Addis Ababa, Ethiopia," *PLoS One*, vol. 14, no. 4, p. e0214235, 2019.

[37] WHO, *WHO Policy on TB Infection Control in Health-Care Facilities, Congregate Settings and Households*, World Health Organization, Geneva, Switzerland, 2009.

[38] Th. H. Th. Thanh, S. D. Ngoc, N. N. Viet et al., "A household survey on screening practices of household contacts of smear positive tuberculosis patients in Vietnam," *BMC Public Health*, vol. 2014, no. 14, p. 713, 2014.

[39] M. Worku, B. Seyum, and H. Kadir, "Assesment of goiter prevalence and associated factors among school age (7–12 years) children of rular primary school of Bedeno Woreda, East Hararghe zone, Ooromia Region, Ethiopia," 2014.

[40] H. Olijira, M. Ifa, and A. Birhanu, "Determinants of active tuberculosis among HIV-positive adults attending clinical care in ambo general hospital and Gedo hospital, West Shoa zone, Oromia regional state, Central Ethiopia," *Journal of Pharmacy and Alternative Medicine*, vol. 10, pp. 72–83, 2016.

[41] S. M. Gelaw, "Socioeconomic factors associated with knowledge on tuberculosis among adults in Ethiopia," *Tuberculosis Research and Treatment*, vol. 2016, Article ID 6207457, 11 pages, 2016.

[42] S. Paramasivam, B. Thomas, J. Thayyil et al., "Knowledge and health seeking behaviour of tuberculosis patients in Kerala, India," *International Journal of Community Medicine and Public Health*, vol. 3, no. 9, pp. 2464–247, 2016.

10

A Comparative Study of Knowledge, Attitude and Determinants of Tuberculosis-Associated Stigma in Rural and Urban Communities of Lagos State, Nigeria

David A. Oladele,[1] **Mobolanle R. Balogun**,[2] **Kofoworola Odeyemi**,[2] **and Babatunde L. Salako**[1]

[1]*Clinical Sciences Department, Nigerian Institute of Medical Research, Lagos, Nigeria*
[2]*Department of Community Medicine and Primary Care, College of Medicine, University of Lagos, Lagos, Nigeria*

Correspondence should be addressed to David A. Oladele; daveohlay@yahoo.com

Academic Editor: Alexander S. Apt

Background. Tuberculosis (TB) is an important public health concern in Nigeria. TB-associated stigma could lead to delayed diagnosis and care, treatment default, and multidrug resistance. Understanding of TB-associated stigma is therefore important for TB control. The study is aimed at determining and comparing the knowledge, attitude, and determinants of TB-associated stigma. *Methodology.* This was a comparative cross-sectional study among adults in urban and rural areas of Lagos State, Nigeria. Respondents were selected through a multistage sampling technique and interviewed using a semistructured questionnaire, which contained the Explanatory Model Interviewed Catalogue (EMIC) stigma scale. IBM SPSS Statistics Software package version 20 was used for analysis. *Results.* A total of 790 respondents were interviewed. High proportions of respondents in rural and urban areas were aware of TB (97.5% and 99.2%, respectively). Respondents in the urban areas had overall better knowledge of TB compared to the rural areas (59.4% vs. 23%; $p < 0.001$), while respondents in the rural areas had a better attitude to TB (60.5% vs. 49.9%; $p = 0.002$). The majority of respondents in rural and urban areas had TB-associated stigma (93% and 95.7%, respectively). The mean stigma score was higher in the urban compared to rural areas (17.43 ± 6.012 and 16.54 ± 6.324, respectively, $p = 0.046$). Marital status and ethnicity were the predictors of TB-associated stigma in the rural communities (AOR-0.257; CI-0.086-0.761; $p = 0.014$ and AOR–3.09; CI-1.087-8.812; $p = 0.034$, respectively), while average monthly income and age of respondents were the predictors of TB-associated stigma in urban areas (AOR–0.274; CI–0.009-0.807; $p = 0.019$ and AOR-0.212; CI–0.057-0.788; $p = 0.021$, respectively). *Conclusion.* TB-associated stigma is prevalent in both rural and urban areas in this study. There is therefore a need to disseminate health appropriate information through the involvement of the community. Also, innovative stigma reduction activities are urgently needed.

1. Introduction

Tuberculosis (TB) is a curable and preventable disease [1]. It is the ninth leading cause of death worldwide and the leading cause of death from a single infectious agent [2, 3]. Nigeria is among the 30 high TB burden countries according to the World Health Organization (WHO). It is also among the eight countries that accounted for two-thirds of the global burden of TB in 2018 [4]. In order to sustain the global fight to end TB, the WHO proposed a paradigm shift in TB control through the "End TB strategy" program [5]. This Global Plan also identifies eight fundamental changes that must be implemented as part of the paradigm shift needed to end TB [5]. One of these changes recommends that countries should prohibit stigma and discrimination against people infected with TB [5].

Health-related stigma could be defined as a "social process that exists when elements of labeling, stereotyping, separation, loss of status, and discrimination occur in a power situation that allows them" [6]. Health-related stigma is known to cause psychological suffering, shame, and isolation in afflicted individuals and families; it could compromise the efforts to provide effective health care and could foster discrimination in societies. Stigma may also directly affect the course and outcome of the stigmatized medical condition [6]. The stigma associated with TB is the least studied among health-related stigmas when compared to other infectious diseases like leprosy and HIV/AIDS [6–9].

The prevalence of stigma associated with TB has been shown to vary from 27% to as high as 82% in different settings across the world [10–13]. It was also found to be associated with nonadherence to treatment and treatment failure [14]; it hampers investigations of household contacts [15] and causes delay in case detection [16] and also associated with high mortality due to late presentation [17]. A study of the trend of TB case notification in Lagos state between 2011 and 2015 showed a decrease in the Case Notification Ratio from 82.9% in 2013 to 72.1% in 2015 [18]. The gap between TB incidence and case notification in Nigeria is 12% [4], making Nigeria one of the 10 countries that accounted for 80% of the estimated global gap between incidence and case notification. This gap is mainly due to underreporting and underdiagnosis, which could result directly or indirectly from TB-associated stigma [4].

Therefore, eradicating the stigma surrounding TB is therefore a crucial component of efforts aimed at encouraging people to seek early diagnosis and treatment, to adhere to treatment guidelines and treatment completion along with psychosocial support or social protection benefits after diagnosis [6–8].

Furthermore, the health-related stigma associated with infectious diseases has been shown to vary among rural and urban dwellings as well as with the knowledge and educational background of the people [19]. For instance, the stigma associated with leprosy was said to differ significantly between rural and urban dwellers [20, 21], and a rural-urban dichotomy has been documented to influence the experience of HIV felt stigma [22, 23]. Also, a systematic review has documented the presence of cultural variations in knowledge, attitudes, and health responses to TB stigma [24]. However, there is a paucity of evidence in the literature comparing the stigma associated with TB among rural and urban dwellers in Nigeria.

The study, therefore, is aimed at assessing and comparing the knowledge, attitude, and determinants of the stigma associated with TB between rural and urban dwellers in Lagos, Nigeria. Understanding of this may lead to improved quality of care of TB patients in rural and urban areas in Nigeria as well as improved health and wellbeing of the general population.

2. Methods

2.1. Study Setting. The study was conducted in Lagos State, which is located in the southwestern part of Nigeria. The state accounts for over five percent of the national estimated population [25]. It has an estimated population of 23,305,971 by 2015 projection [26]. Lagos State is divided into 20 Local Government Areas (LGAs) of which 16 comprise the urban LGAs and the remaining four LGAs are classified as rural LGAs. The study took place at Lagos Mainland LGA (Urban) and Badagry LGA (Rural).

2.2. Study Design and Population. The study was a comparative cross-sectional study, and the respondents were adults 18 years and above in the urban and rural areas in Lagos state. Adult community members that had lived in the community for at least 6 months in the 12 months period preceding the interview were included in the study while those who had been diagnosed with TB or currently on TB treatment were excluded.

2.3. Sample Size Determination. The sample size for the study was determined by using the formulae for comparison of proportions [27]:

$$n = \frac{(Z\alpha + Z\beta)^2\{P1(1 - P1) + P2(1 - P2)\}}{(P1 - P2)^2}. \quad (1)$$

After adjusting for a 10% nonresponse rate, the final sample size was 380 for each of the rural and urban communities was used.

2.4. Sampling Methodology. A multistage sampling technique was used for respondents' selection. In stage one, 2 LGAs were selected by simple random sampling. Stage two involved the selection of 2 wards each from the urban and rural LGAs through simple random sampling. In stage three, 10 streets were randomly selected from each of the selected wards in the urban and rural communities, and in stage four, 20 houses were selected on each street. The habitable houses in each street or settlement were counted and the total number divided by 20 to obtain the sampling interval. The first house on each street was selected by balloting, and the subsequent n^{th} house was sampled until 20 houses had been selected in each of the 20 streets or settlements. In stage five, households for sampling were chosen from the houses selected. In each house, when more than one household exists, a list of all the households was created, and one household was selected by balloting. However, whenever only one household is present in the selected house, the household was selected. When a selected house had no eligible respondent, then the next house was used.

2.5. Data Collection Tool and Technique. A pretested, interviewer-administered questionnaire was used to collect data from house to house between July and October 2017. The study also makes use of a stigma scale, which has been validated to assess health-related stigma for various diseases including TB [28, 29].

The questionnaire was divided into four sections: Section A focused on the sociodemographic characteristics of the respondents and their household. Section B focused on the respondents' knowledge about TB cause, mode of transmission, prevention, and care adapted from WHO advocacy, communication, and social mobilization for TB control: a guide to developing knowledge, attitude, and practice surveys [30]. Section C focused on the respondents' attitude to TB. A three-point Likert scale that assessed the respondent's attitude with regards to susceptibility to TB infection, the severity of TB infection, benefits of TB treatment, and barriers to TB treatment was used [31]. Section D contained the adaptation of the Explanatory Model Interview Catalogue (EMIC) stigma scale for the community [28, 29]. It was designed to evaluate the potential stigmatizers in the community. It assesses perceived stigma and the attitudes of community members towards persons affected with TB. The outcome was determined by summing up the scores per each question. The higher the score, the more the likelihood of TB associated stigma.

2.6. Pretesting and Validation of Study Instrument. The questionnaire was pretested among 30 adults (18 years and above) each in urban and rural communities similar to the study sites. The internal consistency of the EMIC scale was assessed using Cronbach's alpha test, and a score of 0.87 was obtained.

2.7. Data Management. Data entry and analysis were done using the IBM Statistical Package for the Social Sciences (SPSS) Version 20.0 (IBM Corp, Armonk, NY). Knowledge of TB was categorized as good versus poor knowledge by evaluating respondents with appropriate knowledge of TB. Appropriate knowledge of TB was defined as the ability to recognize 5 knowledge domains as follows: able to recognize germ/bacteria as the cause of TB, know that TB is spread through the air, know that cough more than 2 weeks a major symptom, prevention by covering mouth, and treated by modern medicine. Individuals who recognized the 5 domains were said to have good knowledge, and those who recognize less than 5 were said to have poor knowledge [32]. Questions on attitude were scored on a 3-point scale graded 1-3 [31], and the minimum and maximum scores obtainable were 15 and 45, respectively. A score below the median (39) was regarded as a negative attitude, and an attitude score above the median was termed a positive attitude.

The total numbers of questions for the EMIC stigma scale were 15. It has the answer options (score) as follows: yes (2), possibly (1), do not know (0), and no (0). The cut-off point of "8" on the EMIC stigma scale was used to assess the stigma associated with TB. Respondents were considered to have existing stigmatization when they answered at least 4 questions with "yes," or 8 questions with "possibly," or the combination of both answers with a sum score at 8. A score of 8 was chosen to increase the specificity of the cut-off point and to avoid false positives [29].

The scores from the tools were categorized into dichotomous variables. Discrete variables were presented as percentages, while continuous variables were expressed as means (± standard deviation). Proportions for categorical variables were compared using Pearson Chi-square, while the difference in means was compared using the Students t-test. The level of significance was predetermined at $p < 0.05$. Variables attaining significance were further subjected to multivariable analysis using simple and multiple logistic regression to determine the predictors for "TB associated stigma." Results were expressed as odds ratios with 95% confidence intervals.

2.8. Ethical Considerations. The Health Research and Ethics Committee of the Lagos University Teaching Hospital (LUTH), Lagos, Nigeria (ethical approval number: ADM/DCST/HREC/1282), and Institutional Review Board of Nigerian Institute of Medical Research, Lagos, Nigeria (ethical approval number: IRB/17/029) reviewed the protocol, the associated informed consent forms, and study-related documents and gave ethical approval. Permission was also obtained from the local government authority and the Ward Health Committee of the selected wards for the community interview. Written informed consent was obtained from each study participant prior to enrolment in the study. All staff involved in this study had appropriate training on research ethics emphasizing the importance of informed consent and confidentiality. Adequate privacy was ensured during study procedures, and effort was made to protect participants' confidentiality to the extent possible. Respondents were also informed of their right to opt-out of the study if they choose to at any point in the study.

3. Results

A total of 790 respondents were interviewed: three hundred and ninety-five (395) respondents in Mainland LGA and another 395 respondents in Badagry LGA of Lagos state.

The mean age of respondents in the rural and urban communities was 32 ± 11.09 years and 36.2 ± 12.58 years, respectively, with the mean age of urban areas significantly higher than rural areas ($p < 0.05$). The other study participants' demographic characteristics are as shown in Table 1.

More than four-fifth 385 (97.5%) of respondents in the rural area had ever heard about TB compared to 392 (99.2%) of respondents in the urban area. However, this difference was not statistically significant. The common sources of information in these settings were radio, television, healthcare worker, family members, and friends. Significantly higher proportions of respondents in the urban areas got information about TB from radio, television, and healthcare workers when compared to rural areas (Table 2).

A significantly higher proportion of urban respondents 233(59.4%) had good knowledge of TB when compared to rural areas 88 (23%) ($p < 0.001$). Also, respondents with good knowledge of TB were about five times more in urban areas compared to rural areas (OR: 4.896; CI: 3.584-6.689) (Table 3).

An assessment of the attitude of respondents to TB revealed that more respondents in rural areas 233 (60.5%) had a positive attitude score towards TB when compared to urban area 196 (49.9%) ($p = 0.002$) (Table 4).

Assessing the stigma in the community using the EMIC scale showed that a greater proportion of respondents in the urban area (27.6%) felt a person infected with TB would like to keep others from knowing they have TB if possible compared to (20.3%) in the rural area ($p = 0.001$). More

Table 1: Sociodemographic characteristics of respondents.

Variable	Rural ($n = 395$) Freq. (%)	Urban ($n = 395$) Freq. (%)	Total ($n = 790$)	χ^2	df	p value
Age						
<25	113 (28.6)	76 (19.2)	189 (23.9)	27.04	5	<0.001*
25-34	142 (35.9)	113 (28.6)	255 (32.3)			
35-44	90 (22.8)	115 (29.1)	205 (25.9)			
45-54	29 (7.3)	57 (14.4)	86 (10.9)			
55-64	15 (3.8)	19 (4,8)	34 (4.3)			
≥65	6 (1.5)	15 (3.8)	21 (2.7)			
Mean age	32 ± 11.079	36.2 ± 12.576		$t = -4.139$		<0.05*
Sex						
Male	207 (52.4)	192 (48.6)	399 (50.5)	1.139	1	0.160
Female	188 (47.6)	203 (51.4)	391 (49.5)			
Ethnicity ($n = 783$)						
Yoruba	147 (37.2)	295 (76.4)	442 (56.6)	284.0	3	<0.001*
Igbo	34 (8.6)	73 (18.9)	107 (13.7)			
Hausa	1 (0.3)	16 (4.1)	17 (2.2)			
Others**	213 (53.9)	2 (0.5)	215 (27.5)			
Religion						
Christianity	295 (74.7)	244 (61.8)	539 (68.2)	16.96	2	<0.001*
Islam	96 (24.3)	149 (37.7)	246 (31.0)			
Others	4 (1.0)	2 (0.5)	6 (0.8)			
Marital status						
Married	261 (66.1)	240 (60.8)	501 (63.4)	11.0	3	<0.001*
Divorced/separated	6 (1.5)	23 (5.8)	29 (3.7)			
Widowed	13 (3.3)	16 (3.8)	28 (3.5)			
Single	115 (29.1)	117 (29.6)	232 (29.4)			
Education status						
No formal education	51 (12.9)	17 (4.3)	69 (8.6)	61.89	3	<0.001*
Primary	97 (24.6)	52 (13.2)	149 (18.9)			
Secondary	208 (52.7)	220 (55.7)	428 (54.2)			
Tertiary	39 (9.9)	107 (26.8)	146 (18.4)			
Employment status						
Employed	363 (91.9)	322 (81.9)	685 (86.9)	20.02	3	<0.001*
Unemployed	31 (8.1)	71(18.1)	102 (13.1)			
Occupation						
Professional/managerial	14 (3.9)	55 (16.9)	69 (10.0)	63.24	4	<0.001*
Clerical	6 (1.7)	11 (3.4)	17 (2.5)			
Sales and services	136 (37.6)	119 (36.5)	255 (37.1)			
Skilled manual	160 (44.2)	72 (22.1)	232 (33.7)			
Unskilled manual	46 (12.7)	69 (21.2)	115 (16.7)			
Income (naira) ($n = 657$)						
<18,000	180 (51.4)	66 (21.4)	246 (37.4)	64.66	2	<0.001*
18000-30000	61 (17.4)	72 (23.4)	133 (20.2)			
>30000	109 (31.1)	170 (55.2)	279 (42.4)			
Mean income	23,057 ± 20,209	41,516 ± 41,110		$t = -7.44$; $p = 0.010$*		
Median income (range)	15000 (1000 to 150000)	30000 (3000 to 400000)				
Type of house ($n = 775$)						
Duplex	4 (1.03)	1 (0.26)	5 (0.64)	45.05	4	<0.001*

TABLE 1: Continued.

Variable	Rural ($n = 395$) Freq. (%)	Urban ($n = 395$) Freq. (%)	Total ($n = 790$)	χ^2	df	p value
3/2 bedroom flat	37 (9.5)	67 (17.3)	104 (13.4)			
Self-contained	77 (19.8)	137 (35.4)	214 (27.6)			
One room shared	270 (69.6)	182 (47.0)	452 (58.3)			
Head of household						
Yes	192 (49.2)	172 (43.8)	419 (53.5)	3.25	2	0.197
No	198 (50.8)	221 (56.2)	363 (46.4)			

TABLE 2: Awareness of tuberculosis and source of information about TB.

Variable	Rural $n = 395$ Freq. (%)	Urban $n = 395$ Freq. (%)	Total $n = 790$ Freq. (%)	χ^2	p value
Ever heard about tuberculosis.					
Yes	385 (97.5)	392 (99.2)	779 (98.6)	2.305	0.112
No	10 (2.5)	3 (0.8)	11 (1.4)		
Source of information^	$n = 385$	$n = 392$			
Family and friends	227 (59.0)	251 (64.0)	479 (61.5)	2.15	0.082
Radio	200 (51.9)	253 (64.5)	455 (58.4)	12.22	0.001*
Television	117 (30.4)	247 (63.0)	365 (46.9)	82.70	0.001*
Healthcare workers	103 (26.8)	229 (58.4)	333 (42.7)	79.18	0.001*
Brochures and posters	20 (5.2)	92(23.5)	112 (14.4)	52.99	0.001*
Religious leaders	39 (10.1)	69 (17.6)	108 (13.9)	9.23	0.002*
Newspapers and magazines	9 (2.3)	89 (22.7)	98 (12.6)	73.54	0.001*
Billboards	14 (3.6)	71 (18.1)	85 (10.9)	42.0	0.001*
Teachers	13 (3.4)	22 (5.6)	35 (4.5)	2.30	0.082

*Multiple responses allowed.

TABLE 3: Participants appropriate knowledge of tuberculosis.

	Good knowledge Freq. (%)	Poor knowledge Freq. (%)	χ^2	df	p value
Rural area ($N = 385$)	88 (23.0)	294 (77.0)	105.62	1	<0.001*
Urban area ($N = 393$)	233 (59.4)	159 (40.6)			
Odds ratio	4.896 (CI: 3.584-6.689)				

TABLE 4: Attitude scores of respondents to tuberculosis infection.

Attitude	Positive attitude Freq. (%)	Negative attitude Freq. (%)	χ^2	df	p value
Rural area ($n = 385$)	233 (60.5)	152 (39.5)	8.912	1	0.002*
Urban area ($n = 393$)	196 (49.9)	197 (50.1)			

Positive attitude ≥ median attitude score of 39; Negative attitude < median attitude score of 39. *Statistical significance.

respondents in the rural area would think less of themselves if a family member is infected with TB ($p = 0.036$). More respondents from the urban area (41.1%) than the rural area (28.2%) felt that knowing that someone has TB would adversely affect other family members ($p = 0.001$), and a higher proportion of respondents in both rural and urban areas felt people in the community would avoid a person with TB just as a higher proportion of urban respondents (52.3%) than rural respondents (43.3%) would likely refuse to visit the home of a person infected with TB ($p = 0.042$).

About 46.5% of urban respondents compared to rural respondents (30.6%) will have concerns about disclosure if one member of their family is infected with TB ($p < 0.001$).

TB was believed could constitute a problem of preventing a person infected in getting married (45.3%) in rural areas compared to urban areas (39.5%) ($p < 0.001$) but more of the respondents form urban area (31.9%) felt that TB could cause a problem in an ongoing marriage and also cause a problem for a relative of TB patient to get married ($p < 0.001$).

A higher proportion of respondents in the rural areas (88.3%) and urban areas (87.5) would not like to buy food from a person affected by TB ($p = 0.035$) (Table 5).

In all, more respondents 375 (95.7%) in the urban area had TB-associated stigma when compared to rural area 357 (93.0%), and this difference was not statistically significant ($p = 0.071$). The mean EMIC scale score for the urban area is 17.45 ± 6.007, which is significantly higher than that of the rural area 16.55 ± 6.317 (Student t-test $= -2.00$; $p = 0.046$) (Table 6).

Table 5

(a) Assessment of respondent's perceived stigma to TB in the community (EMIC items 1-8)

Variables	Rural $n = 385$ Freq. (%)	Urban $n = 392$ Freq. (%)	Total $n = 778$	χ^2	p value
A person with TB will keep others from knowing, if possible.					
No/do not know	265 (68.7)	191 (48.7)	456 (58.6)	36.05	<0.00
Possibly	42 (10.9)	93 (23.7)	135 (17.4)		1*
Yes	78 (20.3)	108 (27.6)	186 (23.9)		
Would think less of self if a family member had TB because of this person's problem.					
No/do not know	240 (62.2)	272 (69.4)	512 (65.8)	6.65	0.036*
Possibly	77 (20.0)	75 (19.1)	152 (19.6)		
Yes	68 (17.6)	45 (11.5)	113 (14.5)		
TB cause shame or embarrassment					
No/do not know	82 (21.2)	85 (21.7)	167 (21.5)	2.18	0.534
Possibly	129 (33.4)	118 (30.1)	247 (31.7)		
Yes	174 (45.2)	189 (48.2)	362 (46.6)		
Others would think less of a person with TB					
No/do not know	91 (23.6)	104 (26.5)	195 (25.1)	2.055	0.561
Possibly	149 (38.6)	141 (36.0)	290 (37.3)		
Yes	145 (37.6)	147 (37.5)	292 (37.5)		
Knowing that someone has TB would have an adverse effect on others					
No/do not know	110 (28.5)	98 (25.0)	208 (26.7)	14.29	0.001*
Possibly	166 (43.1)	133 (33.9)	299 (38.5)		
Yes	109 (28.2)	161 (41.1)	270 (34.7)		
Other people in this community would avoid a person affected by TB					
No/do not know	45 (11.7)	54 (13.8)	99 (12.7)	3.74	0.154
Possibly	153 (39.6)	130 (33.2)	283 (36.4)		
Yes	187 (48.6)	208 (53.1)	395 (50.8)		
People would refuse to visit the home of a person affected by TB					
No/do not know	56 (14.5)	45 (11.5)	101 (13.0)	6.33	0.042*
Possibly	162 (42.0)	142 (36.2)	304 (39.1)		
Yes	167 (43.3)	205 (52.3)	371 (47.7)		
People in this community would think less of the family of a person with TB					
No/do not know	132 (34.3)	122 (31.1)	254 (32.7)	1.85	0.605
Possibly	129 (33.4)	139 (35.5)	268 (34.4)		
Yes	124 (32.1)	131 (33.5)	255 (32.7)		

*Statistical significance.

(b) Assessment of respondent's perceived stigma to TB in the community (EMIC items 9-15)

Variables	Rural $n = 386$ Freq. (%)	Urban $n = 392$ Freq. (%)	Total $n = 778$	χ^2	p value
TB would cause problems for the family					
No/do not know	81 (21.0)	95 (24.2)	176 (22.6)	5.95	0.051
Possibly	152 (39.5)	122 (31.1)	274 (35.3)		
Yes	152 (39.4)	175 (44.6)	327 (42.0)		

Table 5: Continued.

Variables	Rural $n = 386$ Freq. (%)	Urban $n = 392$ Freq. (%)	Total $n = 778$	χ^2	p value
Family would have concern about disclosure if one of their members had TB					
No/do not know	110 (28.5)	77 (19.6)	187 (24.0)	22.03	<0.001*
Possibly	157 (40.7)	133 (33.9)	290 (37.3)		
Yes	118 (30.6)	181 (46.2)	299 (38.5)		
TB could be a problem for a person to get married.					
No/do not know	68 (17.7)	120 (30.6)	188 (24.2)	17.81	<0.001*
Possibly	142 (36.9)	117 (29.8)	259 (33.3)		
Yes	174 (45.3)	155 (39.5)	329 (42.2)		
TB could cause problems in an on-going marriage.					
No/do not know	226 (58.5)	129 (32.9)	355 (45.6)	55.86	<0.001*
Possibly	100 (26.2)	138 (35.2)	238 (30.6)		
Yes	59 (15.3)	125 (31.9)	184 (23.7)		
TB could cause a problem for a relative of a patient to get married.					
No/do not know	182 (47.3)	161 (41.1)	343 (44.1)	13.68	0.003*
Possibly	118 (30.6)	99 (25.3)	217 (27.9)		
Yes	85 (10.9)	132 (33.7)	217 (27.9)		
TB could cause difficulty for a person to find work.					
No/do not know	9 (2.3)	29 (7.4)	38 (4.9)	19.54	<0.001*
Possibly	61 (16.1)	91 (23.2)	152 (19.6)		
Yes	315 (81.6)	272 (69.4)	587 (75.4)		
People could dislike buying food from a person affected by TB					
No/do not know	7 (1.8)	19 (4.8)	26 (3.3)	6.71	0.035*
Possibly	38 (9.8)	29 (7.4)	67 (8.6)		
Yes	340 (88.3)	344 (87.8)	684 (88.0)		

*Statistical significance.

Table 6: TB-associated stigma in the community.

EMIC score	TB stigma present Freq. (%)	TB stigma absent Freq. (%)	χ^2	df	p value
Rural area ($n = 384$)	357 (93.0)	27 (7.0)	2.63	1	0.071
Urban area ($n = 392$)	375 (95.7)	17 (4.3)			
Odds ratio	1.673 (0.896-3.122)				
Mean EMIC scale score					
Rural	16.54 ± 6.324	Students t test -2.00; $p = 0.046$*			
Urban	17.43 ± 6.012				

Perceived stigma absent = EMIC score < 8; Perceived stigma present = EMIC score ≥ 8. *Statistical significance.

Ethnicity was found to have a statistically significant association with TB-associated stigma in rural and urban communities. Respondents belonging to minority ethnic groups (particularly Egun ethnicity) in the rural areas had a significant proportion of perceived TB-associated stigma compared to the urban areas (Table 7).

Respondents with good knowledge (97.4%) of TB had a higher proportion of TB-associated stigma when compared to those with poor TB knowledge (93.1%) in the urban communities. This difference was found to be statistically significant ($p = 0.038$) (Table 8).

Multivariable analysis to assess the predictors of TB-associated stigma revealed that in the rural areas, ethnicity (p value = 0.014) and marital status (p value = 0.034) predicted TB-associated stigma. Thus, there was a 74.3% reduced likelihood of TB-associated stigma among non-Yoruba people as compared to the Yorubas, (AOR = 0.257, 95% CI: 0.0865-0.761, p value = 0.014), Also, there was a 3-fold odds of TB-associated stigma among unmarried respondents as compared

Table 7

(a) Association between sociodemographic characteristics of respondents and tuberculosis associated stigma in the communities

Variables	Rural (n = 384) TB stigma (%) present (n = 357)	Total	Urban (n = 392) TB stigma (%) present (n = 375)	Total	χ^2	p value
Sex						
Male	184 (91.5)	201	182 (95.8)	190	0.77	0.439
Female	173 (94.5)	183	193 (95.5)	202		
Age						
<25	104 (95.4)	109	73 (97.3)	75	6.96	0.223
25-34	129 (93.5)	138	100 (89.3)	112		
35-44	78 (88.6)	88	113 (98.3)	115		
45-54	27 (96.4)	28	56 (98.2)	57		
55-64	14 (93.3)	15	19 (100)	19		
≥65	5 (83.3)	6	15 (100)	15		
Ethnicity						
Yoruba	142 (97.3)	146	280 (95.2)	294	9.25	0.026*
Igbo	29 (87.9)	33	69 (97.2)	71		
Hausa	1 (100)	1	16 (100)	16		
Others**	185 (90.7)	204	1 (50)	2		
Religion						
Christianity	263 (92.3)	285	233 (96.3)	242	1.64	0.440
Islam	91 (95.8)	95	140 (94.6)	148		
Others	3 (75.0)	4	2 (100)	2		
Marital status						
Married	231 (91.3)	253	228 (95.4)	239	3.55	0.315
Divorced/separated	6 (100)	6	22 (95.7)	23		
Widowed	12 (100)	12	14 (100)	14		
Single	108 (95.6)	113	111 (95.7)	116		

*Statistical significance.

(b) Association between other sociodemographic characteristics of respondents and tuberculosis-associated stigma in the communities

Variables	Rural (n = 384) stigma to TB (%) present (n =357)	Total	Urban (n = 392) stigma to TB (%) present (n = 375)	Total	χ^2	p value
Education						
No formal	49 (98.0)	50	16 (94.1)	17	3.85	0.278
Primary	84 (90.3)	93	49 (94.2)	52		
Secondary	191 (94.1)	203	210 (96.3)	218		
Tertiary	33 (86.8)	38	101 (95.3)	106		
Employment						
Employed	329 (93.5)	352	313 (96.0)	326	1.24	0.249
Unemployed	28 (87.5)	32	63 (94.0)	67		
Occupation (n = 675)						
Professional/managerial	12 (85.7)	14	54 (98.2)	55	2.06	0.725
Clerical	6 (100)	6	11 (100)	11		
Trading	124 (93.9)	132	114 (96.6)	118		
Skilled manual	144 (94.1)	153	65 (91.5)	71		
Unskilled manual	42 (91.3)	46	67 (97.1)	69		
Type of housing						

Table 7: Continued.

Variables	Rural ($n = 384$) stigma to TB (%) present (n =357)	Total	Urban ($n = 392$) stigma to TB (%) present ($n = 375$)	Total	χ^2	p value
Duplex	4 (100.0)	4	1 (100)	1	0.70	0.873
3/2 bedroom flat	34 (94.4)	36	64 (95.5)	67		
Self-contained	70 (90.9)	77	132 (97.1)	136		
One room shared	242 (93.4)	259	171 (94.5)	181		
Income amount (naira) ($n = 647$)						
<18000	165 (93.8)	176	58 (87.9)	66	2.84	0.242
18000-30000	52 (91.2)	57	68 (95.8)	71		
>30000	100 (92.6)	108	165 (97.6)	169		

*Statistical significance.

Table 8

(a) Association between respondent knowledge and attitude and perceived TB-associated stigma in rural communities

Variables	Perceived TB stigma present (%)	Perceived TB stigma absent (%)	Total	χ^2	p value
Attitude to TB					
Positive	219 (94.4)	13 (5.6)	232	1.83	0.176
Negative	138 (90.8)	14 (9.2)	152		
Knowledge of TB					
Good	82 (94.3)	5 (5.7)	87	0.31	0.579
Poor	272 (92.5)	22 (7.5)	294		

(b) Association between respondent knowledge and attitude and perceived TB-associated stigma in urban communities

Variables	Perceived TB stigma present (%)	Perceived TB stigma absent (%)	Total	χ^2	p value
Attitude to TB					
Positive	188 (95.9)	8 (4.1)	196	0.06	0.812
Negative	188 (95.4)	9 (4.6)	197		
Knowledge of TB					
Good	227 (97.4)	5 (2.6)	233	4.30	0.038*
Poor	148 (93.1)	11 (6.9)	159		

*Statistical significance.

to the married ones (AOR = 3.096, 95% CI: 1.087-8.812, p value = 0.034) (Table 9).

In the urban area, average monthly income ($p = 0.019$) and age of respondents ($p = 0.021$) predicted TB-associated stigma. There was a 72.6% reduced likelihood of TB-associated stigma among individual earning less than $50 monthly as compared to those earning more than $50, (AOR = 0.274, 95% CI: 0.093-0.807, p value = 0.019), Also, there was a 78.8% reduced likelihood of TB-associated stigma among individuals less than 35 years old as compared to those older than 35 years (AOR = 0.212, 95% CI: 0.057-0.788, p value = 0.021) (Table 10).

4. Discussion

In this study, 790 adults were interviewed to determine knowledge, attitude, and determinants of TB-associated stigma in rural and urban communities in Lagos State.

Our study is the first study to the best of our knowledge that has examined TB-associated stigma and its disparities in rural and urban communities in Nigeria.

TB is not an unknown illness in communities studied as the majority of respondents in rural and urban areas (97.5% and 99.2%, respectively) had ever heard about the disease. This could be due to the good health information and public enlightenment program in this part of Nigeria. This finding is comparable to that of studies from Libya and Ethiopia that reported 96.5% and 94.9% awareness of TB in the community, respectively [33, 34]; it is also similar to a local study from Ogoja in Cross River State, Nigeria, that reported TB awareness of 97% in the study population [35]. Our finding on awareness of TB in the community was however higher than other Nigerian studies: 93% in Enugu state [36] and 86.5% in Edo state [37].

Our study also revealed a better appropriate knowledge of TB in urban areas compared to rural areas using the

TABLE 9: Simple and multiple logistic regressions of TB-associated stigma and associated factor in rural communities.

Predictor variable	Simple logistic regression				Multiple logistic regression			
	p value	Crude odds ratio	95% CI lower	upper	p value	Adjusted odds ratio	95% CI lower	upper
Ethnicity								
Other ethnic groups	0.018*	0.263	1.716	4.241	0.014*	0.257	0.086	0.761
Yoruba		1				1		
Marital status								
Unmarried	0.085	2.4	0.887	6.491	0.034*	3.09	1.087	8.812
Married		1				1		
Age								
≥35 years	0.165	1.745	0.795	3.828				
<35 years		1						
Sex								
Male	0.255	1.598	0.712	3.587				
Female		1						
Employment								
Employed	0.215	0.489	0.158	1.514				
Unemployed		1						
Attitude								
Negative	0.181	1.709	0.779	3.745				
Positive		1						

TABLE 10: Simple and multiple logistic regressions of TB-associated stigma on associated factors in urban communities.

Predictor variable	Simple logistic regression				Multiple logistic regression			
	p value	Crude odds ratio	95% CI lower	upper	p value	Adjusted odds ratio	95% CI lower	upper
Income (naira)								
<18000	0.005*	0.217	0.075	0.625	0.019*	0.274	0.093	0.807
>18000		1				1		
Age								
<35 years	0.008*	`0.182	0.052	0.645	0.021*	0.212	0.057	0.788
≥35 years		1				1		
Knowledge								
Good	0.046*	2.812	1.018	7.767	0.33	1.72	0.575	5.165
Poor		1				1		
Sex								
Male	0.914	0.947	0.357	2.508				
Female		1						
Ethnicity								
Yoruba	0.566	1.45	0.407	5.162				
Non-Yoruba		1						

*Significant.

respondent's ability to respond to 5 cardinal knowledge questions ($p < 0.001$). This is comparable to a study among prisoners in Ethiopia in which those in urban areas had better overall knowledge compared to those in rural areas [32, 38]. The respondents in rural communities had a better overall positive attitude compared to urban areas but there was no statistically significant association between attitude and sociodemographic factors in the rural and urban communities.

An evaluation of the specific items on the EMIC stigma scale revealed that a higher proportion of urban respondents (27.6%) believed that a person who has TB would desire to keep others from knowing if possible compared to 20.3% among rural respondents ($p < 0.001$). This could be because communal living in rural areas could limit the ability to conceal the disease in this area compared to the urban areas. This could influence the rate of TB diagnosis in these communities as well as adherence to medication. However, the proportion of participants who will desire to conceal TB diagnosis in our study is higher than what was reported from a previous study in rural Ethiopia but lower than 75% reported from a study in rural India [39] and 37.3% reported from another study from Thailand [29].

Also, more respondents in the rural area 17.6% compared to urban area 11.5% would feel inferior to other community members if someone in their family had TB. This could be due to the fact that most people in rural know each other because of living in close proximity compared to an independent lifestyle that is characteristics of urban areas of Lagos metropolis. This finding is similar to a study from Thailand that reported that 17.4% of respondents would think less of themselves if a family member had a TB diagnosis [39]. But lower than the findings of a study from the Indian rural community with 85% rural dwellers who would have diminished self-esteem if a family member was infected with TB [29].

This present study also corroborated the fact that TB infection could cause shame and embarrassment in the community as reported by respondents from rural 45.2% and urban 48.2% communities. This is similar to 48% reported from a study in rural India [39], but higher than 20.3% reported from Thailand [29], 31% reported among prisoners in Ethiopia [37], and 39% reported from a community study in Ethiopia [40]. However, it is lower than 76.3% reported among community respondents in Pakistan that believe TB causes shame [41].

Another stigmatizing behavior in the community to TB patients is that persons in the community usually look down on them. An equal proportion of respondents in rural 37.6% and urban 37.5% areas alluded to this behavior. This finding is however lower than 51% reported among rural dwellers in Ethiopia [40] but higher than that of Thailand study that reported that 22.5% of community members would think less of TB patients [29].

Just like it was reported for other infectious diseases like leprosy, about half of the rural 48.6% and urban 53.1% of respondents believed that people in their communities would avoid a person infected with TB. This is mainly due to the fact that respondents were afraid of contracting the infection if they associate closely with community members who are infected with TB. Also, rural respondents in this study believed that TB infection could reduce the prospect of getting marital partners compared to urban respondents ($p < 0.001$). This could be because people in communities in rural areas hold on to more traditional values in their approach to choosing a marital partner to compare to people living in urban areas. This also could be a reflection of the cultural practice prevalent in our setting in which diseases are perceived to be hereditary, and families do not want to be associated with individuals with chronic diseases [42]. The proportion of those reporting TB could reduce the prospect of finding a marital partner is higher than 20% reported rural Ethiopian study [40] and 30.1% reported from Thailand [29].

TB was also believed to also cause problems in existing marriages. About 31.9% of respondents in urban areas alluded to this when compared to 15.3% among the respondents from the rural areas ($p < 0.001$). This could be due to the fact that persons living in rural areas are more cohesive and likely to be engaged in family and communal support than individuals living in urban areas. However, TB has been reported as a possible cause of marital difficulty in other studies too. For instance, the study of cultural epidemiology of TB in Bangladesh, India, and Malawi reported that divorce and isolation could occur in marriage due to TB infection [43]. Also, another study from Thailand reported that 22.5% of respondents believed that TB could cause a problem in an ongoing marriage [29].

A significantly higher proportion of respondents from rural areas 81.6% believed that TB could cause difficulty in finding a job and earning a living compared to 69.4% among urban respondents ($p < 0.001$). This could be due to the fact that potential employers might avoid the persons infected with TB due to fear of being infected. However, our findings on the difficulty of getting a job for a person infected with TB are higher than 34.75% reported from a Thailand study. The implication of this will include poor economic power and the extreme difficulty of persons infected with TB to manage the catastrophic direct and indirect cost of treating the illness [44].

Generally, the majority of respondents in our study could dislike buying food from a person affected by TB (rural 88.3% and urban 87.3%). This could be because members of communities in these areas have the fear that they can be infected with TB through the food they buy. This finding is however higher than 41.5% reported from a Thailand study [29]. This finding could also be a reflection of the cultural practice in the study settings in which there must be societal acceptance of a person selling food before their food is considered fit for consumption.

Overall, our study reported a high prevalence of TB-associated stigma in the communities studied, and the majority of respondents in the rural areas (93%) and urban areas (95.7%) had TB-associated stigma. However, the mean EMIC stigma scale score is higher among the urban respondents 17.43 ± 6.012 compared to rural respondents 16.54 ± 6.324, and the difference is statistically significant (Student t-test-2, $p = 0.046$). However, the proportion of TB-associated stigma in our study is higher than those reported by different previous studies. A study in India reported a 73% prevalence of stigmatizing attitudes in the community [11], and another study from Pakistan believed that 47.9% of TB patients are stigmatized [41]. Also, a study in the rural community of Ethiopia reported 51.2% had stigma [40], and another study among the pastoralist population in Ethiopia reported 61.8% perceived TB-associated stigma [45] just as a study of Tunisia reported 54.9% of TB-associated stigma [46]. The high proportion of respondents with perceived TB-associated stigma in this study could be due to diverse cultural practices and lack of adequate and correct health information on TB [24].

A major determinant of TB-associated stigma in the rural community was ethnicity and marital status. Respondents who belong to ethnic groups other than the Yoruba tribe had about 74% reduced likelihood of having TB-associated stigma in the community when compared to those of Yoruba ethnicity. Also, unmarried individuals had about 3 times the odds of TB-associated stigma when compared to married individuals. There might be a need to target stigma reduction activities at unmarried individuals in the rural communities because the social support provided by marriage could have contributed to the reduced odds of TB-associated stigma in the rural community.

However, good knowledge of TB, age ≥ 35 years, and monthly income ≥ $50 were found to be associated with TB-associated stigma in the urban community in bivariate analysis. After adjusting for confounders, however, individuals earning more than $50 had about 4 times the odds of TB-associated stigma. So also, individuals who are less than 35 years had about 79% reduced likelihood of TB-associated stigma in the community compared to respondents older than 35 years. This finding is similar to a study in southern Thailand that reported that older age is associated with TB stigma [39]. It is also similar to a community study in India [11] and Pakistan [41] that reported that high-income groups have a higher chance of TB-associated stigma than low-income earners. However, this present study did not find any relationship between gender and TB-associated stigma in contrast to a previous report by the study of the explanatory model of TB stigma in Bangladesh, India, Columbia, and Malawi [43].

An important recommendation to mitigate the negative effect of TB-associated stigma on TB control in Nigeria is that the Ministry of Health at the national and subnational level in line with WHO End TB Strategy should strengthen the stigma reduction component of the existing National Strategic Plan for Tuberculosis Control (2015-2020) that focuses on improving universal access to TB treatment through the creation of a supportive environment, free of stigma and discrimination [47].

A major limitation to generalizing the outcome of the study could be because it was conducted in rural and urban communities of Lagos State, Nigeria. The state is a cosmopolitan state, which has better healthcare indices, compared to other states in Nigeria with arguably better health coverage and better healthcare provider to patient's ratio. Hence, the findings of this study could be different from other states in Nigeria. However, a further study with participants recruited from the six geopolitical zones of Nigeria will provide nationally representative data.

5. Conclusion

There is a high prevalence of TB-associated stigma in rural and urban communities in this study. Ethnicity and marital status were found to be determinants in the rural community while age ≥ 35 years and average monthly income ≥ $50 were found to be determinants of TB-associated stigma in urban communities. There is therefore a need to increase access to appropriate information on TB and TB-associated stigma through print, radio, television, and social media. This information should be age-appropriate and culturally acceptable in local languages. Also, further research into stigma reduction intervention measures will help to provide insight into the appropriate public health approach aimed at mitigating the impact of TB-associated stigma to the national TB control program.

Acknowledgments

The author will like to acknowledge the contribution of research assistance that helped with the data collection as well as the Medical Officer of Health of Badagry and Lagos Mainland Local Government Area, Lagos.

References

[1] D. Maher, "The global plan to stop TB, 2006-2015. Actions for life: towards a world free of tuberculosis," *The International Journal of Tuberculosis and Lung Disease*, vol. 10, no. 3, pp. 240-241, 2006.

[2] World Health Organization, *Global Tuberculosis Report 2017* World Health Organization, Geneva, 2017, Licence: CC BY-NCSA 3.0 IGO.

[3] World Health Organization, *Global Tuberculosis Report 2015* WHO, Geneva Switzaland, 20th edition, 2015, Available from: http://apps.who.int/medicinedocs/documents/s22199en/s22199en.pdf.

[4] World Health Organization, *Global Tuberculosis Report 2019* World Health Organization, Geneva, 2019, Licence: CCBY-NC-SA3.0IGO.

[5] T. B. Stop and U. Partnership, *The Paradigm Shift 2016-2020, Global Plan to End TB [Internet]*, Geneva, Switzerland, 2016January 2018, http://www.stoptb.org/assets/documents/global/plan/GlobalPlanToEndTB_TheParadigmShift_2016-2020_StopTBPartnership.pdf.

[6] W. W. Mak, F. Cheung, J. Woo et al., "A comparative study of the stigma associated with infectious diseases (SARS, AIDS, TB)," *Hong Kong Medical Journal*, vol. 15, no. SUPP8, pp. 34–37, 2009.

[7] B. Hatherall, *Understanding TB-Related Stigma in Asia. R4DDfidGovUk [Internet]*, pp. 1–30, 2009, http://r4d.dfid.gov.uk/pdf/outputs/esrc_dfid/60425_tb-related_stigma_in_asia_nepal1.pdf.

[8] A. van Rie, S. Sengupta, P. Pungrassami et al., "Measuring stigma associated with tuberculosis and HIV/AIDS in southern Thailand: exploratory and confirmatory factor analyses of two new scales," *Tropical Medicine & International Health* vol. 13, no. 1, pp. 21–30, 2008.

[9] J. Macq, A. Solis, and G. Martinez, "Can we make TB control more pro-poor by addressing the sticky business of stigma?," in *36th Union World Conference on Lung Health-" Scaling up TB control to meet the needs of the poor"((France) Paris, du 18/10/2005 au 22/10/2005). In: International Journal of Tuberculosis and Lung Disease,*, Paris, France, 2005.

[10] A. Courtwright and A. N. Turner, "Tuberculosis and stigmatization: pathways and interventions," *Public Health Reports*, vol. 125, 4_suppl, pp. 34–42, 2010.

[11] K. D. Sagili, S. Satyanarayana, and S. S. Chadha, "Is knowledge regarding tuberculosis associated with stigmatising and discriminating attitudes of general population towards tuberculosis patients? Findings from a community based survey in 30 districts of India," *PLoS One*, vol. 11, no. 2, article e0147274, 2016.

[12] S. S. Ali, F. Rabbani, U. N. Siddiqui et al., "Tuberculosis: do we know enough? A study of patients and their families in an outpatient hospital setting in Karachi, Pakistan," *The International Journal of Tuberculosis and Lung Disease*, vol. 7, no. 11, pp. 1052–1058, 2003, http://www.ingentaconnect.com/content/iuatld/ijtld/2003/00000007/00000011/art00007.

[13] A. L. Cremers, M. M. de Laat, N. Kapata, R. Gerrets, K. Klipstein-Grobusch, and M. P. Grobusch, "Assessing the consequences of stigma for tuberculosis patients in urban Zambia," *PLoS One*, vol. 10, no. 3, article e0119861, 2015.

[14] B. Duko, A. Bedaso, G. Ayano, and Z. Yohannis, "Perceived stigma and associated factors among patient with tuberculosis, Wolaita Sodo, Ethiopia: cross-sectional study," *Tuberculosis Research and Treatment*, vol. 2019, Article ID 5917537, 5 pages, 2019.

[15] J. Ngamvithayapong-Yanai, S. Luangjina, S. Thawthong, S. Bupachat, and W. Imsangaun, "Stigma against tuberculosis may hinder non-household contact investigation: a qualitative study in Thailand," *Public Health Action*, vol. 9, no. 1, pp. 15–23, 2019.

[16] E. Osei, P. Akweongo, and F. Binka, "Factors associated with DELAY in diagnosis among tuberculosis patients in Hohoe Municipality, Ghana," *BMC Public Health*, vol. 15, no. 1, 2015.

[17] A. L. Adamu, M. A. Gadanya, I. S. Abubakar et al., "High mortality among tuberculosis patients on treatment in Nigeria: a retrospective cohort study," *BMC Infectious Diseases*, vol. 17, no. 1, p. 170, 2017.

[18] O. A. Adejumo, O. J. Daniel, H. A. Abdur-Razzaq et al., "Trend of tuberculosis case notification and treatment outcome in Lagos State, Nigeria: a 5-year retrospective study," *Transactions of the Royal Society of Tropical Medicine and Hygiene*, vol. 111, no. 7, pp. 300–307, 2017.

[19] S. Costelloe, J. Kemppainen, J. Brion et al., "Impact of anxiety and depressive symptoms on perceptions of stigma in persons living with HIV disease in rural versus urban North Carolina," *AIDS Care*, vol. 27, no. 12, pp. 1425–1428, 2015.

[20] J. R. Naidoo, L. R. Uys, M. Greeff et al., "Urban and rural differences in HIV/AIDS stigma in five African countries," *African Journal of AIDS Research*, vol. 6, no. 1, pp. 17–23, 2007.

[21] N. Roosta, D. S. Black, and T. H. Rea, "A comparison of stigma among patients with leprosy in rural Tanzania and urban United States: a role for public health in dermatology," *International Journal of Dermatology*, vol. 52, no. 4, pp. 432–440, 2013.

[22] V. N. Yebei, J. D. Fortenberry, and D. O. Ayuku, "Felt stigma among people living with HIV/AIDS in rural and urban Kenya," *African Health Sciences*, vol. 8, no. 2, pp. 97–102, 2008.

[23] Y. Hong, X. Li, B. Stanton et al., "Expressions of HIV-related stigma among rural-to-urban migrants in China," *AIDS Patient Care and STDs*, vol. 22, no. 10, pp. 823–831, 2008.

[24] S. Chang and J. K. Cataldo, "A systematic review of global cultural variations in knowledge, attitudes and health responses to tuberculosis stigma," *The International Journal of Tuberculosis and Lung Disease*, vol. 18, no. 2, pp. 168–173, 2014.

[25] National Population Commission (NPC) and [Nigeria] and ICF, "Macro (2009)," *National Population Commission, Nigeria. Nigerian Demographic and Health Survey*, 2008.

[26] Lagos Bureau of Statistic, *Lagos State Government Digest of Statistics 2015*, Lagos State Government, Alausa, Ikeja Lagos, 2015, http://mepb.lagosstate.gov.ng/wp-content/uploads/sites/29/2017/01/Digest-of-Statistics-2015.pdf.

[27] G. Prabhakara, *Biostatistics*Jaypee Brothers Medical Publishers (P) Ltd.July 2016, http://www.jaypeedigital.com/bookdetails.aspx?id=9788180616594&sr=1.

[28] W. van Brakel, C. Voorend, B. Ebenso, H. Cross, and V. Augustine, "Guidelines to reduce stigma [Internet]," in *How to Assess Health-Related Stigma*The International Federation of Anti-Leprosy Associations (ILEP) and the Netherlands Leprosy Relief, London2011, http://www.ilep.org.uk/technical-advice/stigma-guidelines/.

[29] S. Sermrittirong, W. H. Van Brakel, N. Kraipui, S. Traithip, and J. Bunders-aelen, "Comparing the perception of community members towards leprosy and tuberculosis stigmatisation," *Leprosy Review*, vol. 86, pp. 54–61, 2015.

[30] WHO, "Advocacy, communication and social mobilization for TB control: a guide to developing knowledge, attitude and practice surveys," WHO/HTM/STB/, 2008.

[31] A. Y. Nur and S. J. Rohde, "Factors influencing delay in seeking tuberculosis treatment in Belet-Weyne district, Somalia [Internet]," University of Western Cape, South Africa, 2008, http://etd.uwc.ac.za/xmlui/bitstream/handle/11394/2778/Nur_MPH_2008.pdf?sequence=1.

[32] K. Adane, M. Spigt, L. Johanna, D. Noortje, S. F. Abera, and G.-J. Dinant, "Tuberculosis knowledge, attitudes, and practices among northern Ethiopian prisoners: implications for TB control efforts," *PLoS One*, vol. 12, no. 3, article e0174692, 2017.

[33] D. Tolossa, G. Medhin, and M. Legesse, "Community knowledge, attitude, and practices towards tuberculosis in Shinile town, Somali regional state, eastern Ethiopia: a cross-sectional study," *BMC Public Health*, vol. 14, no. 1, p. 804, 2014.

[34] M. A. Solliman, M. A. Hassali, M. Al-Haddad et al., "Assessment of knowledge towards tuberculosis among general population in North East Libya," *Journal of Applied Pharmaceutical Science*, vol. 2, no. 4, pp. 24–30, 2012.

[35] O. O. Kalu and E. E. Jimmy, "Assessment of knowledge, attitude and tuberculosis-related social stigma among school adolescent in a semi-urban town in Cross River State, Nigeria," *International Journal of Education and research*, vol. 3, no. 2, pp. 81–90, 2015.

[36] U. U. Onyeonoro, J. N. Chukwu, D. C. Oshi, C. C. Nwafor, and A. O. Meka, "Assessment of tuberculosis-related knowledge, attitudes and practices in Enugu, South East Nigeria," *Journal of infectious Diseases and Immunity*, vol. 6, no. 1, pp. 1–9, 2014.

[37] E. A. Tobin, P.-W. Okojie, and E. C. Isah, "Community knowledge and attitude to pulmonary tuberculosis in rural Edo state, Nigeria," *Annals of African Medicine*, vol. 12, no. 3, pp. 148–154, 2013.

[38] I. A. Abioye, M. O. Omotayo, and W. Alakija, "Socio-demographic determinants of stigma among patients with pulmonary tuberculosis in Lagos, Nigeria," *African Health Sciences*, vol. 11, no. 3, pp. S100–S104, 2011.

[39] S. Atre, A. Kudale, S. Morankar, D. Gosoniu, and M. G. Weiss, "Gender and community views of stigma and tuberculosis in rural Maharashtra, India," *Glob Public Health*, vol. 6, no. 1, pp. 56–71, 2011.

[40] G. Abebe, A. Deribew, L. Apers et al., "Knowledge, health seeking behavior and perceived stigma towards tuberculosis among tuberculosis suspects in a rural community in southwest Ethiopia," *PLoS One*, vol. 5, no. 10, pp. 1–7, 2010.

[41] M. U. Mushtaq, U. Shahid, H. M. Abdullah et al., "Urban-rural inequities in knowledge, attitudes and practices regarding tuberculosis in two districts of Pakistan's Punjab province," *International journal for Equity in Health*, vol. 10, no. 1, p. 8, 2011.

[42] B. Hatherall, J. N. Newell, N. Emmel, S. C. Baral, and M. A. Khan, ""Who will marry a diseased girl?" Marriage, gender, and tuberculosis stigma in Asia," *Qualitative Health Research*, vol. 29, no. 8, pp. 1109–1119, 2019.

[43] M. G. Weiss, D. Somma, F. Karim et al., "Cultural epidemiology of TB with reference to gender in Bangladesh, India and Malawi [Special section on gender and TB]," *The International Journal of Tuberculosis and Lung Disease*, vol. 12, no. 7, pp. 837–847, 2008.

[44] D. M. Barter, S. O. Agboola, M. B. Murray, and T. Bärnighausen, "Tuberculosis and poverty: the contribution of patient costs in sub-Saharan Africa – a systematic review," *BMC Public Health*, vol. 12, pp. 1–21, 2012.

[45] B. T. Sima, T. Belachew, and F. Abebe, "Knowledge, attitude and perceived stigma towards tuberculosis among pastoralists; do they differ from sedentary communities? A comparative cross-sectional study," *PLoS One*, vol. 12, no. 7, article e0181032, 2017.

[46] N. Bensalah, M. Hsairi, H. Snene et al., "Community knowledge, attitude, and practices towards tuberculosis in Tunisia," *European Respiratory Journal*, vol. 50, article PA2612, 2017.

[47] *The National Strategic Plan for Tuberculosis Control 2015-2020: Towards Universal Access to Prevention, Diagnosis and Treatment*, National Tuberculosis and Leprosy Control Programme, Department of Public Health, Federal Ministry of Health, Nigeria, Abuja, Nigeria, 2014, http://ntblcp.org.ng/strategic-plan.

11

The Presence of Cough and Tuberculosis: Active Case Finding Outcomes in the Philippines

Siwon Lee,[1] Lincoln Lau,[1,2] Krisha Lim,[1] Jansel Ferma,[1] Warren Dodd,[3] and Donald Cole[2]

[1] *International Care Ministries Foundation Inc., Philippines*
[2] *Dalla Lana School of Public Health, University of Toronto, ON, Canada*
[3] *School of Public Health and Health Systems, University of Waterloo, ON, Canada*

Correspondence should be addressed to Lincoln Lau; lincoln.lau@caremin.com

Academic Editor: Edward A. Graviss

The results of a tuberculosis (TB) active case finding (ACF) program, implemented by International Care Ministries (ICM) in the Philippines, were examined to understand how the presence of physical symptoms might influence ACF outcomes among extreme low-income Filipinos. ICM health staff implemented symptom screening in villages and suspected cases were referred to the closest rural health unit (RHU) for TB testing. ACF was carried out in Mindanao and the Visayas, across 16 different provinces. All participants were interviewed pre/postprogram, and screening outcomes were collected. A multilevel regression model was constructed to explore the effect of factors on the likelihood of getting tested. A total of 4635 individuals were screened; 1290 (27.8%) were symptom positive and referred. From those referred, 336 (7.2%) were tested for TB and 53 (1.1%) were TB positive. "Cough for more than two weeks" was associated with a 1.09 (95% CI 1.01, 1.15) times increase in likelihood of getting tested. The finding that the presence of cough is associated with higher rate of testing suggests that individuals in these settings might not know or believe that the lack of cough does not equate to lack of TB infection. While technologies and screening algorithms give us the ability to refine the 'supply' side of the TB screening, addressing the knowledge gap should improve 'demand'.

1. Introduction

Tuberculosis is not a newly emerging disease in the Philippines [1]. Philippines is one of the five countries in the world that share 56% of the global TB patient burden, along with China, India, Indonesia, and Pakistan [2]. Philippines was a pioneer in making state-of-the-art MDR-TB treatment available and the level of awareness of TB in the country is high [3]. Nevertheless, a gap persists in understanding how a TB suspect, experiencing extreme low-income, perceives and responds to common TB symptoms. As a result of their geographic isolation, rural TB patients often face greater financial and transportation burdens associated with accessing healthcare and TB treatment compared to their urban counterparts [4]. More specifically, these financial burdens often include out of pocket expenses for nonmedical costs associated with seeking care, in addition to lost days of work or unemployment from debilitating side effects of the disease and subsequent treatment [5].

According to the WHO, TB symptoms and signs may include cough for two weeks or more, fever, unexplained weight loss, weakness or fatigue, night sweats, and chest pain [6]. Among these symptoms, long-term cough is one of the most commonly identified symptoms by TB patients [7]. Fever and unexplained weight loss are also noted as common symptoms [8]. Based on the Health Behaviour model, an individual's health-seeking behaviour is shaped by an individual's perception of his or her susceptibility to and severity of a specific disease, in addition to barriers to take action [9]. Knowledge about different diseases, accessibility to healthcare facilities, behaviour, and personal background also play a part in an individual's decision making process [8]. According to the model, when an individual is more familiar with a disease, this individual should have greater awareness and capacity to address the disease.

Nevertheless, relying on patients to identify TB via self-reported symptoms is problematic for several reasons. These symptoms are neither specific nor exclusive to TB [10] and their interpretation could vary from person to person, depending on their tolerance [7]. Furthermore, prolonged cough (i.e., cough for more than two weeks) has a sensitivity of only 35% for TB [9]. Although individuals who experience cough may have an increased likelihood to be concerned and seek testing, those with symptoms that resolve might lack motivation to seek a consultation. This is an issue as the 2016 prevalence study conducted by the National Tuberculosis Control Program (NTP) of the Philippines showed that 14.2% of TB positive patients were asymptomatic, and only 6% of TB positive patients presented with a cough that lasted less than 2 weeks and did not belong to a high-risk group [11]. NTP definition of high-risk group included: men, elderly, those in poverty, dwellers in urban slums, smokers, previous TB patients, and diabetic individuals [11]. Therefore, while the presence of cough, most commonly identified symptom (79.7%), can be beneficial by motivating TB suspects to seek screening and testing, the lack of obvious symptoms does not necessarily signify the lack of TB infection or convalescence. The high percentage of asymptomatic TB positive patients suggests that systematic active case finding (ACF) in high prevalence areas might be required to increase case detection. With a recent rise in TB incidence (554/100,000/year) in the country, all high-risk groups in the Philippines should be considered for ACF.

International Care Ministries (ICM), a Philippine-based nongovernmental organization (NGO) that provides poverty alleviation programs to extreme low-income households, has been carrying out ACF in resource-limited settings for eight years. The intervention examined will be referred to as the "ICM TB Screening Program" (TSP) and from June 2014 to May 2015, 1290 participants were identified by this program to be TB symptom positive. In this study, we assessed how TB symptoms affected ACF outcomes in extreme low-income households.

2. Materials and Methods

2.1. ICM TB Screening Program (TSP). The TB Screening Program (TSP) is part of ICM's 16-week poverty reduction program called Transform. This program identifies households experiencing extreme low-income using propensity scoring, and gathers approximately 30 participants in each community for a series of weekly health and livelihood lessons. These lessons are designed to equip the participants to remain healthy and to improve or secure alternative sources of income. During one of these lessons, an ICM health staff carried out ACF and facilitated follow-up in each of the communities in four stages (Figure 1). The communities that ICM works with are geographically spread out over the Visayas and Mindanao in the Philippines (Figure 2). Approximately 325 communities covering 16 different provinces are included in each cycle (16 weeks).

On week three of the Transform program, and following a health lesson on TB, all participants completed a prescreening card (Figure S1 in Supplementary Material) that gathered personal level information on TB symptoms. Adults, aged 15 and above, were categorized to be a TB suspect if they had a cough that lasted for two or more weeks. Children, 15 years and below, were suspected to have TB if found with any one of the following symptoms: (a) cough/wheezing of at least two weeks or more, (b) unexplained fever of two weeks or more, (c) significant and unintentional weight loss, (d) fatigue, lethargy, general malaise, (e) failure to respond to appropriate antibiotic therapy after two weeks, and (f) failure to regain previous state of health after two week following a presumed viral infection. Occasionally, at the ICM health staff's discretion, adults without cough but presenting with other symptoms were also referred for testing.

Individuals with TB symptoms from the prescreen progressed to Stage 1. During weeks five and six of the Transform program, patients continuing to meet the definition of suspected TB were considered Stage 1 positive. In Stage 2, a rural health unit (RHU) referral form was provided to all Stage 1 positive individuals. During weeks seven and eight, and with patient permission, ICM health staff contacted or visited each RHU to provide a list of potential TB patients identified during Stage 1. Each referred participant was asked to attend the RHU for testing. ICM staff provided TB related health knowledge and encouraged those who were hesitant or unwilling to get tested. In a few cases, transportation assistance was provided to those who were willing to visit the RHU on the days ICM staff were present in the community.

At Stage 3, and again with patient permission, ICM handed over all TB patient information to RHUs. This stage was initiated once the patient attended a RHU for sputum testing, and all patients who successfully completed the sputum test were given a RHU reply slip. Patients with a positive TB sputum result were enrolled into a directly observed treatment, short-course (DOTS) program. Patients with persistent symptoms but negative sputum results were further screened by chest X-ray (CXR). For a few participants, financial assistance was provided by ICM for the CXRs. Those determined to be TB positive by CXR were then enrolled in the DOTS program.

During weeks 9-16, RHU reply slips were returned and three kilograms of a micronutrient fortified soy-blended rice product was given to each participant who successfully attended a RHU. ICM staff followed up with those who have not visited the RHU for testing and collected results on those who were tested.

2.2. Data Collection. Program monitoring data was collected at each stage from every patient enrolled into the TSP. At Stage 1, potential TB patients' symptoms were recorded. Outcomes were collected by ICM staff at Stage 3 via follow-up calls with RHU staff and from reply slips completed by doctors (Figure S2 in Supplementary Material). ICM staff collected referral data on paper logbooks and updated this collected data on Google Spreadsheet (Figure S3 in Supplementary Material).

As part of ICM's program, baseline and endline questionnaires were administered at the beginning and end of the

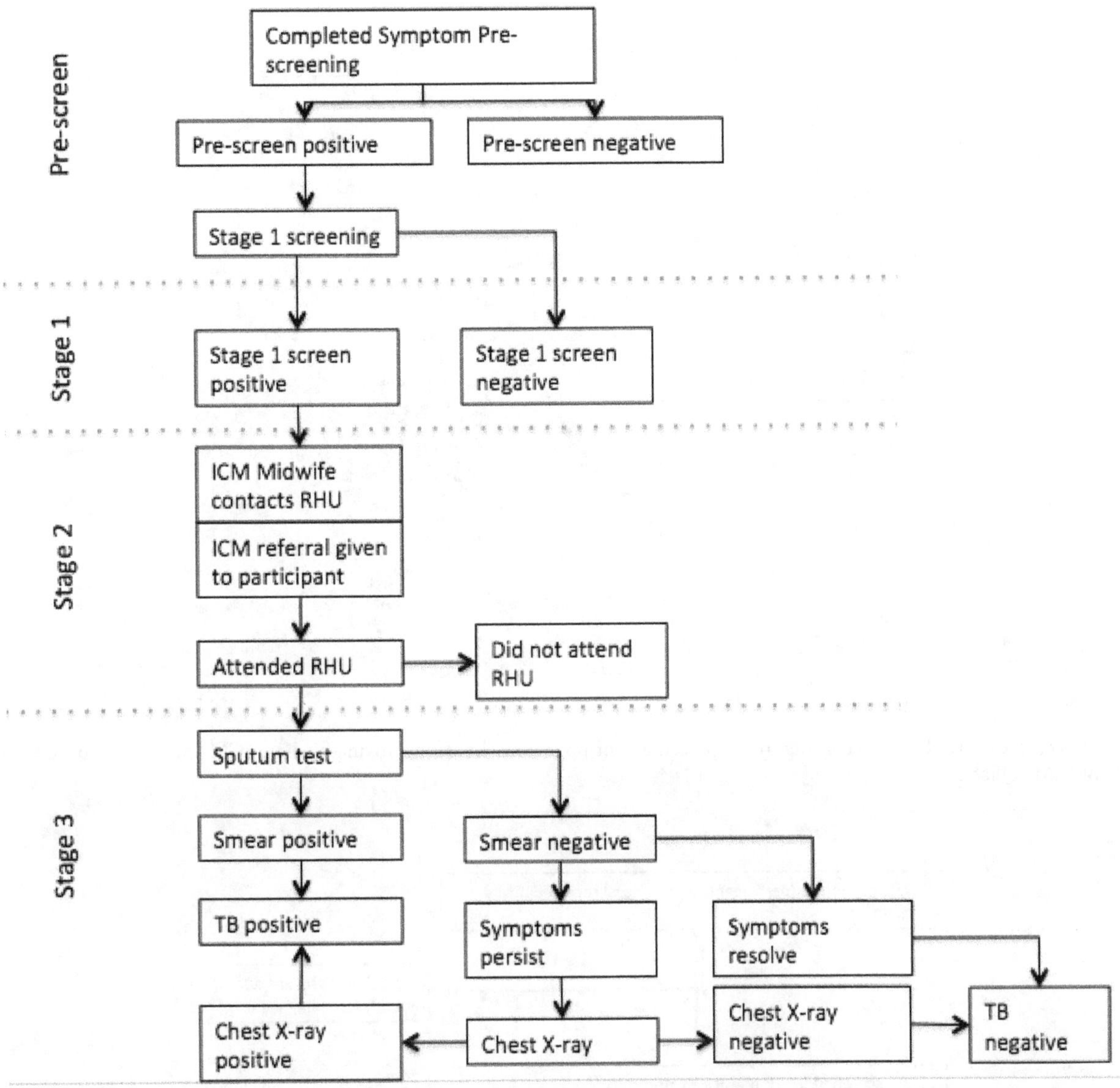

FIGURE 1: Flow chart of ICM TB Screening Program. Prescreening: over the course of 16 weeks, participants of ICM's Transform program go through poverty alleviation lessons. Participants were asked about TB physical symptoms at prescreening. Stage 1: those who were prescreened positive were asked again, the same questions, at this stage to filter out any false positive participants. Stage 2: ICM's health trainers, local staff, who are fully capable of communicating in regional dialects, refer TB suspects to the closest rural health unit (RHU) for TB testing. This is where we monitored participants' health-seeking behaviour through their decision to visit an RHU for testing or not. Stage 3: depending on the RHU, TB suspects are asked to provide a sputum sample and some would be required to have a chest X-ray taken for a more accurate diagnosis.

Transform program. Questions included general demographics, general health, measures of social capital, and asset-based measures of poverty. On physical symptoms, participants were asked if they had experienced: cough/wheezing of two weeks or more; unexplained fever of two weeks or more; significant and unintentional weight loss; fatigue, lethargy, general malaise; failure to respond to two weeks of appropriate antibiotic therapy; failure to regain previous state of health two weeks after a presumed viral infection. These two datasets, baseline questionnaire and physical symptoms, were linked through a unique ID tag where available. Records that could not be linked were excluded from this study. Of the 25,735 Transform program participants, who were surveyed, 13,010, including family members, were screened for TB symptoms and 4635 (36.4%) participants' records were linked (Figure 3). There was no significant difference in age, sex or RHU attendance between the group that was linked and the group that was not linked.

2.3. Analysis. In this study, our objective was to understand which factors were important in contributing to a successful referral which resulted in testing at a RHU. Variables such as symptoms and social capital characteristics of our study population were compared between the groups that

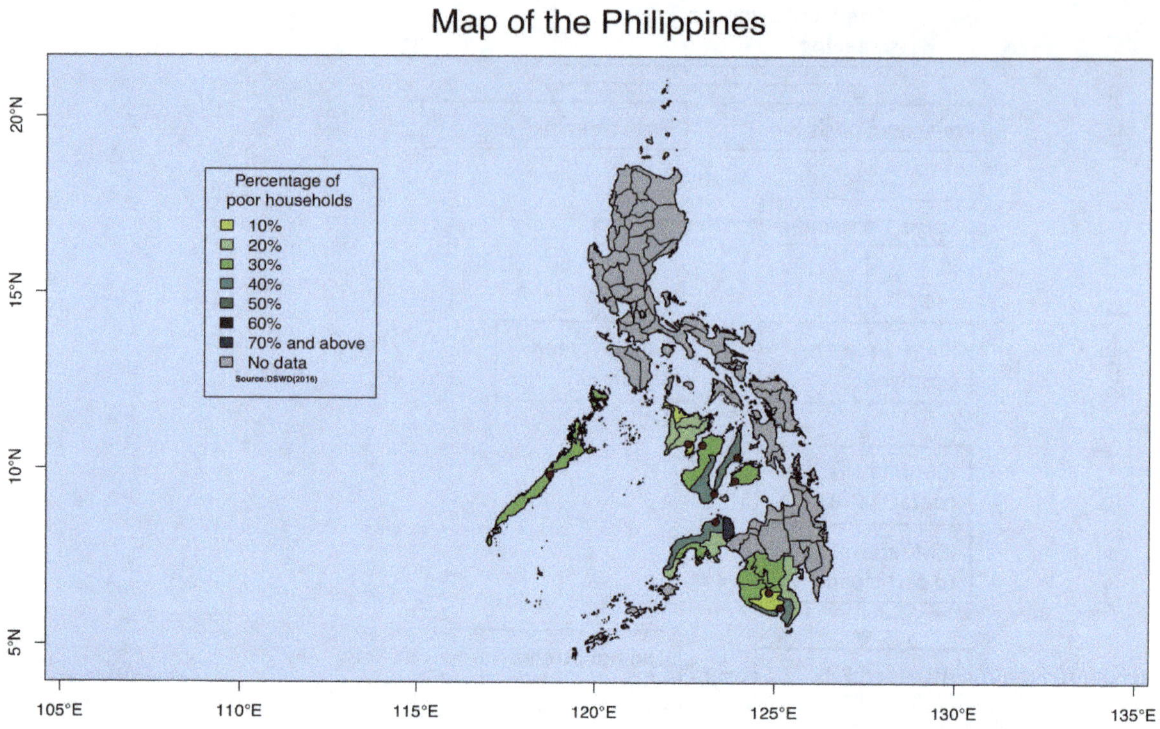

FIGURE 2: Green areas are shaded according to the percentage of poor households in provinces where ICM works in. Red dots indicate locations of ICM's offices.

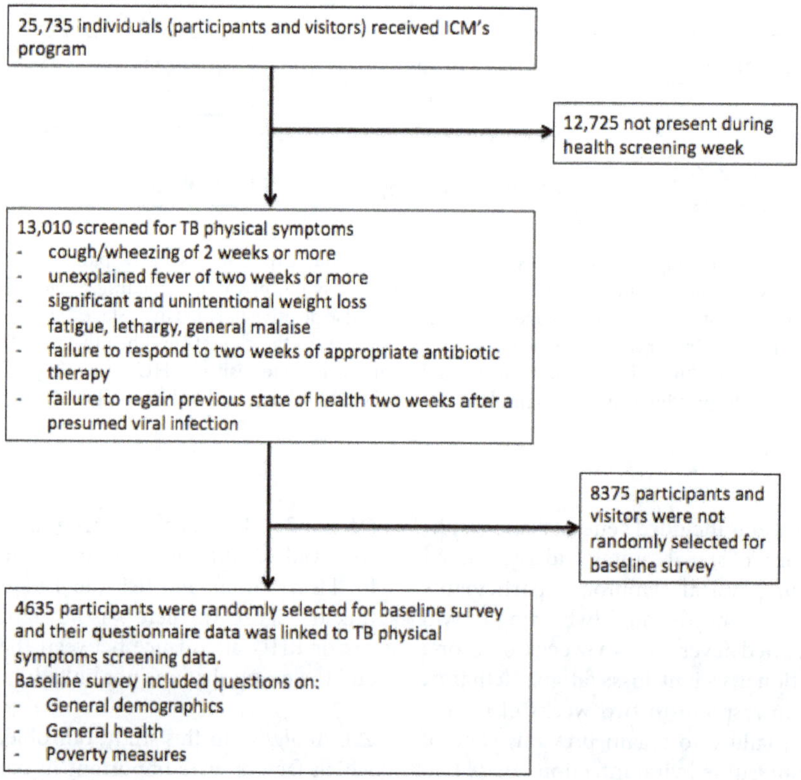

FIGURE 3: Number of participants at each step of the ACF process.

completed testing at a RHU and of those who did not go for testing. The covariates selected for data analysis are common TB symptoms, based on Philippines NTP manual of procedures and WHO systematic screening for active TB, that were asked during our symptom screening [6, 12]. Statistical significance, defined as $p<0.05$, was calculated using Student's t-test and Pearson's chi-square test. To examine the effect of physical symptoms on whether a patient attended the RHU, intraclass correlations (ICC) were examined before multilevel regression modeling, to account for nesting of individuals within communities. Using the 'MCMCglmm' package, the multilevel models were generated, and Markov chain Monte Carlo (MCMC) was used to generate p-values [13]. MCMC techniques promote convergence of such models and provide estimates of p-values and confidence intervals. All analyses were conducted using R version 3.3.3.

This study was approved by the Health Sciences Research Ethics Board of the University of Toronto (Protocol Ref #30943).

3. Results

3.1. Sociodemographics. In total, 4635 participants were screened. 1241 patients were screened from June to September 2014, 2109 patients screened from October 2014 to January 2015, and 1285 patients were screened from February to May 2015. After Stage 1 screening, 2696 were identified as TB suspects, 1290 of them were referred to a RHU, and 333 of the referred participants successfully visited a RHU for TB testing. The literacy rate of screened and referred and those who visited the RHU were similar at 53%, 55%, and 52%, respectively.

Among the individuals that visited a RHU, 189 (56%) were female participants and 147 (44%) were male participants. Additionally, 172 (51%) were registered with the national health insurance program (PhilHealth), and 53 (16%) participants tested positive for pulmonary TB (Table 1(a)). The average age of our ACF participants was 37.7 years, 38.2 years among those who were tested at a RHU, and 44.9 years among those with a confirmed TB diagnosis (see Supplementary Table S5 for breakdown by children and adults). Average household size also did not substantially differ among these three groups: 4.8, 4.6, and 5 members, respectively. Differences were noted by referral status (see Table 1(b)) for age among adults, for gender, and for PhilHealth affiliation.

3.2. Symptoms. Most participants reported at least one symptom (see histogram Fig S.5). Among our study population, 297 (89.2%) of the 333 study participants who were TB tested at a RHU reported having cough or wheezing for at least two weeks or more compared to a slightly lower proportion, 724 of 957 (75.7%), who failed to get tested (Table 2). Although the prevalence of other symptoms tended to be higher among those who attended the RHU (i.e., sicker participants), the differences were not statistically significant: unexplained fever of two weeks or more (6.9%; 4.6%), significant and unintentional weight loss (9.6%; 7.3%), fatigue, lethargy, general malaise (6.3%; 3.9%), failure to respond to two weeks of appropriate antibiotics therapy (2.1%; 1.7%), and failure to regain previous state of health two weeks after viral infection (0.6%; 1.7%). Of those who tested positive for TB, 45 (84.9%) were identified as having cough for two weeks or more.

On univariate analysis, only cough for two or more weeks was associated with attendance at the RHU (see Table S7). The multilevel regression results (Table 3) also showed that cough for two or more weeks was associated with successful attendance at a RHU for testing ($p=0.001$; OR = 1.09). The symptom of 'failure to regain previous state of health two weeks after viral infection' was also found to be statistical relevant ($p=0.032$; OR=0.80). Due to the homogeneity of general demographics factors in our study population, and despite inclusion of these factors and additional social capital factors in the multilevel regression modeling, we did not find them statistically significant.

4. Discussion

One of the biggest challenges faced by our study participants is access to health services. ICM has continuously carried out active case finding over the last eight years in approximately 900 communities each year, and accessibility to health facilities has consistently been a challenge. For our study participants who live in a low socioeconomic position, this challenge may be made up of different factors including distance from the RHU, stigma associated with TB, lack of financial resources, inability to take sick leave, and restricted hours of health service operation. This study explored the physical symptoms that extreme low-income Filipinos identified to influence health service-seeking behaviour.

4.1. Limitations in the System. From this experience, we find that passive case finding systems alone, where a TB symptomatic individual presents himself/herself to a healthcare facility, would not adequately capture suspected TB cases in high prevalence and resource-limited settings. Even for those who make it to the RHU for testing, their diagnosis might not be accurate. For our study participants, sputum smear microscopy is commonly used to provide preliminary information for a TB diagnosis. While the cost for this diagnostic test is low, it also has a low sensitivity (0.61). Additionally, those participants who were diagnosed using sputum smear microscopy were asked to return another day to receive their results. Thus, receiving a positive TB diagnosis often involves taking at least two days off from work and finding money for transportation to make two trips to the RHU. Past studies have shown that negative stigmatization of TB exists in the Philippines [12]. Since TB symptom screening was conducted before education on TB, stigma may have prevented more people from disclosing their TB symptoms.

4.2. Prolonged Cough as a Symptom of TB. Based on our findings, it could be inferred that the study participants associated coughing with TB. Prolonged cough was the only physical symptom found to be significantly different between those who were referred and tested, and those who were referred and not tested. A similar finding was reported by a study conducted in Palawan, Philippines, with a larger study

TABLE 1

(a) General demographics at each step of the TB Screening Program.

	Stage 1: Suspected Cases (N= 2696)		Stage 2: Needed Referral (N=1290)		Stage 3: Attended RHU (N=333)		TB Positive (N=53)	
	n	(%)	n	(%)	n	(%)	n	(%)
% of prior stage	2696/4635	58.2	1290/2696	47.8	333/1290	26	53/333	15.9
Female	1476	0.6	689	0.5	187	0.6	28	0.5
Male	1220	0.5	601	0.5	146	0.4	25	0.5
Registered in PhilHealth[1]	1420	0.5	694	0.5	172	0.5	30	0.6
	Mean	(SD)	Mean	(SD)	Mean	(SD)	Mean	(SD)
Average Age	37.7	21.4	36.5	22.4	38.2	23.2	44.9	18.5
Average Household Size	4.8	2.4	4.8	2.4	4.6	2.5	5	2.8
Average Household Income (PHP per person per day)	22.9	25.8	20.4	20.3	20.7	22.1	18.6	10.2

[1] PhilHealth is the Philippine government-owned nation health insurance program.

(b) Demographic characteristics of referred and not referred participants

Characteristic	Referred RHU (n = 1290)		Not referred (n = 1406)		P-value	Significance*
	mean	SD	mean	SD	For difference in means	
Age	36.5	22.9	27.3	23.1	<0.001	* * *
Child	5.4	4.0	5.2	3.8	0.6338	
Adult	46.6	16.5	43.5	17.2	<0.001	* * *
HH.size	4.8	2.4	4.9	2.2	0.1859	
HH.income	2649.3	2570.6	3353.6	3571.6	<0.001	* * *
	Number	Denominator	Number	Denominator	For difference in proportions	
Male	601	2116	1515	2116	<0.001	* * *
Female	689	2519	1830	2519	<0.001	* * *
Phil. health	694	4635	1865	4635	<0.001	* * *

*P value of <0.001 was considered to be statistically highly significant.

TABLE 2: TB symptoms and signs of study participants divided by those who attended RHU for TB testing and those who did not attend RHU and did not get tested for TB.

TB Symptoms & Signs	Attended RHU (N=333) n	(%)	Did Not Attend RHU (N=957) n	(%)	p-value[1]
Cough/Wheezing of 2 weeks or more	297	89.2	724	75.7	<0.001
Unexplained fever of 2 weeks or more	23	6.9	44	4.6	0.14
Significant and unintentional weight loss	32	9.6	70	7.3	0.22
Fatigue, lethargy, general malaise	21	6.3	37	3.9	0.09
Failure to respond to 2 weeks of appropriate antibiotic therapy	7	2.1	16	1.7	0.79
Failure to regain previous state of health 2 weeks after viral infection	2	0.6	16	1.7	0.24

[1] P-values calculated using Chi-sq test.

TABLE 3: Factors associated with successful attendance at a Rural Health Unit (Markov chain Monte Carlo (MCMC) generalized linear mixed-model).

Outcome: Attended RHU	Posterior mean (95% CI)	Odds Ratio (95% CI)	p-value
Fixed			
(Intercept)	0.16 (0.08, 0.22)	1.17 (1.08, 1.25)	<0.001
Cough/Wheezing of 2 weeks or more	0.08 (0.01, 0.14)	1.09 (1.01, 1.15)	0.01
Unexplained fever of 2 weeks or more	0.01 (-0.10, 0.11)	1.01 (0.91, 1.12)	0.78
Significant and unintentional weight loss	0.03 (-0.06, 0.12)	1.03 (0.94, 1.12)	0.55
Fatigue, lethargy, general malaise	0.05 (-0.06, 0.18)	1.06 (0.94, 1.20)	0.40
Failure to respond to 2 weeks of appropriate antibiotic therapy	0.14 (-0.05, 0.32)	1.14 (0.95, 1.37)	0.15
Failure to regain previous state of health 2 weeks after viral infection	-0.22 (-0.43, -0.03)	0.80 (0.65, 0.97)	0.03
Random			
σ (community)	0.05 (0.01,0.11)		
σ (base)	0.03 (0.02, 0.04)		
Deviance (DIC)			1278.30

population which included 12907 rural poor, 1625 urban poor, and 2145 indigenous people [14]. Among their TB positive participants, 53.9% reported having cough (of any duration) and 25.8% reported having cough for more than two weeks. Comparatively in our study, 85% (45 out of 53) of subjects who tested positive for TB infection presented with prolonged cough. In our study the odds ratio of a referred participant visiting a health centre for TB testing due to prolonged cough symptom was smaller than expected.

Since this ACF was designed based on the most up-to-date symptom screening guidelines of Philippines' National Tuberculosis Control Program in 2013, the primary algorithm referred those who coughed for more than two weeks to a RHU for TB testing. Though ICM staff asked about other symptoms of TB during the screening process, those without prolonged cough were not referred to the RHU for testing.

Cough for two weeks or more was also the most common symptom (79.7%) identified by those presenting any TB symptom in the 2016 survey [2]. Only 2815 (4.82%) of all the NTP 2016 survey participants presented any TB symptom, and of these participants, 2250 (80%) of them had cough for two weeks or more. Of those who were TB confirmed, 298 (64%) did not present prolonged cough, but were CXR positive.

4.3. Expected vs. Observed ACF Results. According to the WHO guidance on planning and implementation of systematic screening for active TB (online tool), not taking our population's relatively higher risk into account, utilizing an algorithm of cough for two or more weeks as the primary symptom and microscopy as the diagnostic tool, we can expect to only identify 20% of all TB cases. This would rise to approximately 38% if Xpert®MTB/RIF (Xpert) is used as the diagnostic tool instead [6].

However, the global detection rate for TB has not significantly improved even with the recent dissemination of Xpert [15]. Inequity in access and dissemination of this new technology is partly responsible, as well as the prevalence of asymptomatic and latent TB cases which has limited drastic improvements. Limitations in access are more pronounced among those who face geographical and socioeconomic barriers [16]. Despite efforts made by the Philippine Department of Health (DOH) and various international funding agencies to make Xpert readily accessible to Filipinos, the participants of this study were mostly unable to benefit from this progress.

We observed a higher prevalence of TB confirmed in the communities included in this study compared to the national rate (approximately 1%). We speculate that the high prevalence is due to our study participants experiencing extreme low-income, which is considered to be a high-risk group for TB in the Philippines. The prevalence in our study population, 53 confirmed cases out of 333 TB tested (15.8%), is substantially higher than that of the study conducted in Palawan (2.2% for rural poor and 2.1% for the urban poor) [14].

Given our study population's difficulty accessing diagnosis with an Xpert, the majority of our participants would have been diagnosed using sputum smear microscopy. This implies that we might have only detected 21% of true positive TB cases or fewer among those who were referred to a RHU for testing and were tested using sputum smear microscopy, based on the WHO's estimation on systematic screening for active TB. Other studies from high prevalence countries have shown that populations experiencing low-income are about 4.5–5.5 times or more vulnerable to TB infection [17–19]. However, with the low testing proportion in our study population, case detection numbers are low [20]. This means that if ACF was performed using Xpert, then there is a possibility that more TB cases would have been detected. Lastly, in the Philippines, HIV prevalence is low at 0.1 for adults, age 15 to 49 [21]. Perhaps this could be another reason why the testing and case detection rate is low. About 54% of Human Immunodeficiency Virus (HIV) positive Filipinos are co-managing HIV and TB [21]. We did not collect HIV/AIDS status of our participants.

5. Conclusion

Based on our study, prolonged cough was recognized as a TB symptom by those in geographically isolated, poor communities, possibly motivating these participants to get tested. Though the odds ratio was only 1.09 (95% CI 1.08, 1.25), we believe that it is still a meaningful finding from our study participants as this could be due to the low proportion of TB patients with noticeable symptoms. ACF strategies in high-risk groups need to be revised so asymptomatic patients are not inadvertently overlooked due to lack of cough. Currently, greater effort is being made to find asymptomatic TB cases by treating latent TB patients globally [22]. Since cough is already recognized as a TB symptom, health promotion activities should aim to educate the public on the high percentage of asymptomatic cases in order to encourage testing even in the absence of prolonged cough. Relying solely on cough as a symptom is precarious since this symptom is highly dependent on severity, and is subjective to each individual's tolerance level. Additionally, detection through symptom screening, prolonged cough, has low sensitivity of 0.247 [6]. Though the results from this paper cannot be generalized for the whole of Philippines, they provide a good understanding of problems that need to be addressed to detect missing TB cases among individuals experiencing low-income, in order to achieve national targets. The study was not able to understand the transmission among close contact groups with TB confirmed participants. ACF using mobile diagnostics tools, widespread screening of high-risk populations, and sputum sample transportation service are possible options for increasing efficiency of ACF in hard to reach areas.

Additional Points

Study Limitations. The authors acknowledge that more statistically significant findings could have been discovered if the study sample size was larger. Through this study we discovered that participants experiencing extreme poverty in the Philippines could be associating cough for 2 or more weeks as a symptom of TB. However, this study was not designed to answer that question and it will be followed up with a more in-depth qualitative study to understand study population's knowledge, attitudes, and practices for health seeking regarding TB.

Disclosure

The abstract of this article was presented orally at the International Health Conference at St Hugh's College, Oxford on the 29th of June 2018.

Acknowledgments

The authors thank all ICM Health Department staff for carrying out active case finding in the communities and data collection. This research received ICM internal program funding.

Supplementary Materials

Four figures and three tables have been provided under the Supplementary Materials to provide visual aid for clearer understanding of the study. Figure S1, S2, and S3 were added to show the forms used for data collection. Table S4 was added as a response to a comment by a reviewer. Table S4 shows the literacy rate of our participants. Table S5 was also added based on a reviewer's comment to show the percentage of adults and children at each stage. Figure S6 shows that having one symptom was the most common among our study participants. Table S7 was added to show univariate analysis of all TB symptoms used during TB screening of the study. *(Supplementary Materials)*

References

[1] C. Auer, J. Sarol, M. Tanner, and M. Weiss, "Health seeking and perceived causes of tuberculosis among patients in Manila, Philippines," *Tropical Medicine & International Health*, vol. 5, no. 9, pp. 648–656, 2000.

[2] World Health Organization, "Global tuberculosis report," 2017.

[3] M. I. D. Quelapio, N. R. C. Mira, R. B. Orillaza-Chi et al., "Responding to the multidrug-resistant tuberculosis crisis: Mainstreaming programmatic management to the Philippine National Tuberculosis Programme," *The International Journal of Tuberculosis and Lung Disease*, vol. 14, no. 6, pp. 751–757, 2010.

[4] N. P. Hoa, A. E. K. Thorson, N. H. Long, and V. K. Diwan, "Knowledge of Tuberculosis and Associated Health-Seeking Behaviour among Rural Vietnamese Adults with a Cough for at Least Three Weeks," *Scandinavian Journal of Public Health*, 2003.

[5] D. G. Storla, S. Yimer, and G. A. Bjune, "A systematic review of delay in the diagnosis and treatment of tuberculosis," *BMC Public Health*, vol. 8, article 15, 2008.

[6] World Health Organization, *Systematic Screening for Active Tuberculosis: Principles and Recommendations*, WHO Press, 2013.

[7] L. G. Miller, S. M. Asch, E. I. Yu, L. Knowles, L. Gelberg, and P. Davidson, "A population-based survey of tuberculosis symptoms: how atypical are atypical presentations?" *Clinical Infectious Diseases*, vol. 30, no. 2, pp. 293–299, 2000.

[8] Z. Li, S. Yang, X. Zhang, E. Fisher, B. Tian, and X. Sun, "Complex relation among Health Belief Model components in TB prevention and care," *Public Health*, vol. 129, no. 7, pp. 907–915, 2015.

[9] H. H. Tola, D. Shojaeizadeh, A. Tol et al., "Psychological and educational intervention to improve tuberculosis treatment adherence in ethiopia based on health belief model: a cluster randomized control trial," *PLoS ONE*, vol. 11, no. 5, Article ID e0155147, 2016.

[10] P. Salgame, C. Geadas, L. Collins, E. Jones-López, and J. J. Ellner, "Latent tuberculosis infection – Revisiting and revising concepts," *Tuberculosis*, vol. 95, no. 4, pp. 373–384, 2015.

[11] Department of Health - Disease Prevention and Control Bureau, "National Tuberculosis Prevalence Survey 2016. Philippines," 2018, http://ntp.doh.gov.ph/downloads/publications/NTPS2016.pdf.

[12] S. H. Chang and J. K. Cataldo, "A systematic review of global cultural variations in knowledge," in *Proceedings of the The International Journal of Tuberculosis and Lung Disease*, vol. 18, pp. 168–173, 2014, https://doi.org/10.5588/ijtld.13.0181.

[13] J. D. Hadfield, "MCMC Methods for multi-response generalized linear mixed models: The MCMCglmm R package," *Journal of Statistical Software*, vol. 33, no. 2, pp. 1–22, 2010.

[14] F. Morishita, A. M. Garfin, W. Lew et al., "Bringing state-of-the-art diagnostics to vulnerable populations: The use of a mobile screening unit in active case finding for tuberculosis in Palawan, the Philippines," *PLoS ONE*, vol. 12, no. 2, p. e0171310, 2017.

[15] H. Cox and M. P. Nicol, "Tuberculosis eradication: renewed commitment and global investment required," *The Lancet Infectious Diseases*, vol. 18, no. 3, pp. 228-229, 2018.

[16] N. Lorent, K. Choun, S. Malhotra et al., "Challenges from tuberculosis diagnosis to care in community-based active case finding among the urban poor in cambodia: a mixed-methods study," *PLoS ONE*, vol. 10, no. 7, p. e0130179, 2015.

[17] O. Oxlade and M. Murray, "Tuberculosis and poverty: why are the poor at greater risk in India?" *PLoS ONE*, vol. 7, no. 11, Article ID e47533, 2012.

[18] S. Hossain, M. A. Quaiyum, K. Zaman et al., "Socio economic position in TB prevalence and access to services: results from a population prevalence survey and a facility-based survey in Bangladesh," *PLoS ONE*, vol. 7, no. 9, Article ID e44980, 2012.

[19] D. M. Barter, S. O. Agboola, M. B. Murray, and T. Bärnighausen, "Tuberculosis and poverty: The contribution of patient costs in sub-Saharan Africa - A systematic review," *BMC Public Health*, vol. 12, no. 1, article no. 980, 2012.

[20] N. Nishikiori and F. Morishita, "Using tuberculosis surveillance data for informed programmatic decision-making," *Western Pacific surveillance and response journal : WPSAR*, vol. 4, no. 1, pp. 1–3, 2013.

[21] UNAIDS, "Country Fact Sheets," 2017, Philippines, https://www.unaids.org/en/regionscountries/countries/philippines.

[22] P. Glaziou, K. Floyd, and M. Raviglione, "Global Epidemiology of Tuberculosis," *Seminars in Respiratory and Critical Care Medicine*, vol. 39, no. 03, pp. 271–285, 2018.

12

Knowledge, Attitude and Practices on Drug-Resistant Tuberculosis Infection Control in Nepal

Sailesh Kumar Shrestha,[1] **Ratna Bahadur Bhattarai**,[2] **Lok Raj Joshi**,[2] **Nilaramba Adhikari**,[3] **Suvesh Kumar Shrestha**,[4] **Rajendra Basnet**,[2] **and Kedar Narsingh K. C.**[2]

[1]*National Academy of Medical Sciences, Bir Hospital, Kathmandu 44600, Nepal*
[2]*National Tuberculosis Control Center, Bhaktapur 44800, Nepal*
[3]*Central Department of Public Health, Institute of Medicine, Kathmandu 44600, Nepal*
[4]*Save the Children/Global Fund, Kathmandu 44600, Nepal*

Correspondence should be addressed to Sailesh Kumar Shrestha; saileshkumarshrestha@gmail.com

Academic Editor: Adwoa Asante-Poku

Drug-resistant tuberculosis (DR-TB) transmission is an important problem, particularly in low-income settings. This study is aimed at assessing the knowledge, attitude, and practices of DR-TB infection control among the healthcare workers under the National Tuberculosis Control Program in Nepal. In this cross-sectional study, we studied the healthcare workers from all the 11 functioning DR-TB treatment centers across Nepal in March 2018. Through face-to-face interviews, trained data collectors collected data on the characteristics of healthcare workers, their self-reported knowledge, attitude, and practice on DR-TB infection control. We entered the data in Microsoft Excel and analyzed in the R statistical software. We assigned a score of one to the correct response and zero to the incorrect or no response and calculated a composite score in each of the knowledge, attitude, and practice domains. We ascertained the healthcare workers as having good knowledge, appropriate attitude, and optimal practices when the composite score was ≥50%. We summarized the numerical variables with median (interquartile range (IQR)) and the categorical variables with proportions. We ran appropriate correlation tests to identify relationships between knowledge, attitude, and practice scores. We regarded a p value of <0.05 as significant. A total of 95 out of 102 healthcare workers responded. There were 46 male respondents. The median age was 33 years (IQR 26-42). Most of them (53, 55.79%) were midlevel paramedics. We found 91 (95.79%) respondents had good knowledge, 49 (51.58%) had an appropriate attitude, and 35 (36.84%) had optimal practices on DR-TB infection control. We found a statistically significant positive correlation between attitude and practice scores ($\rho = 0.37$, $p \leq 0.001$). The healthcare workers at the DR-TB treatment centers in Nepal have good knowledge of DR-TB infection control, but it did not translate into an appropriate attitude or optimal practices.

1. Background

Drug-resistant tuberculosis (DR-TB), a form of tuberculosis (TB) resistant to one or more antitubercular drugs, has emerged as a major public health challenge. Globally, in 2018 alone, there were an estimated 484000 new cases of TB caused by the bacilli resistant to Rifampicin (RR TB), out of which 78% were additionally resistant to Isoniazid (Multidrug Resistant TB (MDR-TB)). Furthermore, the bacilli infecting 6.2% of the MDR-TB cases were additionally resistant to at least a Fluoroquinolone and a second line injectable antitubercular agent (Extensively Drug-Resistant Tuberculosis (XDR-TB)). More than 90% of these cases are from 30 countries that belong to low or middle-income settings [1]. In Nepal, of the 1400 estimated cases of RR/MDR-TB, 635 cases of MDR-TB were notified to the National TB Control Program (NTP) in 2018 [2].

Until recently, the provision of effective first-line treatment was hoped to prevent the emergence of DR-TB. However, growing evidence suggests that person-to-person transmission, not just inadequate treatment, is driving the spread of DR-TB. A dynamic transmission modeling analysis using national tuberculosis notification data estimated that person-to-person transmission rather than *de novo* acquisition accounts for a median of 95.9% of all incident MDR-TB and 61.3% of incident MDR-TB in previously treated individuals [3]. In a prospective study of 404 patients with XDR-TB in South Africa, investigators combined genotyping methods with social-network and epidemiologic analysis and found that at least 69% of the cases of XDR-TB were attributable to transmission [4]. In another study on 324 patients with MDR-TB in China, investigators combined traditional genotyping, whole-genome sequencing, and epidemiological investigation and found that transmission of MDR strains accounted for 73% of cases of MDR-TB [5].

Healthcare centers represent one of the important sites where DR-TB transmission occurs, particularly in settings where the infection control measures are often poor, and the burden of TB is high [6]. A study from Moldova, a high MDR-TB burden country, evaluated 67 patients with MDR-TB being treated as in-patients and followed them up. It was found that 50 patients (74.6%) had a strain in the follow-up that was different from that of the baseline suggesting a high proportion of MDR-TB possibly transmitted during in-patient treatment [7].

Standard guidelines on TB infection control could help minimize healthcare-based DR-TB transmission and should form an indispensable part of DR-TB care. Optimal utilization and implementation of such guidelines could be facilitated by the information on the knowledge gaps, attitudes, and practices on TB infection control of the healthcare workers. However, in many resource-limited settings, TB infection control measures are absent or suboptimal. In Nepal, dedicated national policy and resources for TB infection control are lacking, and a few studies have assessed healthcare workers' knowledge, attitudes, and practices on TB infection control. A study among 190 healthcare workers from 28 TB treatment facilities in Nepal found that the overall knowledge and practices of healthcare workers on TB infection control were not satisfactory [8]. This study, however, was limited to only the urban centers, and the knowledge, attitudes, and practices questionnaire did not extend to include the issues specific to DR-TB. Such information could help in the tailored implementation of the guidelines and thus, more effective take-up of the recommendations. In this study, we aimed to assess the knowledge, attitude, and practices of DR-TB infection control among the healthcare workers under the National Tuberculosis Control Program in Nepal.

2. Materials and Methods

2.1. Study Settings and Participants. We conducted this cross-sectional study among the healthcare workers at the DR-TB treatment centers in Nepal in March 2018. DR-TB treatment in Nepal is ambulatory care provided through DR-TB treatment centers under the NTP. Depending upon the volume of patients and their geographic distributions, the NTP identifies different health centers across the country to introduce the DR-TB treatment services. After orientation training of the healthcare workers on DR-TB care and the provision of required logistics, these centers then start functioning as the DR-TB treatment centers. They evaluate the presumptive cases of DR-TB in close collaboration with the national TB reference laboratories, provide the DR-TB treatment to the diagnosed patients, and monitor them as per the national guidelines. All the patients diagnosed with DR-TB are enrolled at one of these centers. There were 18 DR-TB treatment centers across the country during the data collection period, of which we included 11 centers that had patients enrolled and were receiving treatment. There were 102 healthcare workers involved in the care of the patients with DR-TB at these 11 centers, and we included all of them in our study.

2.2. Data Collection. In a one-day training session, we trained six paramedics on the details of selecting study participants, the process of obtaining informed consent, and data collection using the structured data collection tool. Because no standardized data collection instrument was available to evaluate the knowledge, attitude, and practice in patients with DR-TB, we developed a tool based on earlier studies [9, 10]. We pretested the tool for any problems in understanding or interpreting the questionnaire and incorporated the feedback in the final version. The pretesting was done in 10 healthcare workers at the TB clinic of the National TB Control Center who did not form a part of the actual study sample in the data collection process of our study. The data collection tool consisted of four parts. The first part collected information on the study participants' demographic and other characteristics related to the delivery of DR-TB services (current position at work, work experience in general and specific to DR-TB care, training received on TB infection control, and whether the study participants had encountered colleagues with TB or DR-TB). The midlevel paramedics referred to the health workers working as community health workers or health assistants and required vocational education at upper secondary or postsecondary, nontertiary levels. However, their actual educational qualification, as entered separately in the variable–education, may be of higher level. We classified the education level according to the International Standard Classification of Education [11]. The second part contained a questionnaire on the knowledge which collected information on the study participants' knowledge on the risk of getting infected with DR-TB and the administrative, environmental, and personal protective measures of TB infection control. The responses were recorded as true, false, and do not know. The third part contained a questionnaire on attitude which collected information on the study participants' attitude towards DR-TB and measures of TB infection control. The responses were recorded as agree, disagree, and no comments. The fourth part contained questions on the study participants' self-reported practices on infection control measures while encountering the patients with DR-TB. The responses were recorded as yes, no, and do not know.

2.3. Data Analysis. We entered the data in Microsoft Excel (Office 365, Microsoft Corporation, Washington, United States) and analyzed in the R statistical software (R Core Team (2020). R: A language and environment for statistical computing. R Foundation for Statistical Computing, Vienna, Austria. https://www.R-project.org/). We summarized the numerical variables with median and interquartile range (IQR) and the categorical variables with proportions. We assigned a score of one to the correct response and zero to the incorrect or no response and calculated a composite score in each of the knowledge, attitude, and practice domains. We ascertained the healthcare workers as having good knowledge, appropriate attitude, and optimal practices when the composite score in each of the domains was at least 50%. We ran appropriate correlation tests to identify relationships between knowledge, attitude, and practice scores. A p value of <0.05 was considered significant.

2.4. Ethical Considerations. We obtained ethical approval for the study from Nepal Health Research Council (registration number 109/2018, approval reference number 2328/2018). The trained data collectors obtained written informed consent from the participants for participation in the study.

3. Results

Of the 102 healthcare workers from 11 DR-TB treatment centers, 95 participated in the study (response rate—93.1%). Altogether, there were 14 missing values across five variables. We assumed that the missing values were missing completely at random and analyzed the remaining data with complete case analysis. The median age was 33 (IQR 26-42) years, and there were 49 (51.58%) female respondents. Most of them (53, 55.96%) were midlevel paramedics, and 44 (46.32%) study participants had received postsecondary nontertiary vocational education (Table 1).

The median work experience was 10 (IQR 3–18) years and that in DR TB was 2 (IQR 1–6) years. Eighty-eight (92.63%) study participants were providing health services to the patients in addition to the patients with DR-TB. Seventy-five (78.95%) study participants reported to have encountered colleagues with TB, and 38 participants (40.00%) reported to have encountered colleagues with DR-TB. The majority (71, 74.74%) of the study participants reported that they had received training on DR-TB infection control.

The majority of the study participants responded correctly to the knowledge questions except for the questions on administrative control measures and use of surgical masks by the patients—close to a third of the study participants failed to appreciate the administrative control and use of surgical masks by the DR-TB patients as the crucial measures of TB infection control (Table 2). Yet, a large proportion of healthcare workers (91, 95.79%) were found to have a good knowledge of DR-TB infection control with the median knowledge score of 14 (IQR 12-14) (Figures 1 and 2).

Just over half of our study participants (49, 51.58%) were found to have an appropriate attitude on DR-TB infection control with a median attitude score of 5 (IQR 4-6) (Figures 1 and 2). More than half of the study participants did not think they needed to use N95 respirators while taking care of DR-TB patients, and close to half of the study participants undermined the role of administrative and environmental infection control measures in DR-TB infection control (Table 3). Many study participants thought that their workplaces neither had adequate resources for DR-TB infection control nor were concerned over the risk of DR-TB transmission to the healthcare workers. Over one-third of the study participants felt that DR-TB cannot be cured, and taking infection control precautions will offer a little help to the healthcare workers since they may have already been infected with DR-TB. However, most of them believed that they had been well trained in TB infection control and showed interest in getting tested for TB periodically.

Overall, only over a third of our study participants (35, 36.84%) were found to have optimal practices of DR-TB infection control with the median practice score of 5 (IQR 4-7) (Figures 1 and 2). Around a third of study participants reported poor practices on administrative measures of infection control, the lack of infection control program along with an infection control committee or a focal person in their

Table 1: Characteristics of study participants.

Characteristics	Frequency (n)	Percentage (%)
Age groups		
16-30 years	42	44.21
31-45 years	39	41.05
46-60 years	14	14.74
Sex		
Female	49	51.58
Male	46	48.42
Education		
Postsecondary, nontertiary, vocational education	44	46.32
Bachelors	28	29.47
Upper secondary vocational	13	13.68
Masters	10	10.53
Position		
Midlevel paramedic	53	55.79
Laboratory personnel	17	17.89
Nurse	13	13.68
Program manager	6	6.32
Doctor	3	3.16
Radiographer	3	3.16
Health facility type		
Government	55	57.89
Nongovernment	40	42.11
Work experience as a healthcare worker		
1-10 years	50	53.76
11-20 years	26	27.96
21-30 years	13	13.98
31-40 years	4	4.30
Work experience in drug-resistant tuberculosis		
5 years or less	64	73.56
6-10 years	11	12.64
11-20 years	12	13.79

Table 2: Knowledge questions on drug-resistant tuberculosis infection control and the responses from the study participants.

Knowledge questions	True		False		Do not know		Total responses
	n	%	*n*	%	*n*	%	
Drug-resistant tuberculosis is an infectious disease.	85	91%	—	—	8	9%	93
Drug-resistant tuberculosis is more infectious than drug-sensitive tuberculosis.	76	80%	10	11%	9	9%	95
Healthcare workers have a higher risk of acquiring tuberculosis than the general population.	89	94%	5	5%	1	1%	95
The risk of tuberculosis to healthcare workers can be minimized by observing appropriate infection control measures.	83	87%	5	5%	7	7%	95
Healthcare facilities should implement an infection control program.	88	94%	5	5%	1	1%	94
Administrative measures are the most effective tuberculosis infection control measures.	57	60%	28	29%	10	11%	95
The actively coughing patients should be identified, and prompt care should be provided to minimize the time spent at healthcare facilities.	87	92%	—	—	8	8%	95
The actively coughing patients should be encouraged to cover their mouth and nose while coughing or sneezing.	87	92%	—	—	8	8%	95
Patients with tuberculosis and their close contacts should be educated on the measures of tuberculosis infection prevention.	86	91%	1	1%	8	8%	95
The waiting area and sputum collection area should be in an open and well-ventilated space.	85	89%	10	11%	—	—	95
The health facility should be renovated in such a way that patient consultation rooms and laboratories are well ventilated.	84	88%	3	3%	8	8%	95
The use of mechanical ventilation and ultraviolet gamma irradiation in health facilities helps to minimize tuberculosis transmission.	86	91%	—	—	9	9%	95
Surgical masks are as good as N95 masks in preventing tuberculosis transmission.	22	23%	70	74%	3	3%	95
Healthcare workers should wear N95 masks.	92	97%	3	3%	—	—	95
Patients should wear surgical masks.	64	67%	29	31%	2	2%	95
Healthcare workers should be screened for tuberculosis periodically.	89	94%	4	4%	2	2%	95

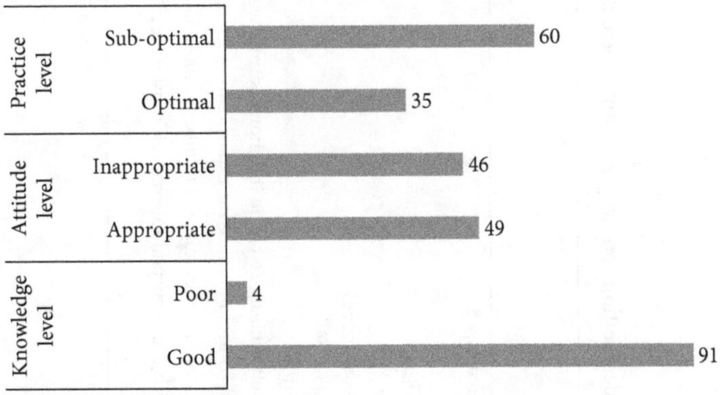

Figure 1: Number of study participants with the knowledge, attitude, and practice levels.

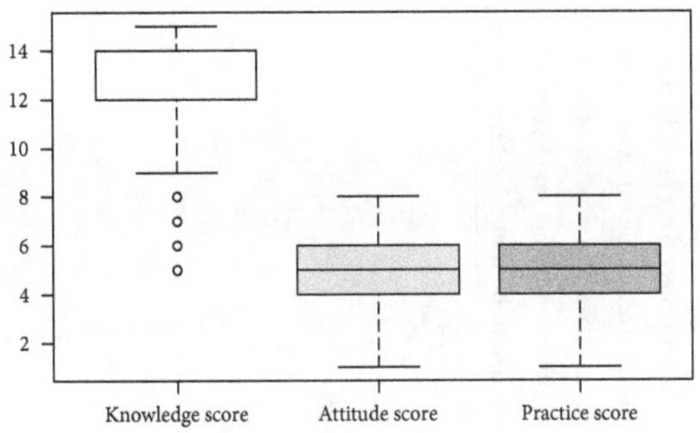

Figure 2: Boxplot of total knowledge, attitude, and practice scores.

workplace, the lack of triaging actively coughing patients to expedite the care they receive in the workplace, and the lack of an appropriate area for sputum collection (Table 4). The resources available for infection control were reportedly inadequate as well. Nearly half of the study participants reported that the ventilation in the patient consultation rooms and laboratories was suboptimal, and exhaust ventilation and ultraviolet radiation were almost nonexistent. Though a significant proportion of study participants reported that they encouraged patients to use surgical masks, less than a quarter of them used N95 respirators themselves when caring for the patients with DR-TB.

Table 3: Attitude questions on drug-resistant tuberculosis infection control and the responses from the study participants.

Attitude questions	Agree		Disagree		No comments		Total responses
	n	%	*n*	%	*n*	%	
I am worried that I may contract drug-resistant tuberculosis.	18	19%	28	29%	49	52%	95
Drug-resistant tuberculosis cannot be cured.	32	34%	60	63%	3	3%	95
My workplace is concerned about the risk of drug-resistant tuberculosis transmission to its staff.	45	47%	40	42%	10	11%	95
My workplace has provisioned adequate resources to minimize the risk of drug-resistant tuberculosis transmission to its staff.	32	34%	59	62%	4	4%	95
I have been well trained in tuberculosis infection control.	50	53%	36	38%	9	9%	95
Healthcare workers have already been infected with tuberculosis, so taking infection control measures will not help.	37	39%	57	60%	1	1%	95
The administrative measures of tuberculosis infection control minimize the exposure to tubercular bacilli.	46	48%	45	47%	4	4%	95
The environmental measures of tuberculosis infection control minimize the number of tubercular bacilli in the environment.	42	45%	44	47%	8	9%	94
The healthcare workers taking care of the patients with drug-resistant tuberculosis must wear N95 masks.	39	41%	56	59%	—	—	95
I would like to be tested for tuberculosis periodically.	56	59%	39	41%	—	—	95

TABLE 4: Practice questions on drug-resistant tuberculosis infection control and the responses from the study participants.

Practice questions	Yes		No		Do not know		Total responses
	n	%	*n*	%	*n*	%	
My workplace has a tuberculosis infection control committee.	36	38%	37	39%	22	23%	95
There is a tuberculosis infection control focal person ascertained in my workplace.	42	44%	32	34%	21	22%	95
There is a tuberculosis infection control program implemented in my workplace.	59	62%	26	27%	10	11%	95
Adequate resources have been allocated for tuberculosis infection control in my workplace.	50	53%	38	40%	7	7%	95
Healthcare workers have been tested for latent tuberculosis infection.	31	33%	50	53%	14	15%	95
The actively coughing patients are identified and provided prompt care to minimize the time spent in my workplace.	61	64%	31	33%	3	3%	95
A separate and open area has been designated as a sputum collection area in my workplace.	55	58%	35	37%	5	5%	95
There are signs of cough etiquette displayed in my workplace.	37	39%	56	59%	2	2%	95
The patient consultation rooms and laboratory in my workplace are well ventilated.	52	55%	41	43%	2	2%	95
There is exhaust ventilation available in my workplace.	—	—	87	92%	8	8%	95
There is ultraviolet irradiation available in my workplace.	—	—	91	96%	4	4%	95
I use an N95 mask most of the time.	22	23%	73	77%	—	—	95
I encourage patients to use surgical masks.	85	89%	10	11%	—	—	95

All the three variable scores (knowledge, attitude, and practice) were not normally distributed, and therefore, we ran Spearman's rank correlations. We found a significant positive correlation between attitude score and practice score ($\rho = 0.37, p \leq 0.001$) but not between knowledge and attitude scores ($\rho = -0.09$, $p = 0.38$) nor between knowledge and practice scores ($\rho = -0.18, p = 0.079$).

4. Discussion

This study is aimed at assessing the knowledge, attitude, and practices of DR-TB infection control among the healthcare workers under the NTP in Nepal and is the first such study in Nepal to be conducted nationwide. We found that most of the study participants had a good knowledge of DR-TB infection control. However, the knowledge score did not correlate with the attitude or practice scores. Only half of the healthcare workers studied had an appropriate attitude, and just over a third had optimal practices on DR-TB infection control. However, attitude score significantly correlated with the practice score.

The NTP in Nepal has been gradually expanding its DR-TB treatment services across the country based on the number of patients reported, their geographic distributions, and available resources. Before introducing the DR-TB treatment services in any health facility, the NTP conducts a five-day-long orientation training on DR-TB care to all the healthcare workers involved. Thereafter, once every three to five years, a three-day-long refresher training is provided as a part of the continuing professional development program. Each of these training programs includes a session on infection control and is, so far, the only formal DR-TB infection control training session available within Nepal NTP. Most of the study participants reported that they had received training on TB infection control. And with the median work experience in DR-TB care of 2 years, most of the study participants had received this training quite recently. These training sessions might have led to a good knowledge of TB infection control in our study participants. In addition, the educational qualification of the study participants could have also contributed to the higher knowledge of DR-TB infection control.

The knowledge scores on DR-TB infection control reported in the earlier studies vary widely. In a national survey of 24 DR-TB facilities involving 499 healthcare workers in South Africa, the average number of correct responses was 3.1 out of 10 knowledge questions [10]. In another study on 377 healthcare workers from two regional referral hospitals in Ethiopia, it was found that the mean knowledge score was seven out of the total possible knowledge score of 10 [12]. Such variation in the knowledge levels reflects the variation in the study settings, including whether the healthcare workers studied were from DR-TB specific facilities as well as the study population, including their educational qualifications, training on TB infection control, and work experience. In both these studies, however, a higher level of clinical training and attending infection control training was associated with significantly higher knowledge scores [10, 12]. Though not conducted on the healthcare workers working exclusively on DR-TB facilities, an earlier study from Nepal has also reported a significant association of education level and training on TB with the respondents having a good knowledge of TB infection control [8]. These findings underscore the importance of training opportunities for the healthcare workers in TB infection control, including engaging the healthcare workers in short-term refresher training and encouraging continuous learning. Such training sessions in the future should reinforce the importance of administrative control as a key strategy for DR-TB infection control. Also, it should be emphasized that the use of surgical masks by the patients is an important measure for source control leading to a fewer number of tubercular bacilli being released into the surrounding.

Our finding that close to half of the study participants had an inappropriate attitude on DR-TB infection control including in the key areas like the role of administrative and environmental infection control measures in DR-TB infection control and the use of N95 respirators by healthcare workers while taking care of DR-TB patients is concerning. These issues put the healthcare workers at an increased risk of acquiring DR-TB infection themselves. Reported attitudes on DR-TB infection control vary between the different studies. In the study in South Africa, nearly one-third of participating healthcare workers from DR-TB facilities reported not using N95 respirators during patient care [10]. On the other hand, almost all the study participants from an earlier study in Nepal agreed that they should wear respirators while caring for TB patients. A higher proportion of them seemed to be concerned about getting infected with TB in comparison to our study participants (Table 3) [8]. Various factors help shape such attitudes on infection control including the educational qualification, whether they have received training specific to TB infection control, and the level of knowledge on infection control [8, 10].

Fewer healthcare workers in our study had optimal practices of DR-TB infection control, particularly on their practices on administrative infection control measures and the use of N95 respirators while caring for the patients with DR-TB. In the earlier studies, the use of N95 respirators during the care of the patients with TB varied from 10% to 39.7% likely reflecting the underlying differences in the study population and their educational qualification as well as the training on TB infection control [8, 10, 12]. While the provision of adequate resources for infection control, including exhaust ventilation and ultraviolet radiation, should be a goal as well, it is the implementation and adherence to relatively cheaper yet more effective measures such as triage of actively coughing patients, reinforcing cough etiquette and a separate well ventilated sputum collection area that should take the precedence.

In our study, a higher score on attitude was associated with a higher score on TB infection control practices, but a higher knowledge score was not associated with higher attitude or practice scores. These findings suggest that good knowledge, though a prerequisite, does not necessarily translate into an appropriate attitude or optimal practices of healthcare workers on DR-TB infection control. The existing training by the NTP has helped the study participants attain a good knowledge on TB infection control, but it has had a little positive impact on the attitude and practices among them. Similar observations have been reported in earlier studies as well. A review on the role of education in infection prevention and control found that while training may improve knowledge, it does not always effectively or sustainably change practice [13]. A systematic review on the barriers and facilitators of tuberculosis infection prevention and control in low- and middle-income countries has also failed to find robust evidence that education improves practice and reduces infection rates in the long run [14]. Two important considerations apply in our study—the current NTP training focuses on the clinical management of the patients with DR-TB failing to highlight the issues on DR-TB infection control and consists of didactic lectures failing to highlight the much needed practical aspects. Training programs that are specifically designed and tailored to educate the healthcare workers on DR-TB infection control need to be implemented that could help build up more appropriate attitudes and improve the DR-TB infection control practices. The need for training sessions specific to TB infection control was also recognized by the earlier study from Nepal [8]. These training programs should help the health workers obtain the skills necessary for optimal infection control practices, for example, the appropriate use of N95 respirators. Besides, the way the NTP delivers the TB infection control training sessions needs to be redesigned as well. We recommend that Nepal NTP take a different approach, for example, using strategies like behavior change communication. This approach is different from the traditional approach of providing information and expecting this to result in changed behavior. Rather, it envisions communications as a horizontal process so that both senders and receivers of the information can take on interchangeable roles through focus group discussions and other methods to reach a mutual understanding and collective decision-making. At least a proportion of health workers, particularly those with good knowledge, could also be motivated to adhere to the TB infection control guidelines with the provision of regular supervision and of penalties/loss of benefits or of rewards depending on whether or not they adhere to the TB infection control recommendations. A study from Russia, which has found loss of benefit payments as an important motivator affecting the TB infection control practices among Russian health workers, supports this hypothesis [15]. This should be reinforced with other measures including ensuring the availability of necessary resources, for example, N95 respirators, creating a supportive environment during supervision visits and interventions to help minimize the stigma surrounding DR-TB. Collectively, these approaches constitute behavior change interventions that are found to be effective to change the practice of health workers to bring about sustained behavioral changes [16].

Our study has some limitations. The questionnaire used in this study has not been assessed for reliability and validity thus limiting the scope of the inferences and conclusions made based on the responses obtained. Besides, the respondents on whom we pretested the study questionnaire belonged to a single center which may not have adequately captured the variation across the study population. Due to time and resource constraints, we recorded TB infection control practices that were self-reported by the study participants and not observed by the data collectors or the investigators. These self-reported practices could differ from actual practices [10]. Therefore, for future studies, we recommend that infection control practices be directly observed by the data collectors and/or investigators. We did not assess the factors that could predict the good knowledge, appropriate attitude, or optimal practices on DR-TB infection control. We recommend that in subsequent studies, such factors and their impact be studied as well, which could help focus the interventions on the key issues on DR-TB infection control.

5. Conclusion

This study has shown that the healthcare workers at the DR-TB treatment facilities in Nepal have good knowledge of DR-

TB infection control. However, it did not translate into the appropriate attitude or optimal practices. This suggests the need to adopt focused TB infection control training for healthcare workers using strategies like behavior change communication, along with several other behavioral change interventions that could bring about positive changes in their attitude and practices.

Disclosure

The funding agency had no role in the study design; collection, management, analysis, and interpretation of data; writing of the manuscript; and the decision to submit the manuscript for publication.

Acknowledgments

This study was supported by the National TB Control Program, Nepal, through Save the Children, Nepal.

References

[1] *Global Tuberculosis Report*, World Health Organization, Geneva, 2019.

[2] *National Tuberculosis Program Annual Report 2018/2019*, National Tuberculosis Control Center, Bhaktapur, Nepal, 2019.

[3] E. A. Kendall, M. O. Fofana, and D. W. Dowdy, "Burden of transmitted multidrug resistance in epidemics of tuberculosis: a transmission modelling analysis," *The Lancet Respiratory Medicine*, vol. 3, no. 12, pp. 963–972, 2015.

[4] N. S. Shah, S. C. Auld, J. C. Brust et al., "Transmission of extensively drug-resistant tuberculosis in South Africa," *The New England Journal of Medicine*, vol. 376, no. 3, pp. 243–253, 2017.

[5] C. Yang, T. Luo, X. Shen et al., "Transmission of multidrug-resistant Mycobacterium tuberculosis in Shanghai, China: a retrospective observational study using whole-genome sequencing and epidemiological investigation," *The Lancet Infectious Diseases*, vol. 17, no. 3, pp. 275–284, 2017.

[6] N. R. Gandhi, D. Weissman, P. Moodley et al., "Nosocomial transmission of extensively drug-resistant tuberculosis in a rural hospital in South Africa," *The Journal of Infectious Diseases*, vol. 207, no. 1, pp. 9–17, 2013.

[7] V. Crudu, M. Merker, C. Lange et al., "Nosocomial transmission of multidrug-resistant tuberculosis," *The International Journal of Tuberculosis and Lung Disease*, vol. 19, no. 12, pp. 1520–1523, 2015.

[8] A. Shrestha, D. Bhattarai, B. Thapa, P. Basel, and R. R. Wagle, "Health care workers' knowledge, attitudes and practices on tuberculosis infection control, Nepal," *BMC Infectious Diseases*, vol. 17, no. 1, p. 724, 2017.

[9] Y. Waheed, M. A. Khan, R. Fatima et al., "Infection control in hospitals managing drug-resistant tuberculosis in Pakistan: how are we doing?," *Public Health Action*, vol. 7, no. 1, pp. 26–31, 2017.

[10] J. E. Farley, C. Tudor, M. Mphahlele et al., "A national infection control evaluation of drug-resistant tuberculosis hospitals in South Africa," *The International Journal of Tuberculosis and Lung Disease*, vol. 16, no. 1, pp. 82–89, 2012.

[11] *International Standard Classification of Education*, United Nations Educational, Scientific and Cultural Organization, Institute for Statistics, Canada, 2011.

[12] K. A. Alene, A. A. Adane, S. Yifiru, B. D. Bitew, A. Adane, and D. N. Koye, "Knowledge and practice of health workers about control and prevention of multidrug-resistant tuberculosis in referral hospitals, Ethiopia: a cross-sectional study," *BMJ Open*, vol. 9, no. 2, article e022948, 2019.

[13] D. J. Ward, "The role of education in the prevention and control of infection: a review of the literature," *Nurse Education Today*, vol. 31, no. 1, pp. 9–17, 2011.

[14] C. Tan, I. I. Kallon, C. J. Colvin, and A. D. Grant, "Barriers and facilitators of tuberculosis infection prevention and control in low- and middle-income countries from the perspective of healthcare workers: a systematic review," *PLoS One*, vol. 15, no. 10, article e0241039, 2020.

[15] W. Woith, G. Volchenkov, and J. Larson, "Barriers and motivators affecting tuberculosis infection control practices of Russian health care workers," *The International Journal of Tuberculosis and Lung Disease*, vol. 16, no. 8, pp. 1092–1096, 2012.

[16] B. F. Chauhan, M. M. Jeyaraman, A. S. Mann et al., "Behavior change interventions and policies influencing primary healthcare professionals' practice-an overview of reviews," *Implementation Science*, vol. 12, no. 1, p. 3, 2017.

13

Tuberculosis Case Finding Cascade and Treatment Outcomes among Male Inmates in Two Prisons in Zimbabwe

Alois Mandizvidza,[1] Riitta A. Dlodlo,[2] Palanivel Chinnakali,[3] Hamufare Dumisani Mugauri,[4] Freeman Dube,[5] Evidence Gaka,[1] Joseph Nembaware,[1] Shepherd Nyambi,[1] Blessing Masunungure,[1] and Davison Garauzive[1]

[1]*Harare Central Prison, Zimbabwe Prison and Correctional Service, Harare, Zimbabwe*
[2]*International Union against Tuberculosis and Lung Disease (The Union), Paris, France*
[3]*Departments of Preventive and Social Medicine, Jawaharlal Institute of Postgraduate Medical Education & Research (JIPMER), Puducherry, India*
[4]*AIDS and TB Unit, Ministry of Health and Child Care, Harare, Zimbabwe*
[5]*National Aids Council (NAC), Harare, Zimbabwe*

Correspondence should be addressed to Alois Mandizvidza; mandizvidzaalois@gmail.com

Academic Editor: Vincent Jarlier

Setting. Zimbabwe is a high tuberculosis (TB) burden country, with an estimated prevalence of 344/100,000 population. Though prisons are known high-prevalence sites for TB, the paucity of data affects the quantification of the disease and treatment outcomes in these settings. We measured the prevalence of TB disease and treatment outcomes among inmates at two major prisons in Harare, Zimbabwe. *Design.* A cohort study using programmatic data was undertaken to assess TB diagnostic cascade in one of the study prisons for 2018. Treatment outcomes among male inmates with TB were assessed over a period of four years, in two study prisons. *Results.* A total of 405 (11%) inmates with presumptive TB were identified, and 370 (91%) of these were evaluated for TB, mostly using rapid molecular testing of sputum specimens. Twenty-five inmates were diagnosed with TB resulting in a prevalence of 649/100,000 population. Of these, 16 (64%) were started on treatment. Nine (36%) were lost to follow-up before treatment initiation. From 2015 to 2018, 280 adult male inmates with TB were started on treatment. Of these, 212 (76%) had pulmonary disease that was bacteriologically confirmed. Almost all (276/280, 99%) had known HIV status, 65% were HIV-infected, and 80% of these were on antiretroviral treatment. The TB treatment success rate (cured or treatment completed) was recorded for 209 (75%) inmates, whilst 14 (5%) died and 11 (4%) were lost to follow-up. The frequency of unfavourable treatment outcomes (death, lost to follow-up, and not evaluated) was higher (54%) among inmates ≥ 60 years than those in the age group of 45-59 years (17%). *Conclusion.* The findings revealed a threefold burden of TB in prisons, compared with what is reported by national survey. To decrease transmission of TB bacilli, it is essential to promote efforts that address missed opportunities in the TB diagnostic cascade, prompt treatment initiation, and ensure that tracking and documentation of treatment outcomes for all inmates are intensified.

1. Introduction

Worldwide prisons are recognised as major congregate institutions with an extraordinarily high burden of tuberculosis (TB), including multidrug-resistant TB, and inadequate resources for health and TB services [1]. It has been estimated that TB in prisons may reach levels that are up to 100 times higher than those among civilian populations. In selected countries, prison populations may account for 25% of national TB burden [2]. Late diagnosis, inadequate treatment, overcrowding, poor ventilation, and repeated prison transfers contribute to rampant transmission of TB bacilli.

Also, HIV infection, malnutrition, alcohol and substance abuse, and other comorbidities are common among inmates and contribute to development of active TB disease [2].

Studies suggest that 50% of inmates with TB may remain undiagnosed and therefore untreated and not notified, creating a source for continuous transmission [3]. Modest TB treatment success of 66% and high proportions of inmates who are lost to follow-up have been reported [4]. Effective TB activities in prisons protect inmates, prison staff, visitors, and community at large [2]. End TB Strategy recognises the need for strengthening TB care and prevention in prisons to attain its ambitious targets [5].

Since the 1990s, Zimbabwe has been devastated by an HIV-associated TB epidemic. In 2017, the estimated TB prevalence was 344 per 100,000 population with an estimated HIV prevalence of 63% among TB patients [6]. A study carried out in 2015-2016 in 24 prisons in the country in a sample of 691 inmates found presumptive TB in 112 (16%) persons who were investigated, and four were found to have TB resulting in TB prevalence of 575/100,000 population [7]. To our knowledge, no studies of TB treatment outcomes among prison inmates in the country have been performed.

This study is aimed at assessing the TB case finding cascade in Harare Central Prison and the programmatic treatment outcomes among inmates in Harare Central Prison and Chikurubi Maximum Prison. The first objective included assessment, among male inmates at admission to Harare Central Prison, to determine the number and proportion of (i) presumptive TB, (ii) presumptive TB evaluated, (iii) bacteriologically confirmed and clinically diagnosed TB, and (iv) initiated on TB treatment. The second objective was to describe, among inmates with TB and initiated on treatment at Harare Central and Chikurubi Maximum Prisons, (i) treatment outcomes and (ii) sociodemographic and disease characteristics associated with unfavourable outcomes.

1.1. Setting

1.1.1. General Setting. Zimbabwe is one of the southern African countries experiencing an HIV-associated TB epidemic with an estimated prevalence of 344/100,000 population [6].

1.2. Background

1.2.1. Zimbabwe Prisons and Correctional Service. The Zimbabwe Prisons and Correctional Service (ZPCS) has a total of 46 established and 24 satellite prisons with an official holding capacity of approximately 17,000 inmates. Most prisons were built several decades ago and have not benefited from renovations resulting in dilapidated buildings with poor ventilation. The prisons are overcrowded, and some of them hold double the number of inmates compared to their recommended maximum holding capacity.

ZPCS has a health directorate responsible for health care services for inmates and staff. There are forty-six established clinics and four prison hospitals staffed by nurses, doctors, and other health professionals. TB diagnostic services are available at Chikurubi Maximum (Harare) and Khami Maximum (Bulawayo) Prison hospitals. One 4-modular XpertMTB/RIF® (Cepheid, Sunnyvale, CA, USA) platform is situated in the laboratory of Chikurubi Maximum Prison where specimens from prisons in Harare are processed. TB treatment is available in all prison clinics. All sputum smear microscopy examinations are done at the National Microbiology Reference Laboratory (NMRL).

1.2.2. Study Sites. Chikurubi Maximum and Harare Central Prisons are among the largest prisons in the country with inmate capacities of 2500 and 2042, respectively. Their health facilities include 30- and 28-bedded hospitals in Chikurubi and Harare Central Prisons, respectively. In the former, there is a laboratory and a radiology facility. Both prison hospitals have an outpatient department attending to 20-40 people a day and a clinic for HIV care. The health staff consists of two medical officers, one clinical officer, 125 nurses, and support staff that include pharmacy, nutrition, dental, laboratory, and rehabilitation officers.

Upon admission to prison, convicted individuals undergo a general medical examination that includes a TB symptom screen that is also undertaken when inmates develop symptoms suggestive of TB during their stay. It includes cough of any duration, weight loss, fever, night sweats, and haemoptysis in the last 12 months and neck swellings. A person with any one of these symptoms is considered a person with presumptive TB and evaluated with the following: sputum examination using XpertMTB/RIF® test and/or chest radiography. All persons with presumptive TB are also offered HIV counselling and testing. They are registered in the presumptive TB register, and the investigation results are documented. Upon diagnosis of TB (bacteriologically confirmed or clinically diagnosed, including extrapulmonary disease), inmates are isolated and started on treatment consisting of six months of isoniazid and rifampicin and, during the initial 2-month intensive phase, of pyrazinamide and ethambutol. This treatment is given daily with support by clinic nurses who administer the fixed-dose combination medication.

The patients are notified to the local health authorities. Monitoring of TB treatment response and recording and reporting follow the national guidelines [8]. If the inmate with TB is released before completion of TB treatment, the relevant local authority is informed through a telephone call so that treatment can be continued at the health facility closest to the person's residence. The NTP transfer out form is also filled in [9]. TB focal nurses and environmental health technicians stationed at the prisons register inmates found to have TB in the TB treatment register and maintain the details of treatment, including the treatment outcomes, in this register following the standardised definitions as listed in the national TB manual [9].

2. Methods

2.1. Study Design. This was a retrospective cohort study using routinely available data on TB services provided by the prison health services.

2.2. Study Population. We included men aged 18 years and above admitted to Harare Central Prison from 1 January

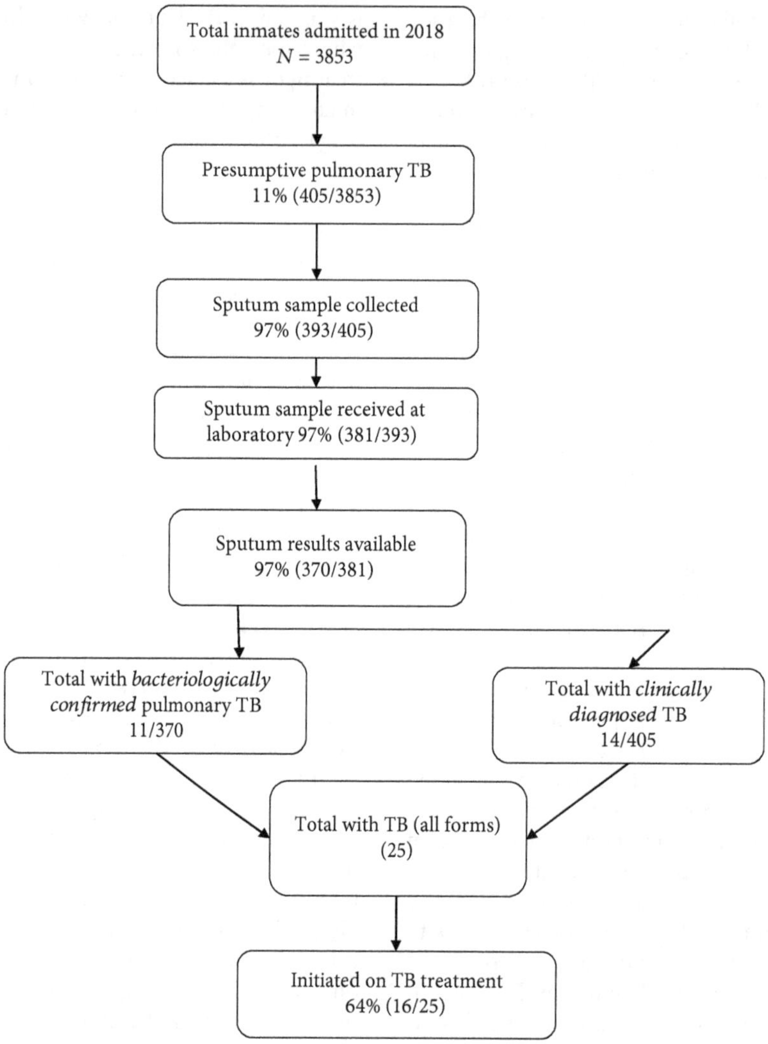

FIGURE 1: Flow chart describing the number of adult inmates admitted and evaluated for tuberculosis in Harare Central Prison, Zimbabwe, 2018.

2018 to 31 December 2018 for assessing the diagnostic cascade. For evaluating treatment outcomes, we included male inmates aged 18 years and above with drug-susceptible TB and started on TB treatment at Harare Central and Chikurubi Maximum Prisons from 1 January 2015 to 31 December 2018.

2.3. Data Variables, Sources of Data, and Data Extraction. For assessment of TB case finding cascade, information on people with presumptive TB, people with their sputum specimens collected, sent to the laboratory, and with results received, and HIV status were extracted from the presumptive TB register. Laboratory registers were used to record, register, and track specimens received as well tracking of sputum results. We obtained the total number of individuals admitted to the prison from the admission register. Data on the number of people with TB by year, their characteristics, type of TB, and TB treatment outcomes were extracted from TB treatment registers.

2.4. Analysis and Statistics. The data were entered using EpiInfo™ software (7.2.3.1, CDC, Atlanta, GA, USA), and analyses were performed in Stata software (version 22.0, Stata Corp LLC, College Station, TX, USA). A descriptive analysis was performed using frequencies and proportions. TB treatment outcomes were described as proportions with 95% CI and categorised into favourable outcomes (cured, completed treatment, and treatment success as combined) and unfavourable outcomes (died, lost to follow-up, failed treatment, and not evaluated). Association of age, residence, site (Harare/Chikurubi), and clinical characteristics (type of TB, site of TB, and HIV status) with unfavourable outcomes was assessed using the chi-squared test and unadjusted relative risk. Multivariable regression analysis (log-binomial model) was done to assess the independent effects of exposure variables on treatment outcomes. All the exposure variables were included in the model. Levels of significance were set at 5%.

2.5. Ethics Approval. The study protocol was reviewed and approved by the Medical Research Council of Zimbabwe (MRCZ/E/252) and The Union Ethics Advisory Group, Paris, France (42/19). The prisons' management gave permission for the access and review of the records of the inmates with presumptive and diagnosed TB.

3. Results

In 2018, a total of 3853 inmates were admitted to Harare Central Prison. Of these, 405 (11%) screened positive for TB symptoms and were registered in the presumptive TB register (Figure 1). A total of 313 (77%) people with presumptive TB were aged 25-44 years and 154 (38%) were HIV-infected (not shown). A total of 370 (91%, 370/405) people with presumptive disease completed TB evaluation, and all but one had a sputum XpertMTB/RIF test. Ten people had *Mycobacterium tuberculosis* detected on XpertMTB/RIF (all rifampicin-susceptible), and one person was diagnosed through sputum microscopy resulting in a positivity rate of 3% (11/370) and a notification rate of 285 cases of bacteriologically confirmed pulmonary TB/100,000 population. In addition, there were 14 clinically diagnosed TB, including one person with extrapulmonary TB. It followed that the TB (all forms) notification rate was 649/100,000 population. Sixteen (64%, 16/25) people were started on TB treatment. The remaining nine (36%, 9/25) could have been transferred or released before commencement on treatment.

From 2015 to 2018, a total of 280 adult male inmates admitted to Harare Central Prison and Chikurubi Maximum Prison were initiated on TB treatment. The median (interquartile range) age was 35 (30-42) years. Their characteristics are presented in Table 1. Two hundred and twelve (75%) were reported to have pulmonary disease, and 121 (43%) had bacteriologically confirmed TB. HIV status was unknown for four (1.4%) of these individuals. Of those with known HIV status, 65% (180/276) were HIV-positive, and of these, 144 (80%, 144/180) were reported to be on antiretroviral treatment.

The TB treatment success rate (cured or treatment completed) was recorded for 209 (75%, 95% CI 69%-80%) individuals. The outcome "not evaluated" was the most frequently (46, 16%) reported unfavourable outcome followed by death (14, 5%) (Table 2).

The factors associated with TB treatment outcomes are described in Table 3. The occurrence of unfavourable outcomes (death, loss to follow-up, and "not evaluated") was higher (54%) among inmates ≥ 60 years than those in the age group of 45-59 years (17%, $P = 0.030$).

Table 1: Sociodemographic and clinical characteristics of adult inmates with tuberculosis admitted at Harare Central Prison and Chikurubi Maximum Prison, Zimbabwe, 2015-2018.

Characteristics	Total	Percentage
Total	280	
Age groups in years		
18-29	63	22.5
30-44	168	60.0
45-59	36	12.9
≥60	13	4.6
Residence		
Urban	151	53.9
Rural	122	43.6
Not recorded	7	2.5
Site of TB		
Pulmonary	212	75.7
Extrapulmonary	15	5.4
Not recorded	53	18.9
Classification by sputum status		
Bacteriologically confirmed	121	43.2
Clinically diagnosed	135	48.2
Not recorded	24	8.6
Classification by history of TB treatment		
New	227	81.1
Previously treated	49	17.5
Not recorded	4	1.4
HIV and ART status		
HIV negative	96	34.3
HIV positive and on ART	144	51.4
HIV positive and not on ART	29	10.4
HIV positive and ART status unknown	7	2.5
HIV status unknown	4	1.4

TB: tuberculosis; ART: antiretroviral therapy.

Table 2: Tuberculosis treatment outcomes among adult inmates admitted at Harare Central Prison and Chikurubi Maximum Prison, Zimbabwe, 2015-2018.

Treatment outcomes*	Number	Percentage with 95% CI
Cured	123	43.9 (38.0-50.0)
Treatment completed	86	30.7 (25.4-36.5)
Died	14	5.0 (2.8-8.2)
Lost to follow-up	11	4.0 (2.0-7.0)
Failure	0	—
Not evaluated	46	16.4 (12.3-21.3)
Total	280	100

*As defined in the national TB manual, Zimbabwe, 2016. CI: confidence interval.

4. Discussion

This is one of the first studies to report on the TB case finding cascade and treatment outcomes in correctional services in Zimbabwe.

Our study in one large prison in Harare showed that 405 (11%) of admissions had presumptive TB and that 12 (3%) people with presumptive TB were lost during TB evaluation. A high TB notification rate was revealed. Pretreatment loss to follow-up was 36%. Assessment of TB treatment outcomes in this and another large prison revealed a treatment success rate (75%) that was lower than the rate (83%, 2017) reported for the country and for male TB patients (90%, 2017) in Harare, and almost one out of four people with TB did not have a TB treatment outcome [9]. The treatment success rate could have been affected by frequent transfers.

Table 3: Factors associated with tuberculosis treatment outcomes among adult inmates admitted at Harare Central Prison and Chikurubi Maximum Prison, Zimbabwe, 2015-2018.

Characteristics	Total	Unfavourable* outcome, *n* (%)	Unadjusted RR (95% CI)	Adjusted RR† (95% CI)	*P* value‡
Total	280	71 (25.4)	—	—	
Age groups in years					
18-29	63	17 (27.0)	1.62 (0.70-3.73)	1.56 (0.67-3.62)	0.298
30-44	168	41 (24.4)	1.46 (0.67-3.18)	1.48 (0.68-3.22)	0.328
45-59	36	6 (16.7)	1	1	
≥60	13	7 (53.9)	3.23 (1.33-7.84)	2.80 (1.1-6.9)	**0.030**
Residence					
Urban	151	40 (26.5)	1.08 (0.72-1.62)	1.19 (0.78-1.81)	0.420
Rural	122	30 (24.6)	1	1	
Not recorded	7	1 (14.3)	0.58 (0.09-3.66)	0.75 (0.13-4.29)	0.748
Site of TB					
Pulmonary	212	49 (23.1)	1	1	
Extrapulmonary	15	3 (20.0)	0.87 (0.31-2.45)	0.77 (0.26-2.27)	0.637
Not recorded	53	19 (35.9)	1.55 (1.00-2.39)	1.41 (0.82-2.4)	0.210
Classification by sputum status					
Bacteriologically confirmed	121	22 (18.2)	1		
Clinically diagnosed	135	39 (28.9)	1.59 (1.00-2.52)	1.36 (0.79-2.32)	0.265
Not recorded	24	10 (41.7)	2.29 (1.25-4.19)	1.99 (1.04-3.81)	**0.038**
Classification by history of TB treatment					
New	227	56 (24.7)	1	1	
Previously treated	49	14 (28.6)	1.16 (0.70-1.90)	1.07 (0.66-1.72)	0.793
Not recorded	4	1 (25.0)	1.01 (0.18-5.61)	0.87 (0.10-7.8)	0.901
HIV and ART status					
HIV negative	96	25 (26.0)	1	1	
HIV positive and on ART	144	36 (25.0)	0.96 (0.62-1.49)	1.04 (0.66-1.64)	0.871
HIV positive and not on ART	29	7 (24.1)	0.93 (0.45-1.92)	0.88 (0.40-1.91)	0.739
HIV positive and ART status unknown	7	2 (28.6)	1.10 (0.32-3.71)	1.22 (0.39-3.83)	0.734
HIV status unknown	4	1 (25.0)	0.96 (0.17-5.42)	1.34 (0.15-12.2)	0.794

RR: relative risk; CI: confidence interval; TB: tuberculosis; ART: antiretroviral therapy. *Unfavourable outcomes include death, loss to follow-up, and "outcome not evaluated." †Adjusted RR is based on the multivariable model (log-binomial regression), and all exposure variables were included in the model. ‡*P* values are from multivariable analysis, and *P* values < 0.05 are highlighted in bold.

The strengths of this study included the use of routinely available programmatic data that were likely to be representative of operational realities in this setting. In addition, the study report adhered to the Strengthening the Reporting of Observational Studies in Epidemiology (STROBE) guidelines [10]. Limitations included the use of the programmatic registers and the recorded data: frequently, data were missing and they could have been inaccurate. Due to unavailability of recorded dates in the registers, we were unable to assess the time taken to make a diagnosis and start TB treatment in those found to have TB that may play an important role in reducing transmission in congregate settings.

The losses (9%) in TB case finding cascade in Harare Central Prison compared favourably with the losses reported for the entire country (24%) in 2018 [9]. The sputum test positivity rate (3%) among inmates on admission and during the stay of inmates was found to be lower than the proportion (6%) among all people with presumptive TB in the country in the same year [9].

The TB prevalence found by our study was threefold compared with the national estimate, and it was in line with the prevalence reported by an earlier assessment [7]. However, it was considerably lower than the rate reported by a study in DRC and was at the lower end of the prevalence reported by a review of studies published from 24 sub-Saharan African countries [11]. This review reported an HIV prevalence of 2%-35% among inmates with TB, and the prevalence we found was considerably higher (64%).

High rates of prediagnosis and pretreatment loss to follow-up have been reported from both the urban and rural areas of Zimbabwe, and these were in line with the finding by our study [9].

Previous studies have reported TB treatment success rates among inmates that ranged from 46% in South Africa and 48% in Uganda to 80% in Ethiopia [12]. The treatment success (75%) in our study compared favourably but was lower than the national rate (83%) in Zimbabwe in 2017 [9]. The proportion of loss to follow-up and/or people with nonevaluated outcomes was reported to be high ranging from 15% in Ethiopia and 16% in our study to 43% in Uganda and 51% in South Africa [3].

This study has the following programmatic implications. First, whilst the rate of presumptive TB was high, it is critical that the missed opportunities in TB case finding cascade in this setting with congestion of inmates and old facilities with a shortage of isolation rooms and inadequate ventilation are reduced. This can be achieved through regular review of the presumptive TB register and ensuring regular specimen transportation to the laboratory and communication of sputum test results back to the clinical staff. It is also possible that some clinically diagnosed TB was missed due to weak access to radiology services.

Second, though the considerable pretreatment loss to follow-up could be partially explained by transfers of inmates to other prisons, the correctional services should set up a system that facilitates tracking of people diagnosed with TB, especially those with infectious forms of the disease. Refresher training for health professionals responsible should be arranged to stress the importance of close observation of sputum test and other investigation results and prompt initiation of appropriate treatment if TB is diagnosed. This is essential to decrease continued transmission of TB bacilli within the correctional services making them "safer".

Third, complete and accurate documentation is critical for data-driven monitoring of TB care and prevention services. It can be enhanced through health staff training in active local use of routinely available TB data for decision-making and ensuring that support supervision is data-driven.

In conclusion, our study findings are suggestive of disproportionate TB burden in the two prisons in the country. The findings have also revealed programmatic gaps, such as losses in the TB case finding cascade and considerable pretreatment loss to follow-up that should be brought to zero. Concerted efforts to ensure that all inmates with TB have a treatment outcome that is correctly documented should also be ensured.

Additional Points

Disclosure

The funders had no role in study design, data collection and analysis, decision to publish, or preparation of the manuscript.

Acknowledgments

This research was conducted through the Structured Operational Research and Training Initiative (SORT IT), a global partnership led by the Special Programme for Research and Training in Tropical Diseases at the World Health Organization (WHO/TDR). The training model is based on a course developed jointly by the International Union against Tuberculosis and Lung Disease (The Union) and Medécins sans Frontières (MSF). The specific SORT IT program which resulted in this publication was implemented by the Centre for Operational Research, The Union, Paris, France. Mentorship and the coordination/facilitation of this particular SORT IT workshop was provided through the Centre for Operational Research, The Union, Paris, France; the Department of Tuberculosis, The Union, Paris, France; The Union, Zimbabwe Office; The Union, South East Asia Office; and AIDS and TB Department, Ministry of Health and Child Care, Harare, Zimbabwe. The following ZPCS health Staff are thanked for their valuable efforts during the data collection process, Manuwere M, Chiremba L, Kunaka D, Bondera ET, and Bvekwa E and Mrs. C Nyahuye. Finally, many thanks are given to the ZPCS management for granting me permission to carry out the study. The training course under which this study was conducted was funded by the UK Department for International Development (DFID) and the World Health Organization Zimbabwe Country Office. The open-access publications costs were funded by the UK Department for International Development (DFID) and LaFondation Veuve Emile Metz-Tesch (Luxembourg).

References

[1] L. Telisinghe, S. Charalambous, S. M. Topp et al., "HIV and tuberculosis in prisons in sub-Saharan Africa," *The Lancet*, vol. 388, no. 10050, pp. 1215–1227, 2016.

[2] World Health Organization, "Tuberculosis in prisons," March 2019, https://www.who.int/tb/areas-of-work/population-groups/prisons-facts/en/.

[3] K. Adane, M. Spigt, S. Ferede, T. Asmelash, M. Abebe, and G.-J. Dinant, "Half of pulmonary tuberculosis cases were left undiagnosed in prisons of the Tigray Region of Ethiopia: implications for tuberculosis control," *PLoS One*, vol. 11, no. 2, article e0149453, 2016.

[4] S. Hatwiinda, S. M. Topp, M. Siyambango et al., "Poor continuity of care for TB diagnosis and treatment in Zambian prisons: a situation analysis," *Tropical Medicine & International Health*, vol. 23, no. 2, pp. 243–250, 2018.

[5] World Health Organization, "Post-2015 Global TB Strategy and targets," March 2019, https://www.who.int/tb/post-2015_TBstrategy.pdf?ua=1.

[6] World Health Organization, *Global tuberculosis report 2018*, World Health Organization, Geneva, Switzerland, 2018, https://apps.who.int/iris/handle/10665/274453. License: CC BY-NC-SA 3.0 IGO.

[7] E. L. Corbett, T. Bandason, Y.-B. Cheung et al., "Prevalent infectious tuberculosis in Harare, Zimbabwe: Burden, risk factors and implications for control," *The International Journal of*

Tuberculosis and Lung Disease, vol. 13, no. 10, pp. 1231–1237, 2009.

[8] Zimbabwe Ministry of Health and Child Care, *Ministry of Health and Child Welfare, National Tuberculosis Program – Strategic Plan (2017-2020)*, Harare, Zimbabwe, 2018, http://www.mohcc.gov.zw/component/content/article/9-uncategorised/359-world-malaria-day-2016-press-conference-talk-points-by-the-honourable-minister-of-health-and-child-care-dr-david-parirenyatwa-2016.

[9] Tuberculosis N, Programme LC, *Ministry of Health and Child Care National Tuberculosis and Leprosy Control Programme*, 2018.

[10] E. von Elm, D. G. Altman, M. Egger et al., "The strengthening the reporting of observational studies in epidemiology (STROBE) statement: guidelines for reporting observational studies," *International Journal of Surgery*, vol. 12, no. 12, pp. 1495–1499, 2014.

[11] M. K. Kayomo, E. Hasker, M. Aloni et al., "Outbreak of tuberculosis and multidrug-resistant tuberculosis, Mbuji-Mayi Central Prison, Democratic Republic of the Congo," *Emerging Infectious Diseases*, vol. 24, no. 11, pp. 2029–2035, 2018.

[12] A. Sharp, J. T. Donahoe, A. Milliken, J. Barocio, S. Charalambous, and Z. M. McLaren, "Do incarcerated populations serve as a reservoir for tuberculosis in South Africa?," *The American Journal of Tropical Medicine and Hygiene*, vol. 99, no. 6, pp. 1390–1396, 2018.

14

Accuracy and Incremental Yield of the Chest X-Ray in Screening for Tuberculosis in Uganda

Joanitah Nalunjogi[1,2] **Frank Mugabe,**[3] **Irene Najjingo,**[1,2] **Pastan Lusiba,**[2] **Francis Olweny,**[2] **Joseph Mubiru,**[4] **Edward Kayongo,**[2] **Rogers Sekibira,**[1] **Achilles Katamba,**[2] **and Bruce Kirenga**[1,5]

[1]*Makerere University Lung Institute, College of Health Sciences, Makerere University, Uganda*
[2]*Clinical Epidemiology Unit, College of Health Sciences, Makerere University, Uganda*
[3]*Uganda National Tuberculosis and Leprosy Program, Ministry of Health, Uganda*
[4]*Accident and Emergency Unit, Mulago National Referral Hospital, Kampala, Uganda*
[5]*Division of Pulmonary Medicine, College of Health Sciences, Makerere University, Uganda*

Correspondence should be addressed to Joanitah Nalunjogi; jmukwaba@gmail.com

Academic Editor: Adwoa Asante-Poku

The WHO END TB strategy requires ≥90% case detection to combat tuberculosis (TB). Increased TB case detection requires a more sensitive and specific screening tool. Currently, the symptoms recommended for screening TB have been found to be suboptimal since up to 44% of individuals with TB are asymptomatic. The chest X-ray (CXR) as a screening tool for pulmonary TB was evaluated in this study, as well as its incremental yield in TB diagnosis using a cross-sectional study involving secondary analysis of data of 4512 consented/assented participants ≥15 years who participated in the Uganda National TB prevalence survey between 2014 and 2015. Participants with a cough ≥2 weeks, fever, weight loss, and night sweats screened positive for TB using the symptoms screening method, while participants with a TB defining abnormality on CXR screened positive for TB by the CXR screening method. The Löwenstein-Jensen (LJ) culture was used as a gold standard for TB diagnosis. The CXR had 93% sensitivity and 65% specificity compared to LJ culture results, while symptoms had 76% sensitivity and 31% specificity. The screening algorithm involving the CXR in addition to symptoms led to a 38% increment in the yield of diagnosed tuberculosis. The number needed to screen using the CXR and symptoms screening algorithm was 32 compared to 45 when the symptoms are used alone. Therefore, the CXR in combination with symptoms is a good TB screening tool and increases the yield of diagnosed TB.

1. Introduction

The WHO 2020 estimates show that tuberculosis (TB) was responsible for 1.4 million deaths [1]. In order to combat tuberculosis, WHO proposed three strategies including intensified case finding (ICF), isoniazid preventive therapy (IPT), and infection control (IC) [2]. In addition, the WHO END TB strategy indicates a need for ≥90% TB case detection among others to combat TB [3].

Uganda has a high TB incidence of 201 per 100,000 population as well as high TB-related mortality of 26 per 100,000 population with a TB case detection rate of 72% [4].

The strategic plan for the Uganda national TB and leprosy programme (NTLP) sought to achieve 85% case detection by 2019/2020; however, confirming TB was difficult. Currently, TB culture is the gold standard, but financial and logistic challenges make it difficult to scale up. There is a need to explore more widely available, low-cost screening and

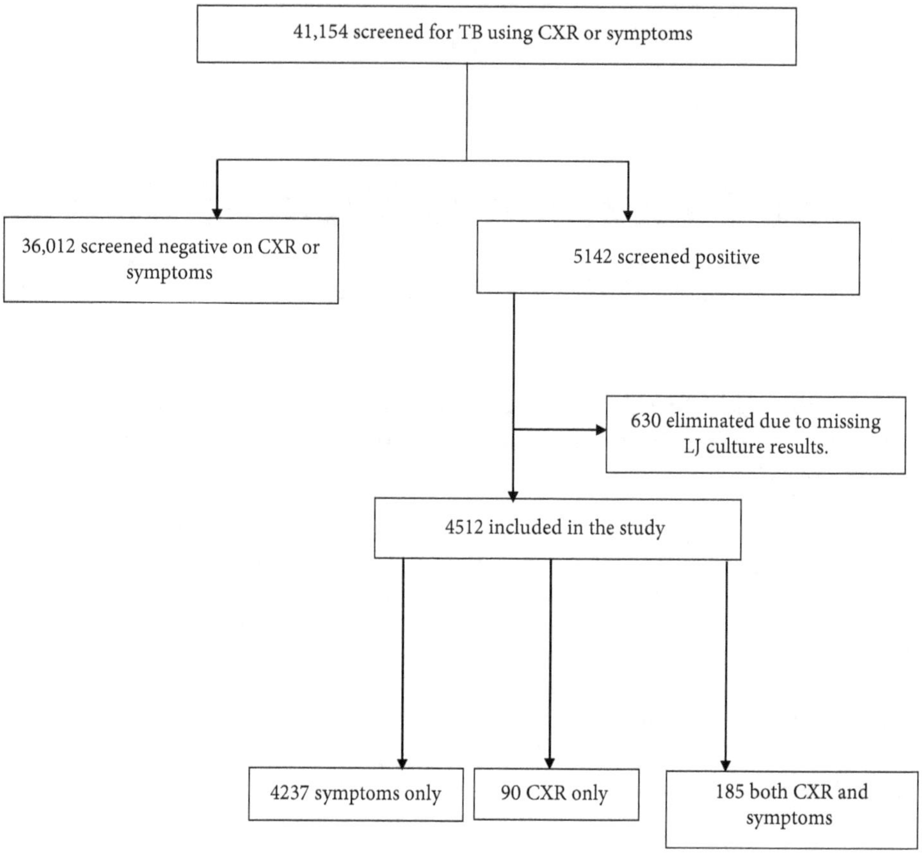

FIGURE 1: Study profile.

diagnostic tools and algorithms to aid TB diagnosis such as the chest radiograph (CXR), as improved TB diagnostics (Gene Xpert) have now become available. Currently, the symptoms screening tool is employed for TB screening in Uganda. This symptoms screening tool has been observed to have 40.7% sensitivity and 81.3% specificity according to a survey done in South Africa considering the presence of any cough, fever, weight loss, or night sweats [5]. Systematic reviews done to assess the performance of the symptoms in high HIV prevalence regions such as Uganda have shown 84% sensitivity and 74% specificity [6]. The symptoms screening tool therefore runs a risk of missing patients with TB as the patients do not seek care and do not have symptoms due to early TB disease. These patients if not diagnosed early by a more specific screening test will continue to spread TB in the community and present with complications due to TB hence poor treatment outcomes.

The recognition that bold new strategies are needed to control TB (END TB Strategy) has led to reconsideration of CXR as a potential TB screening tool, as innovative, lower costs strategies for performing CXR (digital radiography) and reading them (computer-aided reading) have become available [7, 8]. The CXR was commonly used in mass screening campaigns in Europe and the USA in the early TB chemotherapy era (1950s) but has not been widely used in screening TB in low-income countries because of high cost and lack of capacity [9, 10]. This CXR has been found to have 98% sensitivity and 75% specificity in a systematic review done among HIV-negative and HIV-positive individuals [6].

The use of more sensitive TB screening tools such as the CXR may increase the pool of presumptive TB cases hence increasing case detection as more individuals are exposed to the confirmatory test (Gene Xpert or Culture) which ultimately leads to a reduction in mortality and morbidity [11]. In order to assess the accuracy of the CXR in screening tuberculosis, there is a need to use a test known to confirm tuberculosis such as Lowenstein Jensen (LJ) culture.

Uganda carried out a national TB prevalence survey (UTPS) from 2014 to 2015 which screened for TB by collecting data on TB symptoms using questionnaires and performed CXR in all consenting participants; in addition, all sputa were cultured on LJ media to confirm tuberculosis [12].

Therefore, using the data from UTPS, we sought to evaluate the accuracy and incremental yield of using the CXR in screening for TB in Uganda.

2. Materials and Methods

2.1. Study Design. We conducted a cross-sectional study by secondary analysis of the data collected during the Uganda National TB prevalence survey (UTPS) [13]. The UTPS was conducted from October 2014 to July 2015 with the primary objective of determining the prevalence of TB in Uganda. Eligible respondents aged ≥15 years were randomly selected in blocks to participate in the study [12, 13].

All eligible consenting/assenting individuals who were ≥15years were screened for TB using a questionnaire which listed the symptoms and a CXR. Parents/guardians of individuals <18 years offered informed consent. Participants with a cough ≥2 weeks, TB defining abnormality on CXR examination/or any abnormality in the lung on CXR examination, and respondents without a CXR were considered presumptive for TB. All presumptive TB respondents were requested to submit two sputum samples (a spot and an early morning sample) for microscopy and culture. All positive samples by microscopy and contaminated culture samples were subjected to Xpert MTB/RIF test to confirm the presence of mycobacterium tuberculosis (MTB). The CXRs were read by 3 independent radiologists. LJ culture was used as a gold standard for the confirmation of tuberculosis among the survey participants. All records in the electronic database that had bacteriological confirmation of TB as per UTPS by culture were analysed for the substudy [12]. Participants with mycobacterium other than tuberculosis (MOTT) were identified using SD Bio line on positive cultures and Xpert MTB/RIF done on positive smears and contaminated cultures. All individuals with MOTT were not reported as MTB cases. In the UTPS, all cases of TB reported as survey TB were confirmed on culture.

The STARD 2015 guidelines [14] were used to report the results of this study. Data was analysed using Stata version 13.0 (College Station, Texas, USA). In our study, records with any of the above symptoms, i.e., cough ≥2 weeks, fever, weight loss, or night sweats were analysed as positive for symptoms. Records indicating CXR abnormalities suggestive of active TB were analysed as positive by the CXR. Records with culture-confirmed TB were considered as the gold standard for determining the performance of the CXR or symptoms in screening tuberculosis.

Variables were summarised using percentages. Performance of the symptoms screening and CXR were reported as sensitivity, specificity, and negative and positive predictive values. The proportion of confirmed TB cases obtained using the CXR screen was reported as the yield due to the CXR in percentages. The proportion of confirmed TB cases obtained using the symptoms screen was reported as yield due to the symptoms screen and reported in percentages. The incremental yield of the CXR was reported as a percentage increase in the total number of TB cases diagnosed through an algorithm involving the CXR versus an algorithm involving the symptoms screen alone.

Table 1: Demographic, clinical, and radiographic characteristics of the study population.

Characteristic	$N = 4512$ N (%)
Age	
15-24 yrs	767 (17)
25-34 yrs	846 (19)
35-44 yrs	860 (19)
45-54 yrs	727 (16)
55-64 yrs	474 (11)
65+ yrs	838 (18)
Female	2266 (50)
Education	
None	1283 (28)
Primary	2135 (47)
Secondary	890 (20)
Tertiary	204 (5)
Employed	3603 (80)
Rural residence	2889 (64)
Smoking	
Never	3277 (73)
Current	640 (14)
Past	595 (13)
HIV*	
Positive	392 (10)
Symptom characteristics$^{\infty}$	
Cough$^{\infty}$	2827 (63)
Fever$^{\infty}$	668 (14)
Weight loss$^{\infty}$	608 (14)
Night sweats$^{\infty}$	394 (9)
CXR characteristics**	
Normal	2784 (63)
Abnormal healed TB	232 (5)
Abnormal active TB	275 (6)
Abnormal not TB	1150 (26)
Culture confirmed TB	
MTB	160 (3)
MOTT	26 (1)
Contaminated	57 (1)
Negative	4269 (95)

*missing 474/4512 (10.1%), **missing 71/4512 (1.6%) participants who declined to have a CXR examination, $^{\infty}$each individual characteristics N = 4512.

3. Results

3.1. Study Profile. A total of 41,154 participants were enumerated for screening in the UTPS. We excluded 36,012 records of participants who screened negative on the CXR and symptoms and therefore were not required to submit sputum for TB diagnosis. 630 records that were missing data on culture results were additionally excluded leaving 4512 records for further analysis as shown below (Figure 1).

3.2. Characteristics of the Study Population. The study included individuals aged 15–65 years. The participants between ages 25 and 34 years were 846 (19%) as well as those in the age group 35–44 years 860 (19%). There was an equal number of females 2266 (50%) and males. Cough was present in 63% of the respondents, while 6% of the respondents had CXR abnormalities consistent with active TB disease. MOTT was present in 1% of the cultures (Table 1).

3.3. Performance of the Chest Radiograph or Symptoms in Screening TB in Uganda. Pulmonary TB was confirmed in 160 (3.6%) participants using LJ culture. The CXR had

TABLE 2: Performance of the CXR or symptoms in screening culture-confirmed pulmonary tuberculosis.

Strategy	Culture-confirmed TB	Total number	Sensitivity (95% CI)	Specificity (95% CI)	Positive predictive value (95% CI)	Negative predictive value (95% CI)
Prevalence	160	4512				
CXR	148	4441	93 (87, 96)	97 (96, 98)	54 (48, 60)	99 (99, 100)
Symptoms	122	4512	76 (69, 83)	31 (30, 32)	4 (3, 5)	97 (96, 98)
CXR+symptoms	160	4512	100 (98, 100)	29 (28, 31)	5 (4, 6)	100 (99, 100)

TABLE 3: Incremental yield and number needed to screen of using the CXR in a TB screening algorithm.

Strategy/algorithm	Screened	Tested	NNS	Number of TB cases	% of confirmed TB	Incremental yield (%)
Symptoms only	5142	4512	42	122	76	Ref
X-ray only	5142	4441	35	149	93	17
Symptoms and X-ray	5142	4441	32	160	100	23

NNS: number needed to screen (number of people needed to screen to diagnose a bacteriologically positive case, who has not been previously diagnosed by the health system). TB: tuberculosis.

sensitivity 93% (95% CI; 87, 96) and specificity 97% (95% CI; 96, 98) compared to symptoms with sensitivity 76 (95% CI; 69, 83) and specificity 31% (95% CI; 30, 32).

The negative and positive predictive values of the CXR were 99% and 54% versus 97% and 4% of the symptoms. The CXR and symptoms combined had 100% sensitivity and 29% specificity. The positive and negative predictive values of this screening algorithm were 5% and 100%, respectively (Table 2).

3.4. Incremental Yield of Using the CXR in Screening TB versus Symptoms Alone. Using the symptoms alone in screening tuberculosis, 122/160 TB patients would have been diagnosed. The addition of the CXR in the TB screening algorithm increased the cases of TB diagnosed by 38 (23.8%). The number needed to screen was 32 individuals. The detailed results are shown in Table 3, below.

4. Discussion

This study compared the accuracy of the CXR or symptoms against culture-confirmed pulmonary TB by the Lowenstein Jensen (LJ) method in a community TB screening setting such as the National TB prevalence survey.

Our results show that the CXR performs better than the symptoms in correlating with positive TB sputum culture results in community settings just like other studies [2, 15–19]. The sensitivity of 93% and specificity of 97% obtained when considering TB defining CXR abnormalities are comparable to the results obtained in a study done in London when a digital CXR was employed in active case finding [18]. These results indicate that the CXR performs better in correlating TB sputum culture results; therefore, the use of the CXR in addition to symptoms in TB screening in community settings increases TB case detection rate [20] in high TB prevalence settings which allows for timely initiation of TB treatment [19] as bacteriological confirmation and drug susceptibility tests are processed to further determine appropriate TB treatment [19]. Additionally, our screening algorithm involving both the CXR and symptoms showed 100% sensitivity and 29% specificity which results differ from those of a systematic review of TB screening algorithms where a screening algorithm involving both the CXR and symptoms showed sensitivity 87% and specificity 90% [6]. This difference could be explained by the fact that only individuals with symptoms and abnormal CXR exam were eligible for sputum evaluation in the UTPS hence overestimation of the sensitivity at the cost of specificity. However, the use of the CXR increases the overall sensitivity hence an increased number of individuals being subjected to the confirmatory tests resulting into increased TB yield [21, 22]. This is especially important in the era of the new advanced TB diagnostic tools such as the GeneXpert with high sensitivity and specificity [23].

In our study, the symptoms screen showed a sensitivity of 76% and specificity of 31%. These estimates are similar to those obtained in a systematic review of TB screening algorithms [6]; however, studies done in Asia, Zambia, and South Africa to evaluate the accuracy of symptoms in screening TB showed slightly different estimates of sensitivity and specificity of symptoms compared to those seen in our study [24, 25]. This could have resulted from the difference in the population under study, since our study only had cultures done from patients who screened positive by CXR or symptoms or did not have a CXR done.

Furthermore, a 38% increment in the number of TB cases diagnosed as well as a low number needed to screen 32 patients when using a screening algorithm involving both the CXR and symptoms is a good step towards interventions leading to increased TB case finding hence TB elimination. This increment was however lower than that reported in a study done in India among household contacts of TB patients [21]. The difference may be explained by the special population under which the study in India was done which is a more high-risk population for TB compared to the general population that we studied as well as the higher prevalence of TB in India compared to Uganda. This finding however provides insight into the innovations that may lead to the achievement of the 90% TB detection for the END TB strategy [3]. The results are also in agreement with a study done in South Africa on symptoms and digital CXR screening which recorded improvement in the yield of TB [26] screening among prisoners when both screening strategies were employed. The addition of the CXR to symptoms in screening TB can be employed to identify potential TB cases that would be missed when using only symptoms for screening. From our study, the algorithm involving the symptoms screening alone would have missed 23% of the patients with TB. Our finding is also supported by earlier reports of similar studies from different TB endemic countries [5, 13, 17, 24]. The strengths of our study include community screening for TB as shown by the use of data collected during the UTPS. The study was reported according to the STARD (Standards for reporting of Diagnostics Accuracy Studies) 2015 guidelines [14].

Our study is however subject to limitations. The fact that sputum culture was only done for participants with abnormal CXR or TB symptoms could have led to selection bias hence overestimation of the sensitivity of the CXR; however, the large sample size improves our estimation of the performance of the CXR. In addition, we only looked at culture-confirmed pulmonary TB but not clinically diagnosed and not culture-negative or extrapulmonary TB which could greatly impact the performance of symptoms screening and/or CXR to identify true TB. Additionally, the failure to use more sensitive TB confirmatory tests such as the Gene Xpert and Liquid culture could have led to underestimation of confirmed TB hence lead to underestimation of the performance of the CXR or symptoms. Finally, the study was performed under community screening conditions, and therefore, the results may not be applicable to hospital-based TB screening.

5. Conclusion

This study made use of data obtained during the Uganda National TB prevalence survey to determine the performance of the CXR in correlating TB culture results. The results indicate that the CXR is a good TB screening tool and may improve TB case detection when used in community TB screening in addition to symptoms assessment. Individuals with knowledge to observe TB defining pathology on the CXR are adequate to provide expertise for CXR interpretation.

Abbreviations

CXR: Chest X-ray
HIV: Human immune virus
IC: Infection control
ICF: Intensified case finding
IPT: Isoniazid preventive therapy
LJ: Lowenstein Jensen
MoH: Ministry of Health
MOOT: Mycobacterium other than TB
NNS: Number needed to screen
NTLP: National TB and leprosy programme
PLHIV: People living with HIV
PTB: Pulmonary tuberculosis
SOMREC: School of Medicine Research and Ethics Committee
TB: Tuberculosis
UTPS: Uganda TB prevalence survey
WHO: World Health Organisation.

Consent

Not applicable.

Authors' Contributions

JN, IN, PL, FO, EK, and JM contributed to conception, design, analysis, methodology, interpretation of data, drafting, and revision. FM contributed to conception, funding acquisition, data acquisition, and writing. RS contributed to the data curation, software acquisition, and revision. AK contributed to conception, funding acquisition, investigation, resources, supervision, validation, drafting, and revision. JBK contributed to conception, funding acquisition, investigation, supervision, validation, drafting, and revision. All authors read and approved the final manuscript.

Acknowledgments

The authors acknowledge the Ministry of Health, Uganda, through the National TB and Leprosy Program for permission to utilise the data from the National TB Survey 2014-2015. The members of the department of clinical epidemiology and biostatistics of Makerere University College of health sciences school of medicine for their assistance in drafting the proposal. The MakCHS–UCBerkeley-Yale Pulmonary Complications of AIDS Research Training (PART) Program, [NIH D43TW009607], from the Fogarty International Center for the PART fellowship awarded to JN under which this work was completed. The funders had no role in study design, data collection and analysis, decision to publish, or preparation of the manuscript.

References

[1] Organization WH, *Global tuberculosis report 2020*, World Health Organization, Geneva (Switzerland), 2020.

[2] WHO, *Systematic screening for active tuberculosis: principles and recommendations*, World Health Organization, Geneva (Switzerland), 2013.

[3] WHO, *The End TB Strategy: global strategy and targets for tuberculosis prevention, care and control after 2015*, WHO, Geneva, Swirzerland, 2015.

[4] WHO, 2018, <WHO_HQ_Reports-G2-PROD-EXT-TBCountryProfile Uganda.pdf>.

[5] M. M. Claassens, C. van Schalkwyk, S. Floyd, H. Ayles, and N. Beyers, "Symptom screening rules to identify active pulmonary tuberculosis: findings from the Zambian South African Tuberculosis and HIV/AIDS Reduction (ZAMSTAR) trial

prevalence surveys," *PLoS One*, vol. 12, no. 3, article e0172881, 2017.

[6] A. Van't Hoog, M. Langendam, E. Mitchell et al., "A systematic review of the sensitivity and specificity of symptom-and chest-radiography screening for active pulmonary tuberculosis in HIV-negative persons and persons with unknown HIV status," *REPORT-Version March 2013*, World Health Organization, Geneva, Switzerland, 2013.

[7] S. Jaeger, A. Karargyris, S. Candemir et al., "Automatic tuberculosis screening using chest radiographs," *IEEE transactions on medical imaging*, vol. 33, no. 2, pp. 233–245, 2014.

[8] S. Den Boon, E. D. Bateman, D. A. Enarson et al., "Development and evaluation of a new chest radiograph reading and recording system for epidemiological surveys of tuberculosis and lung disease," *The International Journal of Tuberculosis and Lung Disease*, vol. 9, no. 10, pp. 1088–1096, 2005.

[9] N. S. Shah, M. H. Anh, T. T. Thuy et al., "Population-based chest X-ray screening for pulmonary tuberculosis in people living with HIV/AIDS, An Giang, Vietnam," *The International Journal of Tuberculosis and Lung Disease*, vol. 12, no. 4, pp. 404–410, 2008.

[10] J. A. Aluoch, O. B. Swai, E. A. Edwards et al., "Study of case-finding for pulmonary tuberculosis in outpatients complaining of a chronic cough at a district Hospital in Kenya," *American Review of Respiratory Disease*, vol. 129, no. 6, pp. 915–920, 1984.

[11] R. K. Gupta, S. D. Lawn, L.-G. Bekker, J. Caldwell, R. Kaplan, and R. Wood, "Impact of human immunodeficiency virus and CD4 count on tuberculosis diagnosis: analysis of city-wide data from Cape Town, South Africa," *The international journal of tuberculosis and lung disease : the official journal of the International Union against Tuberculosis and Lung Disease.*, vol. 17, no. 8, pp. 1014–1022, 2013.

[12] MoH, *Uganda National TB prevalence Survey 2014- 2015 Uganda Ministry of Health Website Ministry of Health 2017*March 2019, http://health.go.ug/content/uganda-national-tuberculosis-prevalence-survey-2014-2015-survey-report..

[13] I. Law, K. Floyd, E. A. B. Abukaraig et al., "National tuberculosis prevalence surveys in Africa, 2008–2016: an overview of results and lessons learned," *Tropical Medicine & International Health*, vol. 25, no. 11, pp. 1308–1327, 2020.

[14] J. F. Cohen, D. A. Korevaar, D. G. Altman et al., "STARD 2015 guidelines for reporting diagnostic accuracy studies: explanation and elaboration," *BMJ Open*, vol. 6, no. 11, article e012799, 2016.

[15] D. T. M. Nguyen, N. D. Bang, N. Q. Hung, R. P. Beasley, L.-Y. Hwang, and E. A. Graviss, "Yield of chest radiograph in tuberculosis screening for HIV-infected persons at a district-level HIV clinic," *The International Journal of Tuberculosis and Lung Disease*, vol. 20, no. 2, pp. 211-217, 2016.

[16] S. Shah, M. Demissie, L. Lambert et al., "Intensified tuberculosis case finding among HIV-infected persons from a voluntary counseling and testing center in Addis Ababa, Ethiopia," *JAIDS Journal of Acquired Immune Deficiency Syndromes*, vol. 50, no. 5, pp. 537–545, 2009.

[17] F. A. Khan, S. Verkuijl, A. Parrish et al., "Performance of symptom-based tuberculosis screening among people living with HIV: not as great as hoped," *AIDS*, vol. 28, no. 10, pp. 1463–1472, 2014.

[18] A. Story, R. W. Aldridge, I. Abubakar et al., "Active case finding for pulmonary tuberculosis using mobile digital chest radiography: an observational study," *The International Journal of Tuberculosis and Lung Disease*, vol. 16, no. 11, pp. 1461–1467, 2012.

[19] Organization WH, "Systematic Screening for Active Tuberculosis," in *Principles and Recommendations*, World Health Organization, Geneva (Switzerland), 2013.

[20] M. R. A. van Cleeff, L. E. Kivihya-Ndugga, H. Meme, J. A. Odhiambo, and P. R. Klatser, "The role and performance of chest X-ray for the diagnosis of tuberculosis: a cost-effectiveness analysis in Nairobi, Kenya," *BMC infectious diseases*, vol. 5, no. 1, 2005.

[21] R. Ananthakrishnan, R. Thiagesan, S. Auguesteen et al., "The impact of chest radiography and Xpert MTB/RIF testing among household contacts in Chennai, India," *PLoS One*, vol. 15, no. 11, article e0241203, 2020.

[22] S. M. Machekera, E. Wilkinson, S. G. Hinderaker et al., "A comparison of the yield and relative cost of active tuberculosis case-finding algorithms in Zimbabwe," *Public health action.*, vol. 9, no. 2, pp. 63–68, 2019.

[23] C. Miller, K. Lonnroth, G. Sotgiu, and G. B. Migliori, "The long and winding road of chest radiography for tuberculosis detection," *European Respiratory Journal*, vol. 49, no. 5, 2017.

[24] J. Cheng, L. Wang, H. Zhang, and Y. Xia, "Diagnostic value of symptom screening for pulmonary tuberculosis in China," *PLoS One*, vol. 10, no. 5, article e0127725, 2015.

[25] K. P. Cain, K. D. McCarthy, C. M. Heilig et al., "An algorithm for tuberculosis screening and diagnosis in people with HIV," *New England Journal of Medicine*, vol. 362, no. 8, pp. 707–716, 2010.

[26] H.-Y. Kim, V. Zishiri, L. Page-Shipp et al., "Symptom and digital chest X-ray TB screening in South African prisons: yield and cost-effectiveness," *The International Journal of Tuberculosis and Lung Disease*, vol. 24, no. 3, pp. 295–302, 2020.

15

Tuberculosis at Farmer-Cattle Interface in the Rural Villages of South Gondar Zone of Northwest Ethiopia

Amir Alelign,[1,2,3] Aboma Zewude,[1] Beyene Petros,[2] and Gobena Ameni[1]

[1]*Aklilu Lemma Institute of Pathobiology, Addis Ababa University, P.O. Box 1176, Addis Ababa, Ethiopia*
[2]*College of Natural Sciences, Department of Microbial, Cellular and Molecular Biology, Addis Ababa University, P.O. Box 1176, Addis Ababa, Ethiopia*
[3]*College of Natural and Computational Sciences, Department of Biology, Debrebrhan University, P.O. Box 445, Debrebrhan, Ethiopia*

Correspondence should be addressed to Amir Alelign; aleamiro2009@gmail.com

Academic Editor: Alexander S. Apt

Background. Tuberculosis (TB) has been an important public health concern in Ethiopia, particularly at areas of human-animal intersection. However, limited epidemiological information is available in this respect in the country. Therefore, the present study was conducted to investigate the transmission of TB at human-cattle interface, associated risk factors and public awareness about the disease at South Gondar Zone, northwest Ethiopia. *Methods.* A cross sectional study was conducted between March 2015 and April 2018 on 186 farmers and 476 cattle in South Gondar Zone, northwest Ethiopia. Bacteriological examination, region of difference (RD) 9-based polymerase chain reaction (PCR), single intradermal comparative tuberculin test (SICTT), and questionnaire were used for undertaking this study. *Results.* Culture positivity in farmers was 59.7% (111/186) and all the culture positive isolates were *M. tuberculosis.* About 68% (74/111) of culture positive respondents did not know about the transmission of TB from cattle to human or vice versa. The animal and herd prevalence of bovine TB were 1.5% (7/476) and 7.4% (7/95), respectively. Although the result was not statistically significant, the odds of bovine TB in cattle owned by TB positive households was slightly higher than those owned by TB free households (adjusted odds ratio, AOR = 1.39; 95% CI: 0.31–7.10; $p = 0.76$). *Conclusion.* Although SIDCTT reactivity was slightly higher in cattle owned by TB positive households, all the human isolates were *M. tuberculosis* and no *M. bovis* was isolated from farmers, which could be due to the low prevalence of bovine TB in the area.

1. Introduction

Tuberculosis (TB) is an infectious disease of humans and animals. The most common cause of human TB is known to be *Mycobacterium tuberculosis* (*M. tuberculosis*), and the main cause of TB in animals is *Mycobacterium bovis* (*M. bovis*). Zoonotic TB is a form of TB that is caused by *M. bovis* and transmitted from animals to humans. While reverse zoonotic TB is the form of TB that is caused by *M. tuberculosis* and is transmitted from humans to animals. *M. bovis* often causes extra pulmonary TB (EPTB) disease and pulmonary TB (PTB) disease, which is clinically indistinguishable from TB caused by *M. tuberculosis*. In 2016, an estimated 147,000 new cases of zoonotic TB were reported globally, and 12,500 deaths from zoonotic TB. The highest burden of zoonotic TB was reported from the African, followed by the South-East Asian region [1].

The transmission of TB from cattle to human is due to consumption of raw/undercooked infected animal products such as milk and meat or through inhalation due to close contact between the cattle and humans. It is estimated that in countries where pasteurization of milk is rare and bovine TB is common, 10%–15% human cases of TB are caused by *M. bovis* [2]. According to some studies from Tanzania, Nigeria, and Uganda, *M. bovis* accounted for 20% or more of the MTBC isolated from human TB cases [3–5].

Data on TB transmission at the human-animal interface are important in designing a "one health" approach for the control of the disease, particularly, rural settings. In the Amhara Region, north-western Ethiopia, information on the public health risk of zoonotic TB is scarce. Few cross sectional studies conducted in cattle reported animal prevalence of

3.55% and 8.7% [6, 7]. In addition, *M. bovis* was isolated from humans in north-western Ethiopia [7, 8].

In South Gondar Zone, Amhara Region, north-western Ethiopia, the practices of inhabitants could promote the transmission of TB from cattle to humans or vice versa. However, there is scarcity of epidemiological data on public awareness, risk factors and transmission of TB between humans and their cattle in the Zone. Hence, the present study was conducted to investigate the public awareness, risk factors to bovine TB (BTB) and the potential transmission of TB from cattle to humans or vice versa in South Gondar Zone of north-western Ethiopia.

2. Materials and Methods

2.1. Study Area. The study was conducted in South Gondar Zone, north-western Ethiopia. The Zone is located in the Amhara Region, 660 km north east of Addis Ababa, the Capital of Ethiopia. The Zone is known for its diverse topography ranging from flat and low grazing land to high cold mountains. The altitude of the Zone ranges from 1500 to 3,600 m above sea level. The average yearly rainfall of the Zone ranged from 700 mm to 1300 mm in while the average daily temperature was 17°C in 2017. South Gondar Zone consisted of 10 districts and covers a total area of 14,320 sq km. According to the Central Statistical Agency of Ethiopia, the Zone has a total population of 2,051,738 and a population density of 145.56 [9]. Majority of the population (90.47%) of the Zone were rural inhabitants. A total of 468,238 households were counted in this Zone, which resulted in an average of 4.38 persons to a household [9].

The majority of the population has depended on subsistence farming and dairy cattle rearing [10]. The Zone has been known for its indigenous milk cattle such as the "Fogera" and "Dera" cattle. Dairying is commonly practiced using small herd size.

2.2. Study Population and Sampling. Human TB cases were recruited randomly from districts health centres, peripheral health posts, zonal and regional government as well as private referal hospitals (Debretabor, Felegehiwot and Gambi hosptals). The human cases included were those active TB patients who visited the health facilities seeking for TB-treatment. The control human subjects were households who did not have TB cases for the last five years and residing in the same villages with the households which have TB cases in their family members. Cattle owned by both TB positive households and TB negative households were tested for bovine TB.

2.3. General Inclusion and Exclusion Criteria. Small scale dairy farmers who were permanently living in the zone for at least two months prior to the study, aged five years and above at the time of the study as well as who were consented and willing to participate in the study were included, whereas, individuals who had no association with cattle, those who were not willing to participate, aged below five years and seriously ill ones were excluded from participating in the study. Both local and cross breed cattle older than six months and owned by households with active TB cases and TB free households were included. Young cattle with age less than six months, clinically sick ones, and cows one month pre-and post partum were excluded from the study.

2.4. Study Design and Sample Size Determination. A comparative cross sectional study was conducted between December 2015 and February 2018. The sample size for this study was calculated with the assumption of a 15% bovine TB prevalence in TB positive households and a 5% bovine TB prevalence among TB free households, a 95% confidence interval (CI) with a power of 80%, a ratio of cases to comparison groups of 3 : 1 (based on findings of 15.3% bovine TB among TB positive households and a 5.9% BTB among TB free households) [8]. Adding a 10% nonresponse rate, the required sample size was 105 for TB positive households and 35 TB for free households. However, in the present study, due to several limitations we have only managed to reach out only 63 TB positive and 32 TB negative households. Based on this, a total of 476 cattle (315 from TB positive households and 161 from TB free households) were tested for bovine TB.

3. Data Collection

3.1. Questioner Survey. All human study participants were interviewed with a questionnaire in order to assess their awareness and practices about the zoonotic transmission of TB, and the possible risk factors for the disease. Their socio-demographic characteristics, knowledge, attitudes, and practices towards TB including their consumption habits of raw milk/meat as well as husbandry practices were asked. Moreover, all herd owners of tuberculin tested cattle were interviewed for possible risk factors of TB positive cattle. Data on age and sex of individual animal, herd size, origin, breed type, recent introduction of new animals into the herd, and keeping of different livestock together were collected. Previous history about BCG vaccination of cattle was recorded.

3.2. Laboratory Methods. After informed consent was obtained, two sputum samples (on-spot and morning) from suspected PTB patients and fine needle aspirate (FNA) samples fromsuspected EPTB cases were collected by trained laboratory technicians and pathologists, respectively.

The samples were first digested and concentrated/decontaminated by the N-acetyl-L-cysteine-Sodium hydroxide (NALC-NaOH) method. Smears of the final deposits from the various specimens were stained by the Ziehl-Neelsen (ZN) method and examined under oil immersion using a binocular light microscope. All smear positive TB samples were stored at +4°C at the study site and then transported to Regional Health Research Laboratory Center (Bahirdar) and kept at +4°C until bacteriological culture was performed.

Similarly, FNA specimens were collected by pathologists and stored in cryo-tubes in phosphate buffer saline (PBS) with pH 7.2. ZN staining was performed. AFB-positive specimens were stored at −20°C until mycobacterial culture was performed.

The samples were processed for culturing according to the standard methods described earlier [11, 12]. Both sputum and FNA samples were cultured at the Bahir Dar Regional Health Research Laboratory Centre.

To differentiate *M. tuberculosis* from other members of the *M. tuberculosis* complex (MTBC) species, RD9-based PCR was performed according to protocols previously described [13]. In addition spoligotyping and *M. tuberculosis* drug resistance (MTBDR*plus* assay) molecular tests were used to differentiate *M. tuberculosis* from other members of mycobacteria. *M. tuberculosis* H37Rv, *M. bovis* bacille Calmette Guérin (BCG) were included as positive controls and water was used as a negative control. Interpretation of the result was based on bands of different sizes (396 base pairs (bp) for *M. tuberculosis* and 375 bp for *M. bovis*) as previously described [14].

4. Animal Study

4.1. Single Intradermal Comparative Tuberculin Test. Single intradermal comparative tuberculin test (SIDCTT) was performed for detecting TB in cattle. SICTT was done using both bovine and avian purified protein derivatives (PPDs) (Prionics Lelystad B. V., The Netherlands). The tuberculin test measures the hypersensitivity reaction on the skin due to the administered antigens (PPDs).

Two sites were shaved in the middle of the side of the neck, one above the other, separated by about 12 cm for injection of the two PPDs. The thickness of the skin fold at both injection sites was measured using a caliper and recorded before injection. The sites were injected with 0.1 ml (2000IU) aliquot of bovine PPD and 0.1 ml (2500IU) of avian PPD intradermally. After 72 h, the two sites were measured for change in skin thickness, and the result was interpreted according to international [15] and local [16] criteria.

5. Data Analysis

Data were entered in to Excel file format and transferred in to SPSS software version 25 for statistical analysis. Descriptive statistics were used to depict the demographic variables. Chi-square (χ^2) test was used to test differences in proportions and the association between categorical variables with raw milk consumption habit. Bivariate and multivariate logistic regressions were used to determine the association between background variables with awareness of zoonotic TB and tuberculin reactivity in cattle. Results were considered statistically significant whenever p -value was less than 5%.

5.1. Ethics Approval and Consent to Participate. Ethical clearance for the study was obtained from the Ethics Committee of Addis Ababa University, College of Natural and Computational Science (Ref. CNSDO/491/07/15). In addition, written permission was sought from the Amhara Regional Health Bureau Research Ethical Committee (Ref. HRTT/1/271/07). Each study participant consented with a written form and agreed to participate in the study after a clear explanation of the study objectives and patient data confidentiality. In case of participants under the age of 18 years, consent was obtained from their parents/guardians. The animals used in this study were privately owned by the study participants, and a written consent was sought from the owners to take samples from the animals. A high standard veterinary care was taken to minimize cattle suffering during tuberculin test.

6. Results

6.1. Tuberculosis in Farmers. Culture positivity was obtained in 59.7% (111/186) of the active TB cases. Of which, 59.5% (66/111) was isolated from EPTB patients. The molecular typing of culture positive isolates using RD9-based PCR revealed that all isolates had intact RD9 locus and were subsequently classified as *M. tuberculosis.* No *M. bovis* was detected (Figure 1). In addition, the spoligotyping and molecular anti-TB drug sensitivity tests also confirmed that all the mycobacterial isolates from human TB patients were *M. tuberculosis* (data not shown).

6.2. Awarness on Zoonotic Transmission of TB and Food Consumption Habit. About 68% (74/111) of the respondents did not know about the transmission of TB from cattle to human or vice versa. About 69% (77/111) of the respondents had the habit of consuming raw milk and other uncooked dairy products (Table 1).

The logistic regression, taking log-odds of awareness about zoonotic transmission as an outcome variable, resulted patient origin, and educational status were observed to be significantly associated ($p < 0.05$) (Table 1). The study participants in Libo kemkem and Simada were 11 and 10 times more aware about the zoonotic tramnsmission of TB as compared to those of Dera District (Libo kemkem vs. Dera AOR = 11.84; 95% CI: 1.67–73.2; $p = 0.003$) and (Simada vs. Dera AOR = 10.47; 95% CI: 0.72–116.3; $p = 0.038$). The odds of having awareness on zoonotic transmission of TB was higher among individuals with secondary school educational level (AOR = 4.16; 95% CI: 1.05–15.57; $p = 0.029$) compared to those of illiterates (Table 1).

However, other patient characteristics such as age groups, sex, TB history in the family, raw milk consumption habit, and patient category (new or retreatment cases) were not significantly associated with particpants' over all awarness about zoonotic transmission of TB (Table 1).

7. Tuberculosis in Cattle

7.1. Characteristics of the Study Cattle. The majority of the cattle were females accounting for 54.2% (258/476) of the study cattle. Cattle within the age range of 5–10 years had the greatest share (47%) from the total cattle tested with a mean age of 5.5 years. Many of the cattle, 447 (94%), were Zebu breed, while only 29 (6%) of them were cross breed (Table 2). None of the study cattle had previous exposure to BCG vaccination.

7.2. Prevalence of TB in Cattle. Animal prevalence was 1.6% (5/315) and 1.2% (2/161) at ≥2 mm cut-off value in TB positive and TB free households, respectively. Using

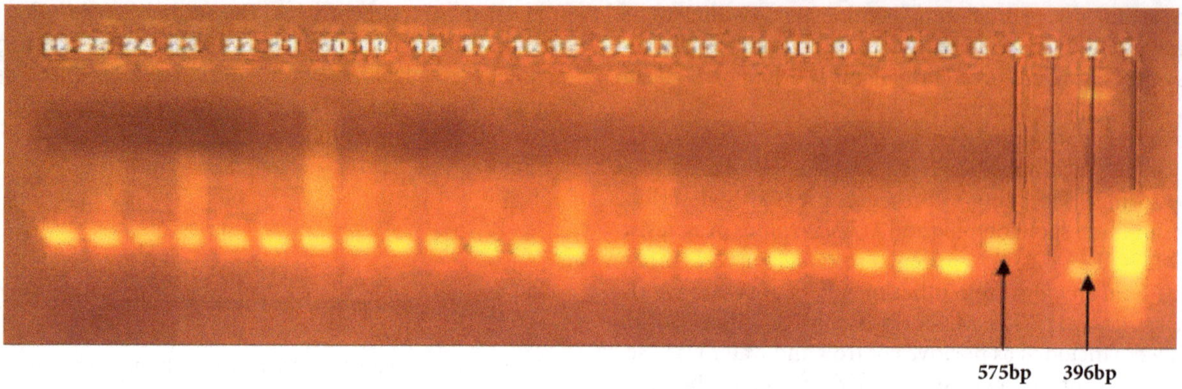

FIGURE 1: Electrophoretic separation of PCR products by RD9 deletion typing. The figure represents only for 22 mycobacteria isolates from sputum and FNA human samples: Lane 1 DNA ladder, 2 *M. tuberculosis* control (396 base pair), 3 molecular grade water (negative control), 4 *M. bovis* control (575 bp), lane 5_26 are culture isolates of *M. tuberculosis* from human tuberculosis patients designated with their sample code as: 5FE1, 6FE2,7FE3,8FE4, 9FE7, 10FE11, 11FE12,12FE15, 13FE16,14FE19,15FE21, 16FE23, 17FE24, 18FE25, 19FE27, 20FE28, 21FE31, 22FE33, 23FE36, 24FE38, 25FE47, 26FE48.

TABLE 1: Association of demographic factors with awarness to zoonotic transmission of TB among AFB culture positive TB patients (N = 111), South Gondar Zone, northwest Ethiopia (2015–2017).

Demographic factors	Number of respondents (%)	Aware of zoonotic TB		COR (95% CI)	AOR (95% CI)	p-value
		Yes (%)	No (%)			
Patient origin						
Dera	26 (23.4)	6 (23.1)	20 (76.9)	1.00	1.00	
Ebinat	10 (9)	2 (20)	8 (80)	0.83 (0.13–5.03)	0.66 (0.39–1.28)	0.842
Este	15 (13.5)	1 (6.7)	14 (93.3)	0.23 (0.02–2.20)	0.25 (0.01–2.53)	0.178
Farta	9 (8.1)	2 (22.2)	7 (77.8)	0.95 (0.15–5. 86)	0.63 (0.02–5.53)	1.00
Fogera	35 (31.5)	13 (37.1)	22 (62.9)	1.96 (0.62–6.16)	1.99 (0.58–8.02)	0.240
Gayint	6 (5.4)	3 (50)	3 (50)	3.33 (0.52–21.03)	3.24 (0.31–21.0)	0.186
Libo kemkem	7 (6.3)	5 (71.4)	2 (28.6)	11.66 (1.89–71.79)	11.84 (1.67–73.2)	0.003
Simada	3 (2.7)	2 (66.7)	1 (39.3)	10.0 (0.87–114.74)	10.47 (0.72–116.3)	0.038
Age group (year)						
<18	10 (9)	5 (50)	5 (50)	1.00	1.00	
18–30	42 (37.8)	17 (40.5)	25 (59.5)	0.68 (0.17–2.71)	0.64 (0.13–2.94)	0.583
31–43	35 (31.5)	8 (22.9)	27 (77.1)	0.29 (0.06–1.28)	0.32 (0.04–1.42)	0.094
44–56	18 (16.2)	5 (27.8)	13 (72.2)	0.38 (0.07–1.92)	0.46 (0.09–2.31)	0.239
>56	6 (5.4)	2 (33.3)	4 (66.7)	0.50 (0.06–4.09)	0.51 (0.07–5.21)	0.515
Sex						
Male	58 (52.3)	18 (31.0)	40 (69.0)	1.00	1.00	
Female	53 (47.7)	19 (35.8)	34 (64.2)	1.24 (0.56–2.73)	1.16 (0.49–2.97)	0.590
Education status						
Illiterate	73 (65.8)	22 (30.1)	51 (69.9)	1.00	1.00	
Adult education	5 (4.5)	1 (0.2)	4 (99.8)	0.57 (0.06–5.48)	0.23 (0.04–5.53)	0.630
Primary level	18 (16.2)	4 (22.2)	14 (77.8)	0.66 (0.19–2.24)	0.62 (0.08–2.62)	0.505
Secondary level	11 (9.9)	7 (63.6)	4 (36.4)	4.05 (1.07–15.28)	4.16 (1.05–15.57)	0.029
Higher level	4 (3.6)	3 (0.75)	1 (0.25)	6.95 (0.68–70.60)	6.52 (0.62–70.71)	0.062
Raw milk consumption						
Yes	77 (69.4)	27 (35.1)	50 (64.9)	1.00	1.00	
No	34 (30.6)	10 (29.4)	24 (70.6)	0.71 (0.29–1.69)	0.71 (0.26–1.88)	0.441
Patient category						
New	91 (82.0)	29 (31.9)	62 (68.1)	1.00	1.00	
*Retreatment	20 (18.0)	8 (40.0)	12 (60.0)	1.42 (0.52–3.86)	1.38 (0.42–3.93)	0.484

*Retreatment: A patient who remained smear positive or became again smear positive at the end of five months or later after commencing treatment. COR: Crude odds ratio, AOR: Adjusted odds ratio, CI: Confidence interval.

Table 2: Association of host risk factors with bovine tuberculin test reactivity in cattle based on a ≥2 mm cut-off value, South Gondar Zone, northwest Ethiopia (2015–2018).

Characteristics	Tuberculin test (N = 476) Positive	Negative	Total (%)	COR (95% CI)	AOR (95% CI)	p-value
Age of cattle (years)						
<5	1	160	161 (33.8)	1		
5–10	5	203	208 (43.7)	4.11 (0.47–35.55)	3.10 (0.35–35.69)	0.16
>10	1	106	107 (22.5)	1.58 (0.09–25.45)	1.69 (0.16–25.93)	0.74
Sex						
Male	2	215	217 (45.6)	1		
Female	5	254	259 (54.4)	2.11 (0.40–11.01)	2.16 (0.35–12.21)	0.36
Breed type						
Local	6	441	447 (94.0)	1		
Cross	1	28	29 (6.0)	2.62 (0.30–22.56)	2.67 (0.25–23.74)	0.36
Source						
Homebred	5	364	369 (77.3)	1		
Purchased	2	105	107 (22.7)	1.38 (0.27–7.25)	1.38 (0.17–7.55)	0.69
Body condition						
Poor	1	196	197 (41.4)	1		
Medium	3	204	207 (43.5)	2.88 (0.29–27.94)	3.00 (0.27–28.38)	0.33
Good	3	69	72 (15.1)	8.52 (0.87–83.29)	8.53 (0.85–83.34)	0.02
Household TB status						
Negative	2	159	161 (33.8)	1		
Positive	5	310	315 (66.2)	1.28 (0.24–6.68)	1.39 (0.31–7.10)	0.76

N: number of total cattle tested. COR: crude odds ratio, AOR: Adjusted odds ratio, CI: confidence interval.

the same cut-off value, 7.9% (5/63) and 6.3% (2/32) herd prevalence was recorded in cattle owned by TB positive and TB free households, respectively. The overall animal and herd prevalence was 1.5% (7/476) and 7.4% (7/95), respectively. However, none of the tested cattle were positive for bovine TB at the international cut-off value of >4 mm.

7.3. Risk Factors for Bovine TB. Risk factor analysis to the occurrence of bovine TB in cattle revealed that age groups between 5 and 10 years were more reactive, but not statistically significant ($P > 0.05$), to tuberculin test than younger age groups (AOR = 3.1; 95% CI: 0.35–35.69; $p = 0.16$). Cattle with apparently good (AOR = 8.53; 95% CI: 0.85–83.34; $p = 0.02$) and medium (AOR = 3.00; 95% CI: 0.27–28.38; $p = 0.33$) body conditions were more likely to be reactive to the tuberculin test as compared to those with apparently poor body condition, and the difference was statistically significant ($p < 0.05$) (Table 2). Although the difference was not statistically significant ($p > 0.05$), the odds of bovine TB that cattle owned by TB positive cases were slightly higher than those owned by TB free households (AOR = 1.39; 95% CI: 0.31–7.10; $p = 0.76$). Despite the observed differences, sex, breed type, source of cattle, and households TB status were not significantly associated ($p > 0.05$) with the occurrence of BTB in the present study (Table 2).

7.4. Zoonotic Transmission of TB. In the present study, molecular typing of culture positive isolates using RD9-based PCR confirmed that all the human isolates were *M. tuberculosis* (Figure 1). Furthermore, no *M. bovis* was detected even from those TB patients who owned tuberculin reactor cattle. Hence, this study did not reveal evidence of direct transmission of tuberculosis from cattle to their closely associated owners.

8. Discussion

The identification of *M. tuberculosis* as the only *Mycobacterium* species in the present study, using RD9-based PCR, was in agreement with previous reports in other parts of Ethiopia in which all or the majority of the isolates found from human TB cases were *M. tuberculosis* [6, 17–19], suggesting a minimal contribution of *M. bovis* to the overall burden of human TB. In contrast, previous studies conducted in large scale commercial farms and pastoral communities suggested the contribution of *M. bovis* to the overall burden of TB in humans [20, 21]. The reason for the difference in *Mycobacterium* species prevalence in this study and previous studies might be due to the low TB infection rate in cattle owned by smallholder farmers that participated in the present study.

Although zoonotic transmission of *M. bovis* from cattle to famers was expected, all the human isolates were *M. tuberculosis*. Nonetheless, previous study conducted in and around Bahir Dar City [8], Borena Zone [20] and Afar Region reported the isolation of *M. bovis* from human TB cases. It has been well established in the literature that the prevalence of human TB caused by *M. bovis* in specific geographic region is directly proportional to the prevalence of bovine TB in that specific geographic region [22]. In the present study, the prevalence of bovine TB was very low and hence the chance of its transmission to humans is minimal.

Nevertheless, the awareness of farmers about zoonotic transmission of TB was low and thus was similar to the magnitude of awareness recorded by previous studies conducted in Ethiopia [8, 21, 23] and in other countries including Zambia and Zimbabwe [24, 25]. The poor awarness of farmers on the transmission of zoonotic TB to them could pose risk of infection by zoonotic pathogens including *M. bovis,* suggesting a need for an awareness creation campaign about zoonotic TB in the study area. On the other hand, in contrast to the low awareness of the farmers included in the present study, farmers in Cameroon and Malawi had good awareness on the zoonotic TB and its transmission [26, 27].

Although *M. bovis* was not isolated from the farmers with active TB, majority of culture posistive TB patients had the habit of consuming raw milk. This observation is similar to the observation of previous studies conducted in different parts of Ethiopia [8, 28–30]. The higher preference of raw milk consumption in Ethiopia could be associated to culture, its taste, availability in the local market, an easy access from a door to door supply by farmers and lower price [31].

The animal and herd prevalence of bovine TB at a severe cut-off value of SICTT were low in South Gondar Zone of north-western Ethiopia. In agreement with the prevalence report of this study, low prevalence of bovine TB was reported in and around Bahir Dar City and Yeki District of southern Ethiopia [6, 32]. On the other hand, higher prevalence of bovine TB was reported in and around other cities of Ethiopia [16, 33–36]. These variations in the prevalence of bovine TB are associated with the breed of cattle kept and the type of husbandry under which the cattle are kept. Previous studies in Ethiopia have indicated that *Bos taurus* breed is more susceptible to bovine TB as compared to *Bos indicus* breed [37]. In the present study about 94% of the study cattle were local Zebu breeds, which might be the reason for the low power detection of tuberculin reactivity even at a cut-off value of 2 mm. Moreover, it was observed that cattle kept in intensive farms are more susceptible to bovine TB as compared to cattle kept in extensive farms [37]. In addition, it was well established that the prevalence of bovine TB is directly associated with the herd size [37]. Thus, the observation of low prevalence bovine TB in the present study is not surprising as all the study cattle were *Bos indicus* and were also kept in extensive farming; both of which do not favour the occurrence and transmission of bovine TB. Furthermore, all the herds included in the present study were small (ranging from 3 to 10 cattle per herd) and thus did not favour the transmission of bovine TB.

Nevertheless, although the overall prevalence of bovine TB recorded by the present study was low, it was relatively higher in cattle owned by TB positive households than cattle owned by TB free households. But the difference of prevalence between the two groups was not statistically significant. Other earlier studies reported higher prevalence of bovine TB in cattle owned by households with active TB cases than TB free households [7, 34, 38, 39]. Such observation could suggest the existence of TB transmission between cattle and their owners. The transmission could be zoonotic (transmission of *M. bovis* from cattle to humans) or reverse zoonotic (transmission of *M. tuberculosis* from humans to cattle). In the present study, isolation of mycobacteria was not done from cattle and diagnosis of bovine TB was made by SICTT. On the other hand, all the human isolates were *M. tuberculosis.* This could imply that *M. tuberculosis* might have been transmitted to cattle from their owners and positivity to SICTT was due to sensitization to infection with *M. tuberculosis* as it was observed earlier by other authors [13, 38, 40].

The present study has some limitations in conducting pathological examination and there by strain identification of mycobacteria isolates from tuberculin reactor cattle, which could give more power to infer TB transmission between humans and cattle.

9. Conclusion

All the human isolates recovered from farmers with active TB cases were *M. tuberculosis* and no *M. bovis* was isolated. Moreover, the overall prevalence of bovine TB in the area was low; but it was slightly higher in cattle owned by households with active TB cases than in cattle owned with active TB free households; which could suggest the presence of zoonotic and or reverse zoonotic transmission of TB between cattle and their owners. This could also be exacerbated by the low level of awareness of the farmers on the transmission of mycobacterial species between cattle and their owners.

Acknowledgments

We would like to thank all laboratory working staff and administrators at the Regional Health research Center, Bahirdar and ALIPB, Addis Ababa University, for their support in the development of this study. We also greatly thank health officials, laboratory workers, and study participants in the study area, without whom this study would have not been completed.

References

[1] World Health Organization, "Global zoonotic tuberculosis report 2017," Geneva, Switzerland, 2017, http://www.who.int/tb/areas-of-work/zoonotic-tb/en.

[2] D. A. Ashford, E. Whitney, P. Raghunathan, and O. Cosivi, "Epidemiology of selected mycobacteria that infect humans and other animals," *Revue Scientifique et Technique de l'OIE*, vol. 20, no. 1, pp. 325–337, 2001.

[3] S. Cleaveland, D. J. Shaw, G. Mfinanga et al., "*Mycobacterium bovis* in rural Tanzania: risk factors for infection in human and cattle populations," *Tuberculosis*, vol. 87, no. 1, pp. 30–43, 2007.

[4] J. D. Mawak, N. E. Gomwalk, C. S. S. Bello, and Y. T. Kandakai-Olukemi, "Human pulmonary infections with bovine and environment (atypical) mycobacteria in Jos Nigeria," *Ghana Medical Journal*, vol. 40, no. 4, pp. 132–136, 2006.

[5] J. Oloya, J. Opuda Asibo, R. Kazwala et al., "Mycobacteria causing human cervical lymphadenitis in pastoral communities in the Karamoja region of Uganda," *Epidemiology and Infection*, vol. 136, no. 5, pp. 636–643, 2008.

[6] A. Nuru, G. Mamo, L. Teshome et al., "Bovine tuberculosis and its risk factors among dairy cattle herds in and around Bahir Dar City, Northwest Ethiopia," *Ethiopian Veterinary Journal*, vol. 19, no. 2, pp. 27–40, 2015.

[7] A. Mengistu, F. Enqusselasie, A. Aseffa, and D. Beyene, "Bovine tuberculosis in rural Ethiopia: a comparative cross-sectional study on cattle owned by households with and without tuberculosis," *Mycobacterial Diseases*, vol. 5, no. 4, 2015.

[8] A. Nuru, G. Mamo, A. Zewude et al., "Preliminary investigation of the transmission of tuberculosis between farmers and their cattle in smallholder farms in northwestern Ethiopia: a cross-sectional study," *BMC Research Notes*, vol. 10, no. 1, Article ID 31, 2017.

[9] Central Statistics Agency (Ethiopia), "Summary and statistical report of the population and housing census: population size by age and sex," Addis Ababa, Ethiopia, 2007, https://www.scribd.com/doc/28289334/Summary-and-Statistical-Report-of-the-2007.

[10] Ethiopia Demographic and Health Survey, "Central Statistical Agency 2011 Ethiopia and ICF International Calverton, Maryland, USA Addis Ababa," https://www.unicef.org/ethiopia/ET_2011_EDHS.pdf.

[11] Federal Ministry of Health (Ethiopia), "Tuberculosis, Leprosy and TB/HIV Prevention and Control Programme. Addis Ababa, Ethiopia," 4th edition, 2008, http://www.who.int/hiv/pub/guidelines/ethiopia_tb.pdf.

[12] World Health Organization, "Laboratory services in tuberculosis control: culture. Part III, Geneva, Switzerland 1998," https://apps.who.int/iris/bitstream/10665/65942/3/WHO_TB_98.258_%28part3%29.pdf.

[13] S. Berg, R. Firdessa, M. Habtamu et al., "The burden of mycobacterial disease in Ethiopian cattle: implications for public health," *PLoS One*, vol. 4, no. 4, e5068 pages, 2009.

[14] L. M. Parsons, R. Brosch, S. T. Cole et al., "Rapid and simple approach for identification of *Mycobacterum tuberculosis* complex isolates by PCR-based genomic deletion analysis," *Journal of Clinical Microbiology*, vol. 40, no. 7, pp. 2339–2345, 2002.

[15] Office International des, "Epizooties Terrestrial manual: World Health Organization for Animal Health, Paris. 2009," https://www.devex.com/organizations/world-organisation-for-animal-health-oie-48619.

[16] G. Ameni, G. Hewinson, A. Aseffa, D. Young, and M. Vordermeier, "Appraisal of interpretation criteria for the comparative intradermal tuberculin test for the diagnosis of bovine tuberculosis in Central Ethiopia," *Clinical and Vaccine Immunology*, vol. 15, no. 8, pp. 1272–1276, 2008.

[17] B. Diriba, T. Berkessa, G. Mamo, Y. Tedla, and G. Ameni, "Spoligotyping ofmultid-rug-resistant *Mycobacteriumtuberculosis* isolates in Ethiopia," *International. Journal of Tuberculosis and Lung Disease*, vol. 17, no. 2, pp. 246–250, 2013.

[18] M. Belay, G. Ameni, G. Bjune, D. Couvin, N. Rastogi, and F. Abebe, "Strain diversity of *Mycobacterium tuberculosis* isolates from pulmonary tuberculosis patients in Afar pastoral region of Ethiopia," *BioMedical Research International*, vol. 2014, Article ID 238532, pp. 1–12, 2014.

[19] T. Debebe, A. Admassu, G. Mamo, and G. Ameni, "Molecular characterization of *Mycobacterium tuberculosis* isolated from pulmonary tuberculosis patients in Felege Hiwot Referral Hospital, northwest Ethiopia," *Journal of Microbiology Immunology and Infection*, vol. 47, no. 4, pp. 333–338, 2014.

[20] B. Gumi, E. Schelling, S. Berg et al., "Zoonotic transmission of tuberculosis between pastoralists and their livestock in South-East Ethiopia," *Eco Health*, vol. 9, no. 2, pp. 139–149, 2012.

[21] M. Tibebu, W. Mekonnen, T. Awoke et al., "A high prevalence of tuberculosis among dairy farm workers in Addis Ababa and its surroundings," *Mycobacterial Diseases*, vol. 4, no. 1, p. 139, 2014.

[22] O. Cosivi, M. Grange, J. Daborn, C. Raviglione, T. Fujikura, and D. Cousins, "Zoonotic tuberculos-is due to *Mycobacterium bovis* in developing countries," *Emerging Infectious Diseases*, vol. 4, no. 1, pp. 59–70, 1998.

[23] B. Temesgen, M. Shigut, T. Hailemariam, and E. Chali, "Assessment of community awareness towards zoonotic tuberculosis in West Shoa, Ethiopia," *Clinical Medicine Research*, vol. 6, no. 2, pp. 37–42, 2017.

[24] M. Munyeme, B. Muma, H. M. Munang'Andu, C. Kankya, E. Skjerve , and M. Tryland , "Cattle owners' awareness of bovine tuberculosis in high and low prevalence settings of the wildlife-livestock interface areas in Zambia," *BMC Veterinary Research*, vol. 6, no. 1, p. 21, 2010.

[25] D. Mosalagae, D. M. Pfukenyi, and G. Matope, "Milk producers' awareness of milk borne zoonoses in selected smallholder and commercial dairy farms of Zimbabwe," *Tropical Animal Health and Production*, vol. 43, no. 3, pp. 733–739, 2011.

[26] J. Ndukum, C. Kudi, G. Bradley, N. Ane-Anyangwe, S. Fon-Tebug, and J. Tchoumboue, "Prevalence of bovine tuberculosis in abattoirs of the littoral and Western highland regions of Cameroon: a cause for public health concern," *Veterinary Medicine International*, vol. 2010, Article ID 495015, pp. 1–8, 2010.

[27] S. F. Tebug, G. R. Njunga, M. G. Chagunda, J. P. Mapemba, J. Awah-Ndukum, and S. Risk Wiedemann, "knowledge and preventive measures of smallholder dairy farmers in northern Malawi with regard to zoonotic brucellosis and bovine tuberculosis," *Onderstepoort Journal of Veterinary Research*, vol. 81, no. 1, 2014.

[28] W. Tigre, G. Alemayehu, T. Abetu, and B. Deressa Gelalcha, "Preliminary study on public health implication of bovine tuberculosis in Jimma town South Western Ethiopia," *Global Veterinaria*, vol. 6, no. 4, pp. 369–373, 2011.

[29] H. K. Abraham, S. Dessalegn, M. Aklilu, and M. Pal, "Knowledge, attitude and practice towards human and bovine tuberculosis among high school students in Addis Ababa, Ethiopia," *International Journal of Livestock Research*, vol. 5, no. 1, pp. 1–11, 2015.

[30] L. G. Gebremichael, B. S. Fanta, S. M. Abay, and C. D. Subas, "Anti-tuberculosis drug resistance in Ethiopia: a mata- analysis," *Journal of Drug Delivery and Therapeutics*, vol. 4, no. 3, pp. 154–163, 2014.

[31] The Netherlands Development Organization, "Dairy investment opportunities in EthiopiaAddis Ababa: 2008," 148 pages, http://www.primeethiopia.org/wpcontent/uploads/2015/03/dairy_investment_opportunities_in_ethiopia.pdf.

[32] P. Admasu, W. Berihun, and A. Niguse, "Prevalence of bovine tuberculosis in dairy cattle of Yeki district, Southern Ethiopia," *African Journal of Basic and Applied Sciences*, vol. 6, no. 5, pp. 135–140, 2014.

[33] G. Ameni and E. Aklilu, "Bovine tuberculosis on small-scale dairy farms in Adama Town, central Ethiopia, and farmer awareness of the disease," *Revue Scientifique et Technique-Office International des Epizooties*, vol. 26, no. 3, pp. 711–719, 2007.

[34] A. Regassa, G. Medhin, and G. Ameni, "Bovine tuberculosis is more prevalent in cattle owned by farmers with active tuberculosis in central Ethiopia," *The Veterinary Journal*, vol. 178, no. 1, pp. 119–125, 2008.

[35] W. Tsegaye, A. Aseffa, A. Mache, Y. Mengistu, B. Stefan, and G. Ameni, "Conventional and molecular epidemiology of bovine tuberculosis in dairy farms in Addis Ababa city, the capital of Ethiopia," *The International Journal of Applied Research in Veterinary Medicine*, vol. 8, no. 2, pp. 143–151, 2010.

[36] R. Firdessa, R. Tschopp, A. Wubete et al., "High prevalence of bovine tuberculosis in dairy cattle in central Ethiopia: implications for the dairy industry and public health," *PLoS One*, vol. 7, no. 12, p. e52851, 2012.

[37] G. Ameni, A. Aseffa, H. Engers, D. Young, G. Hewinson, and M. Vordermeier, "Cattle husbandry in Ethiopia is a predominant factor affecting the pathology of bovine tuberculosis and gamma interferon responses to Mycobacterial antigens," *Clinical and Vaccine Immunology*, vol. 13, no. 9, pp. 1030–1036, 2006.

[38] G. Ameni, K. Tadesse, E. Hailu et al., "Transmission of *Mycobacterium. tuberculosis* between farmers and cattle in central Ethiopia," *PLoS One*, vol. 8, no. 10, e76891 pages, 2013.

[39] F. Tamiru, M. Hailemariam, and W. Terfa, "Preliminary study on prevalence of bovine tuberculo-sis in cattle owned by tuberculosis positive and negative farmers and assessment of zoonotic awareness in Ambo and Toke Kutaye districts, Ethiopia," *Journal of Veterinary Medicine and Animal Health*, vol. 5, pp. 288–295, 2013.

[40] G. Ameni, M. Vordermeierb, R. Firdessa et al., "*Mycobacterium tuberculosis* infection in grazing cattle in central Ethiopia," *The Veterinary Journal*, vol. 188, no. 3, pp. 359–361, 2011.

16

Predictors of Treatment Outcomes among Multidrug Resistant Tuberculosis Patients in Tanzania

Tamary Henry Leveri,[1,2] **Isack Lekule,**[2] **Edson Mollel,**[1,3] **Furaha Lyamuya,**[1] **and Kajiru Kilonzo**[1]

[1]*Kilimanjaro Christian Medical University College, P.O. Box 2240, Moshi, Tanzania*
[2]*Kibong'oto Infectious Diseases Hospital, P.O. Box 12, Sanya Juu, Tanzania*
[3]*Western Zone Blood Transfusion Center, P.O. Box 1782, Tabora, Tanzania*

Correspondence should be addressed to Tamary Henry Leveri; tamaryhenry@yahoo.com

Academic Editor: Isamu Sugawara

Background. According to World Health Organization (WHO) the final multidrug resistant tuberculosis (MDRTB) treatment outcome is the most important direct measurement of the effectiveness of the MDRTB control program. Literature review has shown marked diversity in predictors of treatment outcomes worldwide even among the same continents. Therefore, findings could also be different in Tanzanian context, where the success rate is still lower than the WHO recommendation. This study sought to determine the predictors of treatment outcomes among MDRTB patients in Tanzania in order to improve the success rate. *Methodology.* This was a retrospective cohort study, which was conducted at Kibong'oto Infectious Diseases Hospital (KIDH) in Tanzania. Patients' demographic and clinical parameters were collected from the MDRTB registry and clinical files. Then, a detailed analysis was done to determine the predictors of successful and unsuccessful MDRTB treatment outcomes. *Results.* Three hundred and thirty-two patients were diagnosed and put on MDRTB treatment during the year 2009 to 2014. Among them, males were 221 (67%), and 317 (95.48%) were above 18 years of age, mean age being 36.9 years. One hundred and sixty-one patients (48.5%) were living in Dar es Salaam. The number of MDRTB patients has increased from 16 in 2009 to 132 in 2014. Majority of patients (75.7%) had successful treatment outcomes. The following predictors were significantly associated with MDRTB cure: presence of cavities in chest X-rays (aOR 1.89, p value 0.002), low BMI (aOR 0.59, p value 0.044), and resistance to streptomycin (aOR 4.67, p value 0.007) and ethambutol (aOR 0.34, p value 0.041). Smoking and presence of cavities in chest X-rays were associated with MDRTB mortality, aOR 2.31, p value 0.043 and aOR 0.55, p value 0.019, respectively. *Conclusion.* The study indicated that overall number of MDRTB patients and the proportion of successful treatment outcomes have been increasing over the years. The study recommends improving nutritional status of MDRTB patients, widespread antismoking campaign, and close follow-up of patients with ethambutol resistance.

1. Introduction

Drug resistant tuberculosis (DRTB) is a form of tuberculosis (TB), which is resistant to any of the first line antituberculosis drugs. There are different types of DRTB such as monoresistant tuberculosis and multidrug resistant tuberculosis (MDRTB). The former is a form of tuberculosis, which is resistant to any single drug of the first line antituberculosis medications while the latter is resistant to key first line antituberculosis drugs, rifampicin, and isoniazid. Polyresistant tuberculosis is resistant to more than one first line drugs, other than both rifampicin and isoniazid. Extensively Resistant Tuberculosis (XDRTB) includes MDRTB and additional resistance to any of the fluoroquinolones and any of the injectable second line medications.

Among all TB cases worldwide, 3.7% of new cases and 20% of previously treated cases have DRTB [1]. Despite an increased DRTB awareness and roll-out of molecular tests such as Xpert MTB for diagnosis of DRTB, which has enabled early treatment initiation, DRTB and especially MDRTB are still a disease of public health concern. This affects the global efforts to control TB [2].

Globally, there were an estimated 480,000 new cases of MDRTB and an additional 100,000 new cases of rifampicin resistant tuberculosis (RRTB) in the year 2015 [1]. Worldwide the MDRTB/RRTB treatment success rate was only 52%, with 17% mortality [1].

In Tanzania the MDRTB treatment success rate is only 68%, which is lower than that recommended by World Health Organization (WHO) of above 75% [1]. Furthermore, the MDRTB/RRTB incidence has been increasing to 4.9 per 100,000 for year 2015 [1].

According to WHO the final MDRTB treatment outcome is the most important direct measurement of the effectiveness of the MDRTB control program [3]. There are six MDRTB treatment outcomes "cured" (which is restricted to pulmonary TB cases only), "completed", "died", "failed", "lost to follow up", and "MDRTB cases on MDRTB treatment regimen with no outcome assigned (transferred, still on treatment, or unknown)" [3]. Successful treatment includes being cured and completing treatment, while unsuccessful treatment includes dying, treatment failure, and loss to follow-up.

Cases that have not been evaluated due to transfer or still not completed treatment at the time of final assessment or missing information are all grouped together. Indicators are measured 24 months after the end of the year of assessment to give sufficient time for most patients to complete their treatment and for the final culture results to be issued and retrieved [3].

Treatment of MDRTB is complicated, takes long duration, is associated with several adverse events, and is very expensive [2]. MDRTB treatment is also associated with unsuccessful outcomes compared to non-MDRTB treatment [4]. In the quest to address some of these challenges the WHO has introduced a short treatment regimen for treating MDRTB patients [5].

Tanzania has adopted the new short regimen and has now decentralized MDRTB diagnosis and treatment to the peripheral hospitals which was initially only done at Kibong'oto Infectious Diseases Hospital (KIDH). Factors that have contributed to decentralization include the high cost of treating these patients in inpatients setting and the overwhelming increase in number of MDRTB diagnosis after the introduction and widespread use of Gene Xpert machines for diagnosis of TB in the country. This has led to a substantial increase in early MDRTB diagnosis and early treatment initiation.

Several studies have been done in other countries to determine the predictors of MDRTB treatment outcomes, in the general population and certain specific groups such as those with HIV coinfection, adults, and children [6]. These studies have shown a wide variation in predictors of treatment outcome among countries worldwide.

Some of the predictors that were found to be associated with successful treatment outcomes include Body Mass Index (BMI) >18.5kg/m^2, use of more than 4 effective drugs, negative baseline sputum smear, and undergoing a surgical resection [7]. Others were the use of fluoroquinolones, or linezolid [8], use of individualized treatment [9], receiving any assistance from TB program, better TB knowledge, and higher level of trust and support from nurses and doctors [10]. Moreover, other studies have focused on the predictors of unsuccessful treatment outcomes, such as extensive drug resistance [8, 11, 12], low BMI [13], hypoalbuminemia [11], comorbidities such as diabetes [11, 14], and cavitary disease [11, 13]. Others were HIV coinfection, positive smear at the start of treatment, and previous history of TB treatment [4, 11, 15], smoking [16, 17], pre-XDRTB, and diabetes mellitus [17],

Other factors include age >44 years [13], resistance to Ofloxacin [8, 15, 18], male sex [16, 19], low body weight at diagnosis < 40 kg [18, 19], and poor drug adherence [19]. Furthermore, smear positivity at month 2 of treatment, use of traditional medicine, and interruption of treatment more than 14 days [14] were also associated with unsuccessful treatment outcome.

In Phillipines, Tupasi and colleagues found that non-HIV immunosuppression, alcohol consumption, lifestyle factors, noncompliance, deficient health education, diabetes, self-rating, and severity of vomiting were the predictors of poor treatment outcome (Loss to follow-up). Other predictors found by other authors include illicit drug use, site of TB [16], ambulatory treatment initiation, having different providers of intensive phase and continuation phase, culture conversion after 4 months [20], and rural residence [18].

However, several studies have shown contradictory findings for some of the factors mentioned above; for example, positive baseline smear and HIV infections were not associated with unsuccessful treatment outcomes [19]. This study aimed to determine the proportions of treatment outcomes and their predictors among MDRTB patients in Tanzania in order to improve the treatment outcomes by combating the predictors or adjusting management protocols accordingly.

2. Methodology

This was a retrospective cohort study. It was done from August 2017 to June 2018. It was conducted at KIDH which is located in Siha District in Kilimanjaro region. It is the national specialized public reference hospital assigned for management of MDRTB patients in Tanzania. All patients who were diagnosed with MDRTB since 2009 in Tanzania mainland and Zanzibar were being treated for 18 to 24 months and admitted at KIDH for the whole duration of initial treatment phase (6 to 8 months depending on sputum culture conversion) until recently when decentralization commenced.

Medical records of all MDRTB patients admitted at KIDH from November 2009 (when the MDRTB program started in Tanzania) to December 2014 were studied. The selection of this timeline was based on the availability of the treatment outcomes as the management of MDRTB by then was 18 to 24 months depending on sputum culture conversion. Sputum culture conversion was defined as two consecutive negative culture results. These patients were treated with the standardized regimen, which included (for the intensive phase of minimum 6 months, or 6 months after culture conversion)

TABLE 1: Patients' sociodemographic characteristics (N=332).

Patient's characteristics	N=332 (% of total)
Age (mean =36.9 years (SD 13.59), median =36 years)	
(i) Below 18	15(4.52)
(ii) Above or equal 18	317(95.48)
Sex	
(i) Male	221(66.6)
(ii) Female	111(33.4)
Residence	
(i) Dar es Salaam	161(48.5)
(ii) Other regions	171(51.5)
Marital status	
(i) Divorced	14(4.20)
(ii) Married	126(38.0)
(iii) Single	176(53.0)
(iv) Widow/widower	16(4.82)

Amikacin or Kanamycin, Ofloxacin or Levofloxacin, Pyrazinamide, Ethionamide, Cycloserine, and Ethambutol. Then continuation phase of minimum 12 months or 18 months after culture conversion included Ofloxacin or Levofloxacin, Ethionamide, Pyrazinamide, Cycloserine, and Ethambutol. Therefore, the outcomes were available two years after finishing treatment, so that proper treatment outcomes can be assigned to the patient. Excluded patients were those who died before initiation of MDRTB treatment and those who were initially diagnosed with MDRTB but were later found to have *Mycobacterium* other than tuberculosis (MOTT).

2.1. Data Collection Method and Tools. Data was collected from the DRTB registry for all patients who were admitted in the KIDH, between November 2009 and December 2014. Data missing in the registry were completed with data from the patients' clinical files. Data collection tool was a data extraction sheet for filling patient's demographic and clinical data.

Study variables were selected in the light of previous studies as shown in the literature review, availability of data, and management protocols in Tanzania context. Available data for the following variables was collected: age, sex, residence, HIV status, history of previously treated TB, smoking status, alcohol use, drug resistance pattern, and the presence of cavities on chest x-rays which was determined by a specialist radiologist. It also included data on baseline BMI, baseline sputum smear and baseline sputum culture.

Treatment outcomes were standardized, as recommended by WHO, as "cured, treatment completed, died, lost to follow-up, and treatment failure" (WHO, 2013). Successful treatment outcomes included declared cured and treatment completion. Unsuccessful treatment outcomes included loss to follow-up, death, and treatment failure.

2.2. Data Analysis Plan. Data was then deidentified and entered in an excel sheet. It was then transferred to a statistical software STATA version 14.2 for analysis. Categorical data were summarized as frequencies and percentages. Continuous data was summarized as mean and standard deviation if normally distributed or median and interquartile range if skewed. Statistical significance was considered at 0.05 level. Predictors of successful treatment outcomes and unsuccessful treatment outcomes were then determined, using chi square test. Logistic regression was used to identify predictors which were independently associated with the treatment outcomes.

2.3. Ethical Considerations. Ethical clearance was sought from Kilimanjaro Christian Medical University College (KCMUCo) Research Ethical Committee, as well as permission to conduct the study from the KIDH administration. Patients' confidentiality and privacy were strictly observed.

3. Results

During the study period data for a total of 332 patients who were admitted at KIDH between 2009 and 2014 was collected. About two-thirds (221 (67%)) of the patients were males, and 317 (95.48%) were above 18 years of age. About half of the patients (161 (48.5%)) had been residing in Dar es Salaam. The mean and median ages of the study population were 36.9 years (SD 13.59) and 36 years (IQR of 27.5 to 46 years), respectively (Table 1). The number of patients being treated at KIDH has been steadily increasing from 2009 when the MDRTB program started (Figure 1).

The majority of patients (273 (82.2%)) had previous TB history while 95 patients (28.6%) and 68 patients (20.5%) had history of alcohol use and smoking, respectively (Table 2). More than one-third of the patients were HIV positive (116 (34.6%)). Out of 212 patients,109 patients (51.42%) had a BMI below 18kg/m^2. A total of 279 X-ray films were available for interpretation and 64 (19.3%) of them had showed cavitary lesions (Table 2). Most of the patients had TB strains resistant to rifampicin (202 patients (60.8%)) and 130 patients (39.2%) were resistant to isoniazid (Table 3). Two hundred and eight patients (62.7%) were cured: 43 (13%) completed treatment,

Table 2: Patients' clinical and radiological features (N=332).

Characteristics	N(% of total)
BMI (N=312)	
(i) Below 18.5 kg/m^2	109(51.42)
(ii) Above or equal to 18.5 kg/m^2	103(48.58)
HIV status	
(i) Positive	116(34.9)
(ii) Negative	216(65.1)
History of previous TB treatment (N=329)	
(i) Yes	273(82.2)
(ii) No	56(16.9)
Smoking history (N=177)	
(i) Yes	68(20.5)
(ii) No	109(32.9)
Alcohol use (N=189)	
(i) Yes	95(28.6)
(ii) No	94(28.3)
Cavitary lesions on Chest x-ray radiography (N=279)	
(i) Yes	64(19.3)
(ii) No	215(64.8)
Diabetes (N=319)	
(i) Yes	5(1.5)
(ii) No	314(94.6)

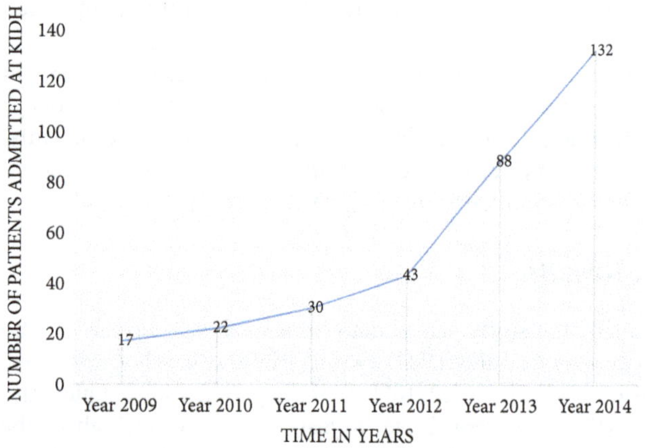

Figure 1: Trend showing increase in patients over years (2009-2014).

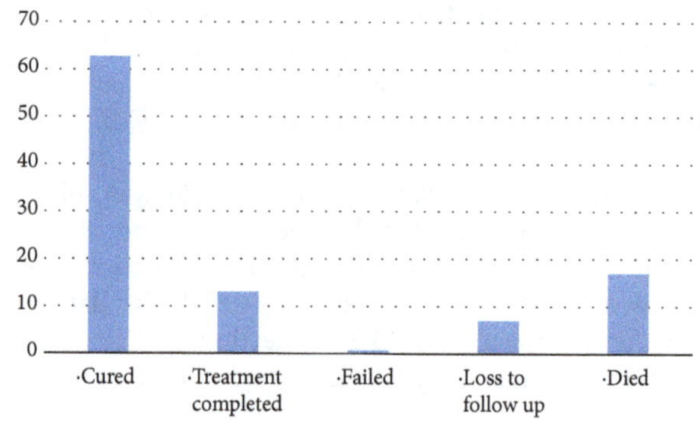

Figure 2: Percentages of patients' treatment outcomes (N=332).

while only 2 (0.6%) had failed treatment (Figure 2) and a total of 252 patients (75.6%) had successful treatment outcome (Figure 3). More than 50% of all patients who have been treated at KIDH were declared cured each year (Figure 4). After multivariate analysis, it was found that low BMI (below 18 kg/m^2) is significantly associated with reduced chance of being cured, aOR=0.59 (95% CI 0.39-0.88), p value of 0.044, while presence of cavitary lesions on chest X-rays had association with being cured of MDRTB (aOR=1.89 (95% CI 1.27-2.81), p value 0.002). Resistance to streptomycin was positively associated with cure, while resistance to ethambutol was negatively associated with cure (aOR =4.67 (95% CI 1.53-14.32), p value 0.007 and 0.34 (95% CI 0.12-0.96), and p value 0.041, respectively), (Table 4). No independent factors were found to be associated with MDRTB treatment completion (Table 5). Resistance to streptomycin and resistance to ethambutol had negatively (aOR =0.14 (95% CI 0.02-1.14), p value 0.066) and positively (aOR=4.65 (95% CI 0.88-24.56), p value 0.070) borderline association with loss to follow-up outcome, respectively (Table 6). Smoking habit and presence of cavitary lesions on chest radiographs were independent factors that became positively and negatively associated with mortality after multivariate analysis, with aORs of 2.31 (95% CI 1.35-5.01), p value of 0.043) and 0.55 (95% CI 0.34-0.91), p value 0.019), respectively, (Table 7).

The sociodemographic characteristics of MDRTB patients admitted at KIDH between 2009 and 2014 (N=332)

Table 3: Patients' drug susceptibility test (DST) results.

Drug name	N(%)
Isoniazid(N=141)	
(i) Resistant	130(39.2)
(ii) Susceptible	11(3.3)
Rifampicin (N=207)	
(i) Resistant	202(60.8)
(ii) Susceptible	5(1.5)
Streptomycin(N=114)	
(i) Resistant	80(24.1)
(ii) susceptible	34(10.2)
Ethambutol (N=110)	
(i) Resistant	73(22.0)
(ii) Susceptible	37(11.1)

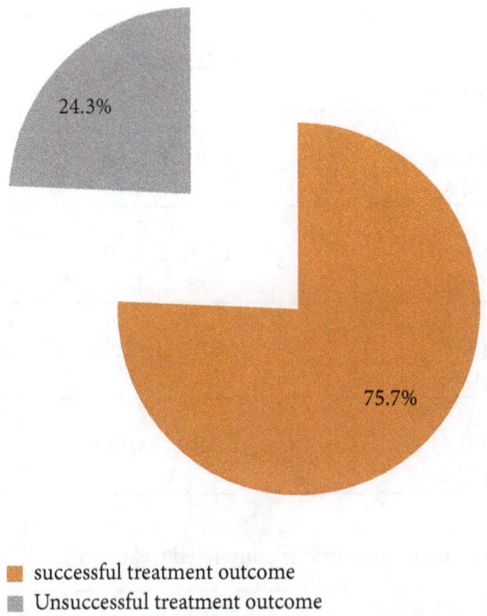

Figure 3: The proportion of successful and unsuccessful treatment outcomes in five years' time. (2009-2014).

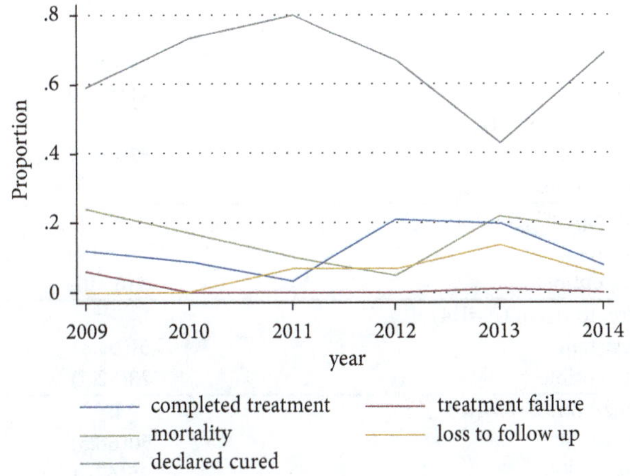

Figure 4: Trends of proportions of patients who were cured, completed treatment, were lost to follow-up, and died from 2009 to 2014.

4. Discussion

This study has found that the absolute numbers of MDRTB patients receiving treatment at KIDH since 2009 has been increasing as well as the number of patients being cured (a total of 208 patients were cured, 62.7% of all patients) (Table 2). Similar findings were observed in South Africa whereby the cure rate was 79% [21]. This could be due to increasing awareness of the MDRTB disease over the time and stability of the services provision by the hospital. Most of the patients, 317 (95.48%) were above 18 years of age, indicating that in Tanzania the most productive age category is the mostly affected with the disease. Forty-eight percent of all these patients were coming from Dar es Salaam, which is the busiest and overcrowded city in the country indicating the potential increased risk of disease transmission in overcrowded cities. Only 116 patients (34.9%) were HIV positive and 273 patients (82.2%) had positive previous TB treatment (Table 2). Only 2 patients (0.6%) had treatment failure during the entire time indicating both effective drug regimens and a stable health system (Figure 2). None of the patient had a missing treatment outcome, also a good indication of the regimen effectiveness and stable health system.

After multivariate analysis, presence of cavities in chest radiographs was associated with cure aOR 1.89. This is different from other findings, for example, a study by Kempker found that cavities were associated with increased drug resistance [22] as well as poor prognosis [11]. It could as well be due to the fact that cavities in the chest radiographs are more common among MDRTB patients compared to drug-sensitive TB patients [23]. But also variations in chest X-rays interpretation could also result in overdetection of cavities among MDRTB patients in our context, as found in Western Europe [24].

Low BMI was found to be significantly related to treatment cure in this study aOR 0.59. Other studies such as the one done by Kwak did not find a significant association between BMI and MDRTB treatment success [8], while

TABLE 4: Adjusted OR after multivariate analysis for predictors of treatment outcome of cure.

Characteristics	Cured N (%)	Other treatment categories N (%)	aOR (95% CI)	p-value
Cavitary lesions on CXR (N=279)				
Yes	45(70.3)	19(29.7)	1.89(1.27-2.81)	0.002
No	143(66.5)	72(33.5)		
BMI				
Below 18.5	9(60.0)	6(40.0)	0.59(0.39-0.88)	0.044
Above or equal 18.5	199(62.8)	118(37.2)		
Residence				
Dar	105(65.2)	56(34.8)	1.03(0.58-1.81)	0.922
Other	103(60.2)	68(39.8)		
Positive baseline sputum culture (N=253)				
Yes	105(68.2)	49(31.8)	1.55(0.79-3.01)	0.200
No	62(62.6)	37(37.4)		
HIV status (N=208)				
Yes	71(61.2)	45(38.8)	1.03(0.57-1.86)	0.933
No	137(63.4)	79(36.6)		
Positive baseline sputum smear (N=253)				
Yes	105 (68.2)	49 (31.8)	0.62(0.30-1.29)	0.203
No	62 (62.6)	37 (37.4)		
Isoniazid (N=141)				
Resistant	87(66.9)	43(33.1)	1.03(0.47-2.26)	0.948
susceptible	7(63.6)	4(36.4)		
Rifampicin (N=207)				
Resistant	128(63.4)	74(36.6)	0.77(0.37-1.59)	0.479
Susceptible	4(80.0)	1(20)		
Streptomycin (N=114)				
Resistant	51(63.8)	29(36.3)	4.67(1.53-14.32)	0.007
susceptible	28(82.4)	6(17.6)		
Ethambutol (N=110)				
Resistant	50(68.5)	23(31.5)	0.34(0.12-0.96)	0.041
susceptible	25(67.6)	12(32.4)		

TABLE 5: Adjusted OR after multivariate analysis for predictors of treatment outcome of completed treatment.

Characteristics	Completed treatment N (%)	Other treatment categories N (%)	aOR(95% CI)	p-value
Baseline sputum smear				
(i) Yes	32(15.2)	178(84.8)	2.09(0.66-6.61)	0.210
(ii) No	7(8.0)	81(92.0)		
Baseline sputum culture				
(i) Yes	22(14.3)	132(85.7)	1.25(0.47-3.29)	0.654
(ii) No	9(9.1)	90(90.9)		
HIV status				
(i) Yes	15(12.9)	101(87.1)	0.99(0.43-2.29)	0.977
(ii) No	28(13.0)	188(87.0)		
Isoniazid				
(i) Resistant	16(12.3)	114(87.7)	1.17(0.41-3.33)	0.765
(ii) susceptible	2(18.2)	9(81.2)		
Rifampicin				
(i) Resistant	26(12.9)	176(87.1)	1.56(0.55-4.43)	0.405
(ii) Susceptible	1(20.0)	4(80.0)		
Streptomycin				
(i) Resistant	9(11.3)	71(88.8)	0.31(0.08-1.26)	0.101
(ii) Susceptible	4(11.8)	30(88.2)		
Ethambutol				
(i) Resistant	7(9.6)	66(90.4)	2.49(0.68-9.03)	0.166
(ii) susceptible	6(16.2)	31(83.8)		

TABLE 6: Adjusted OR after multivariate analysis for predictors of treatment outcome of loss to follow-up.

Characteristics	Loss to follow up N (%)	Other treatment categories N (%)	aOR(95% CI)	p-value
Residence				
(i) Other	7(4.3)	154(95.7)	2.41(0.84-6.91)	0.102
(ii) Dar	16(9.4)	155(90.6)		
Diabetes				
(i) Yes	1(20.0)	4(80.0)	0.29(0.04-2.08)	0.216
(ii) No	19(8.9)	295(91.1)		
Smoking				
(i) Yes	6(7.7)	72(92.3)	0.74(0.32-1.77)	0.509
(ii) No	5(4.6)	104(95.4)		
HIV status				
(i) Yes	8(6.9)	108(93.1)	0.96(0.34-2.76)	0.943
(ii) No	15(6.9)	201(93.1)		
Alcohol use				
(i) Yes	9(9.5)	86(90.5)	1.61(0.72-3.56)	0.244
(ii) No	5(5.3)	89(94.7)		
Isoniazid				
(i) Resistant	9(7.4)	121(92.6)	1.22(0.32-4.68)	0.768
(ii) Susceptible	1(9.1)	10(90.9)		
Rifampicin				
(i) Resistant	14(6.9)	188(93.1)	0.93(0.25-3.44)	0.909
(ii) Susceptible	0(0.0)	5(100.0)		
Streptomycin				
(i) Resistant	7(8.8)	73(91.2)	0.14(0.02-1.14)	0.066
(ii) Susceptible	1(2.9)	33(97.1)		
Ethambutol				
(i) Resistant	4(5.5)	69(94.5)	4.65(0.88-24.56)	0.070
(ii) Susceptible	4(10.8)	33(89.2)		

a study done by Tang and colleagues found a significant association between low BMI (less than 18.5kg/m^2) and poor treatment [11].

Resistance to streptomycin and ethambutol was each associated with MDRTB treatment cure. Our study found out that patients with TB strains resistant to streptomycin had an increased chance of being cured (aOR 4.67) while resistance to ethambutol was associated with decreased chance of being cured (aOR 0.34). Other studies have found other MDRTB drug, such as ofloxacin resistance which was inversely associated with MDRTB cure [18].

Dhingra identified the other factors as predictors of MDRTB treatment cure: weight gain at six months, sputum culture conversion, radiological improvement during treatment, resistance to strains less than or up to three antituberculosis drugs, use of less than or up to three second line drugs, and no change of treatment regimen during MDRTB treatment [25].

None of the independent factors predicted completion of treatment even after multivariate analysis but 43 patients (13%) had treatment completion as an outcome. The reason for not testing sputum culture and smear after completion of MDRTB treatment could be due to high number of consecutive negative sputum smear and culture at the final months during continuation phase of treatment, as well as the cost involved in these terminal follow-up visits. Most of these patients were discharged after an intensive phase of treatment and would be required to come back monthly for sputum cultures and smears as well as taking their monthly medications during the continuation phase of treatment. The last visit would only require them to come for sputum test to determine their cure status, without provision of any additional medications. Most of these patients would regard themselves as cured after several negative sputum smear and culture results towards the end of treatment and so would miss the last visit. Though none of the predictors had any association with completion of treatment, a study in South Africa found that HIV patients on ARVs were more likely to complete MDRTB treatment compared to HIV negative patients [12]. Both cure and treatment completion are defined by the WHO as successful treatment outcomes [3]. Other factors related to successful treatment outcomes include intensive treatment of adverse effects, nutritional supplementation, adherence interventions, and collaboration between the Ministry of Health and other nongovernmental organizations [26]. Others include the use of fluoroquinolones or

TABLE 7: Adjusted OR after multivariate analysis for predictors of treatment outcome of mortality/death (N=332).

Characteristics	Died N (%)	Other treatment categories N (%)	aOR(95% CI)	p-value
Cavitary lesions on CXR (N=279)				
(i) Yes	8(12.5)	56(87.5)	0.55(0.34-0.91)	0.019
(ii) No	29(13.7)	182(86.3)		
Smoking (N=177)				
(i) Yes	24(31.6)	52(68.4)	2.31(1.35-5.01)	0.043
(ii) No	14(12.8)	95(87.2)		
Baseline positive sputum smear (N=268)				
(i) Yes	33(16.0)	173(84.0)	1.24(0.48-3.21)	0.661
(ii) No	13(14.9)	74(85.1)		
Baseline positive sputum culture (N=253)				
(i) Yes	16(10.5)	136(89.5)	0.55(0.23-1.34)	0.190
(ii) No	17(17.3)	81(82.7)		
HIV status				
(i) Yes	22(19.5)	91(80.5)	1.10(0.49-2.50)	0.815
(ii) No	34(15.9)	180(84.1)		
Diabetes (N=319)				
(i) Yes	1(20.0)	4(80.0)	1.49(0.33-6.71)	0.609
(ii) No	52(16.8)	258(83.2)		
Isoniazid				
(i) Resistant	17(13.3)	111(86.7)	0.77(0.24-2.46)	0.661
(ii) susceptible	1(9.1)	10(90.9)		
Rifampicin				
(i) Resistant	33(16.7)	165(83.3)	1.27(0.50-3.22)	0.614
(ii) Susceptible	0(0.0)	5(100.0)		
Streptomycin				
(i) Resistant	12(14.8)	67(85.2)	0.54(0.10-2.78)	0.459
(ii) Susceptible	1(3.0)	32(97.0)		
Ethambutol				
(i) Resistant	11(15.3)	61(84.7)	0.97(0.20-4.68)	0.974
(ii) Susceptible	2(5.6)	34(94.4)		

bacteriostatic drugs [27], also having no previous history of TB treatment [28], BMI > 18.5kg/m^2 [7], and individualized treatment [9].

None of the predictors had a significant association with loss to follow-up, but other studies have found other factors that were related to loss to follow-up such as alcohol abuse and developing adverse reactions while protective factors include receiving assistance from TB program, patients' better knowledge of TB, and trust in treating physicians and nurses [10]. A study by Javaid and colleagues found that living in rural areas had an increased risk of being loss to follow-up [18].

Smoking, which lowers immunity against TB, was associated with mortality (aOR 2.31). Similar findings have been observed by Mollel and colleague whereby cigarette smoking and HIV positive status were both positively associated with MDRTB mortality [29]. Presence of cavities on chest X-rays was inversely associated with mortality. This is different from other studies such as that done by Kempker [22] and Tang [11]. Other predictors of MDRTB mortality include drug resistance pattern [30], diabetes history [31], anemia, positive sputum smear, hepatitis and drug use, resistance to ofloxacin [18], HIV positive infection, and low CD4 count [29]. A study in Egypt indicated that being diabetic is associated with unsuccessful MDRTB treatment outcome [32]; this could be related to the effect of diabetes on delaying sputum culture conversion in TB patients [33], leading to treatment failure and death [34].

Being a retrospective study, this study had some limitations, including missing data for some parameters such as smoking and alcohol use, but also diabetic patients were few. This may have had an impact on the results belonging to this category.

5. Conclusion

While streptomycin resistance and presence of cavity on chest radiographs are positively associated with MDRTB cure, ethambutol resistance and low BMI were inversely associated with MDRTB cure. Smoking and presence of cavities in chest radiographs were positively and negatively associated with MDRTB mortality, respectively. The study recommends, improving nutritional status of MDRTB patients, widespread antismoking campaign, and close follow-up of patients with ethambutol resistance.

Authors' Contributions

Tamary Henry Leveri, Edson Mollel, Furaha Lyamuya, and Kajiru Kilonzo contributed to the design of the study, Tamary Henry Leveri and Isack Lekule collected the data, Edson Mollel analysed the data, and all authors participated in writing the paper and approved the final version.

Acknowledgments

Thanks are due to all staff of Kibong'oto Infectious Diseases Hospital and Kilimanjaro Christian Medical Center who gave their inputs and contributed in the making and completion of this work. The authors did not receive any financial support to conduct the study.

References

[1] WHO, GLOBAL TUBERCULOSIS REPORT 2016, 2016.

[2] WHO, "The Global Plan to Stop TB: 2011-2015," 2010, http://www.stoptb.org.

[3] WHO, "Multidrug-Resistant Tuberculosis (MDR-TB) Indicators," 2010, https://apps.who.int/iris/bitstream/handle/10665/70484/WHO_HTM_TB_2010.11_eng.pdf;jsessionid=5E41E5961BFB7D932AA29BAE85D057DC?sequence=1.

[4] O. S. Elmi, H. Hasan, S. Abdullah, M. Z. Mat Jeab, Z. BA, and N. N. Naing, "Treatment outcomes of patients with multidrug-resistant tuberculosis (MDR- TB) compared with Non-MDR-TB infections in peninsular malaysia," *Malaysian Journal of Medical Sciences*, vol. 23, no. 4, pp. 17–25, 2016.

[5] WHO, "WHO treatment guidelines for drug-resistant tuberculosis," 2016.

[6] P. Isaakidis, E. C. Casas, M. Das, X. Tseretopoulou, E. E. Ntzani, and N. Ford, "Treatment outcomes for HIV and MDR-TB co-infected adults and children: systematic review and meta-analysis," *The International Journal of Tuberculosis and Lung Disease*, vol. 19, no. 8, pp. 969–978, 2015.

[7] Y. Kwon, Y. Kim, G. Suh et al., "Treatment outcomes for HIV-uninfected patients with multidrug-resistant and extensively drug-resistant tuberculosis," *Clinical Infectious Diseases*, vol. 47, no. 4, pp. 496–502, 2008.

[8] N. Kwak, H. Kim, C. Yoo, Y. W. Kim, S. K. Han, and J. Yim, "Changes in treatment outcomes of multidrug-resistant tuberculosis," *The International Journal of Tuberculosis and Lung Disease*, vol. 19, no. 5, pp. 525–530, 2015.

[9] K. T. Kibret, Y. Moges, P. Memiah, and S. Biadgilign, "Treatment outcomes for multidrug-resistant tuberculosis under DOTS-Plus: a systematic review and meta-analysis of published studies," *Infectious Diseases of Poverty*, vol. 6, no. 1, p. 7, 2017.

[10] T. E. Tupasi, A. M. Garfin, E. V. Kurbatova et al., "Factors associated with loss to follow-up during treatment for multidrug-resistant tuberculosis, the philippines, 2012–2014," *Emerging Infectious Diseases*, vol. 22, no. 3, pp. 491–502, 2016.

[11] S. Tang, S. Tan, L. Yao et al., "Risk factors for poor treatment outcomes in patients with MDR-TB and XDR-TB in China: retrospective multi-center investigation," *PLoS ONE*, vol. 8, no. 12, Article ID e82943, pp. 1–8, 2013.

[12] K. Schnippel, K. Shearer, D. Evans, R. Berhanu, S. Dlamini, and N. Ndjeka, "Predictors of mortality and treatment success during treatment for rifampicin-resistant tuberculosis within the South African National TB Programme, 2009 to 2011: a cohort analysis of the national case register," *International Journal of Infectious Diseases*, vol. 39, pp. 89–94, 2015.

[13] M. A. Khan, S. Mehreen, A. Basit et al., "Predictors of poor outcomes among patients treated for multidrug- resistant tuberculosis at tertiary care hospital in Pakistan," *American-Eurasian Journal of Toxicological Sciences*, vol. 7, no. 3, pp. 162–172, 2015.

[14] B. Sawadogo, K. S. Tint, M. Tshimanga, L. Kuonza, and L. Ouedraogo, "Risk factors for tuberculosis treatment failure among pulmonary tuberculosis patients in four health regions of Burkina Faso, 2009: case control study," *Pan African Medical Journal*, vol. 21, pp. 1–14, 2015.

[15] K. Kliiman and A. Altraja, "Predictors of poor treatment outcome in multi- and extensively drug-resistant pulmonary TB," *European Respiratory Journal*, vol. 33, no. 5, pp. 1085–1094, 2009.

[16] G. Kuchukhidze, A. M. V. Kumar, P. de Colombani et al., "Risk factors associated with loss to follow-up among multidrug-resistant tuberculosis patients in Georgia," *Public Health Action*, vol. I(4), pp. 249–251, 2014.

[17] A. Periasamy and K. A. P. Viswanatham, "Pulmonary & respiratory medicine predictors of outcome in drug resistant tuberculosis patients," *Journal of Pulmonary and Respiratory Medicine*, vol. 7, no. 7, pp. 1–4, 2017.

[18] A. Javaid, Z. Shaheen, M. Shafqat, A. H. Khan, and N. Ahmad, "Risk factors for high death and loss-to-follow-up rates among patients with multidrug-resistant tuberculosis at a programmatic management unit," *American Journal of Infection Control*, vol. 45, no. 2, pp. 190–193, 2017.

[19] E. Elliott, H. R. Draper, P. Baitsiwe, and M. M. Claassens, "Factors affecting treatment outcomes in drug-resistant tuberculosis cases in the Northern Cape, South Africa," *Public Health Action*, vol. 4, no. 3, pp. 201–203, 2014.

[20] K. S. Shringarpure, P. Isaakidis, K. D. Sagili, R. K. Baxi, and N. Mistry, "Loss-to-follow-up on multidrug resistant tuberculosis treatment in Gujarat, India: the when and who of it," *PLoS ONE*, vol. 10, no. 7, Article ID e0132543, pp. 1–10, 2015.

[21] J. C. Brust, A. R. Berman, B. Zalta et al., "Chest radiograph findings and time to culture conversion in patients with multidrug-resistant tuberculosis and hiv in tugela ferry, south africa," *PLoS ONE*, vol. 8, no. 9, Article ID e73975, pp. 1–8, 2013.

[22] R. R. Kempker, A. S. Rabin, K. Nikolaishvili et al., "Additional drug resistance in *Mycobacterium tuberculosis* isolates from resected cavities among patients with multidrug-resistant or extensively drug-resistant pulmonary tuberculosis," *Clinical Infectious Diseases*, vol. 54, no. 6, pp. e51–e54, 2012.

[23] A. Icksan, M. Sonang Napitupulu, M. Nawas, and F. Nurwidya, "Chest X-ray findings comparison between multi-drug-resistant tuberculosis and drug-sensitive tuberculosis," *Journal of Natural Science, Biology and Medicine*, vol. 9, no. 1, pp. 42–46, 2018.

[24] Y. Balabanova, R. Coker, I. Fedorin et al., "Variability in interpretation of chest radiographs among Russian study," *Peer-Reviewed Medical Journal*, vol. 331, pp. 1–4, 2005.

[25] V. K. Dhingra, S. Rajpal, A. Mittal, and M. Hanif, "Outcome

of multi-drug resistant tuberculosis cases treated by individualized regimens at a tertiary level clinic," *The Indian Journal of Tuberculosis*, vol. 55, no. 1, pp. 15–21, 2007.

[26] D. Meressa, R. M. Hurtado, J. R. Andrews et al., "Achieving high treatment success for multidrug-resistant TB in Africa: initiation and scale-up of MDR TB care in Ethiopia—an observational cohort study," *Thorax*, vol. 70, no. 12, pp. 1181–1188, 2015.

[27] L. Anderson, S. Tamne, J. Watson et al., "Treatment outcome of multi-drug resistant tuberculosis in the United Kingdom: retrospective-prospective cohort study from 2004 to 2007," *Eurosurveillance*, vol. 18, no. 40, pp. 1–10, 2013.

[28] V. Milanov, D. Falzon, M. Zamfirova et al., "Factors associated with treatment success and death in cases with multidrug-resistant tuberculosis in Bulgaria, 2009–2010," *International Journal of Mycobacteriology*, vol. 4, no. 2, pp. 131–137, 2015, 2014 Asian African Society for Mycobacteriology. Production and hosting by Elsevier Ltd. All rights reserved.

[29] E. W. Mollel and J. O. Chilongola, "Predictors for mortality among multidrug-resistant tuberculosis patients in tanzania," *Journal of Tropical Medicine*, vol. 2017, Article ID 9241238, 6 pages, 2017.

[30] N. R. Gandhi, J. R. Andrews, J. C. M. Brust et al., "Risk factors for mortality among MDR- and XDR-TB patients in a high HIV prevalence setting," *The International Journal of Tuberculosis and Lung Disease*, vol. 16, no. 1, pp. 90–97, 2012.

[31] K. Chung-Delgado, S. Guillen-Bravo, A. Revilla-Montag, and A. Bernabe-Ortiz, "Mortality among MDR-TB cases: comparison with drug-susceptible tuberculosis and associated factors," *PLoS ONE*, vol. 10, no. 3, Article ID e0119332, pp. 1–10, 2015.

[32] M. A. Gadallah, A. Mokhtar, M. Rady, E. El-Moghazy, M. Fawzy, and S. K. Kandil, "Prognostic factors of treatment among patients with multidrug-resistant tuberculosis in Egypt," *Journal of the Formosan Medical Association*, vol. 115, no. 11, pp. 997–1003, 2016.

[33] A. D. Salindri, M. Kipiani, R. R. Kempker et al., "Diabetes reduces the rate of sputum culture conversion in patients with newly diagnosed multidrug-resistant tuberculosis," *Open Forum Infectious Diseases*, vol. 3, no. 3, pp. 1–10, 2016.

[34] Y. A. Kang, S. Y. Kim, K. Jo et al., "Impact of diabetes on treatment outcomes and long-term survival in multidrug-resistant tuberculosis," *Respiration*, vol. 86, no. 6, pp. 472–478, 2013.

17

Tuberculosis among Patients Undergoing Solid Organ Transplantation or Dialysis in a Low-Endemic Country, 2004-2017

Marie Helleberg,[1,2] Daniel Cho,[2] Christina Ekenberg,[2] Søren Sørensen,[3] Marianne Rix,[3] Finn Gustafsson,[4] Allan Rasmussen,[5] Michael Perch,[4] Peter H. S. Andersen,[6] Jens D. Lundgren,[1,2] and Aase Bengaard Andersen[1]

[1]*Department of Infectious Diseases, Copenhagen University Hospital, Rigshospitalet, Blegdamsvej 9, 2100 Copenhagen Ö, Denmark*
[2]*Centre of Excellence for Health, Immunity and Infections (CHIP), Copenhagen University Hospital/Rigshospitalet, Blegdamsvej 9, 2100 Copenhagen Ö, Denmark*
[3]*Department of Nephrology, Copenhagen University Hospital, Rigshospitalet, Blegdamsvej 9, 2100 Copenhagen Ö, Denmark*
[4]*Department of Cardiology, Copenhagen University Hospital, Rigshospitalet, Blegdamsvej 9, 2100 Copenhagen Ö, Denmark*
[5]*Department of Surgery C, Copenhagen University Hospital, Rigshospitalet, Blegdamsvej 9, 2100 Copenhagen Ö, Denmark*
[6]*Department of Infection Epidemiology and Prevention, The State Serum Institute, Artillerivej 5, 2300 Copenhagen S, Denmark*

Correspondence should be addressed to Marie Helleberg; marie.helleberg@regionh.dk and Aase Bengaard Andersen; aase.bengaard.andersen@regionh.dk

Academic Editor: Edward A. Graviss

Background. The risk of active TB among solid organ transplant (SOT) recipients and patients initiating chronic dialysis in a country with low incidence of TB is not well elucidated. *Methods.* Patients aged >18 years who were transplanted with a solid organ or initiated chronic dialysis at Copenhagen University Hospital in the period 2004-2017 were followed from date of transplantation or initiation of dialysis. Data on demographics and outcomes were obtained from nationwide registries. *Results.* We included 1,989 SOT recipients and 1,305 patients initiating chronic dialysis, who were followed for a total of 9,785 and 4,196 person-years (PY), respectively. Only a minority of patients had been screened for latent TB prior to SOT or initiation of dialysis. The incidence rates (IRs)/100,000 PY of TB among patients from medium/high TB endemic areas were 358 (95% CI 115-1,110) and 1,266 (95% CI 681-2354) for SOT and dialysis patients, respectively, whereas IRs among patients of Danish origin were 11 (95% CI 2-81) and 31 (95% CI 4-218). *Conclusion.* The incidence of TB among immunosuppressed immigrants from medium/high TB endemic countries was very high, while the risk of TB among patients from low-endemic countries was minimal.

1. Introduction

Compromised immune function increases the risk of developing active tuberculosis (TB). Apart from HIV, two important risk factors for TB reactivation are solid organ transplantation (SOT) and chronic renal failure requiring dialysis [1]. Progression to active TB is a serious condition in patients with impaired renal function and in SOT recipients. Extrapulmonary disease is common, symptoms and signs are often unspecific which causes difficulties in timely diagnosis, and rates of disseminated disease at time of diagnosis are high [2]. Treatment is a challenge due to drug-drug interactions with rifampicin and the various immunosuppressant drugs. Dosing is difficult in patients with renal impairment, and it is reported that >50% of patients on dialysis have significant side effects to anti-TB drugs [3].

WHO guidelines and the Infectious Diseases Society of America recommend screening of high-risk populations for latent TB infection and prescribe preventive therapy [4, 5].

Denmark, like most European and so-called western countries, has a low and declining incidence of TB. However, TB high-risk subpopulations exists, especially in people originating from high TB endemic areas like Africa, Asia, and Greenland. In a "globalized world," large population groups migrate due to political instability to Europe and northern America, but the contact pattern to their country of origin often remain close with a high level of travelling activity also by the young 2nd-generation immigrants. Some patients may even present to the health system with a recently transplanted organ, acquired in a TB endemic country. The magnitude of the problem of TB reactivation in patients undergoing immunosuppressive therapy in a country with a low TB incidence is not well elucidated.

The aim of this study was to estimate the risk of developing active TB among SOT recipients and patients requiring chronic dialysis in a country with a low incidence of TB.

2. Methods

2.1. Setting. Denmark has a total population of 5.8 mil inhabitants, and 493.468 are immigrants or 1st-degree descendants from nonwestern countries as of 2018 [6]. In 2017, the incidence of TB in Denmark was 4.8 per 100,000 population, and 75% of TB cases were among immigrants [7].

"Rigshospitalet" is a third-level, referral university hospital located in Copenhagen, the capital of Denmark. The hospital serves as a national transplantation center for liver and lung transplantations and a regional center for kidney and heart transplantations.

2.2. Study Population. We included all consecutive patients, aged >18 years, who were transplanted with a solid organ or who initiated chronic dialysis at Rigshospitalet, Copenhagen University Hospital, in the period 2004-2017.

2.3. Data Sources. Data on ethnic origin, immigrations, emigrations, and dates of death were obtained from the Danish Civil Registration System. A local data warehouse, entitled "The PERSIMUNE data warehouse," provided data on laboratory tests, dialysis, and date and type of SOT [8]. Nationwide data on laboratory tests are only complete from 2010 and onwards. We obtained nationwide data on diagnoses of active TB from the Danish National TB registry and from the Danish National Patient Registry [9].

Data were linked using the unique 10-digit civil registration number which is assigned to all people living in Denmark at birth or at immigration.

2.4. Definitions. Greenland and countries in Eastern Europe, Africa, Asia, and South America were categorized as medium/high TB endemic countries; and countries in Northern and Western Europe, Northern America, and West Pacific were categorized as low TB endemic countries, i.e., <10 cases per 100,000 population. Second-generation immigrants were categorized as of Danish origin in the analyses as they were too few to be included as a separate category.

2.5. Statistics. Patients were followed from date of SOT or date of initiation of chronic dialysis until date of diagnosis of active TB, death, emigration, or 28 February 2017, whichever came first. Patients who initiated dialyses and later received a SOT were censored at the time of SOT and were

TABLE 1: Characteristics of the study population, *n* (%).

	Solid organ transplant recipients ($n = 1{,}989$)	Patients on chronic dialysis ($n = 1{,}305$)
Male	1,182 (59.4)	844 (64.7)
Age, median (IQR)	48 (36-58)	64 (52-73)
Year of study inclusion		
2004-2009	763 (38.4)	603 (46.2)
2010-2017	1,226 (61.6)	702 (53.8)
Origin		
Denmark*	1,756 (88.3)	1,044 (80.0)
Greenland	33 (1.7)	33 (2.5)
Other low TB endemic countries	49 (2.5)	48 (3.7)
Other medium/high TB endemic countries	151 (7.6)	180 (13.8)
SOT type		
Kidney	917 (46.1)	
Liver	530 (26.7)	
Lung	365 (18.5)	
Heart	158 (7.9)	
Pancreas-kidney	12 (0.6)	
Liver-kidney	3 (0.2)	

*43 SOT and 17 dialysis patients were second-generation immigrants with parents from TB endemic countries. SOT: solid organ transplant; IQR: interquartile range; TB: tuberculosis.

included in the group of SOT patients at the date of transplantation. Patients who received a SOT and later initiated chronic dialysis accrued follow-up time in the SOT group irrespective of dialysis.

Time to development of active TB was estimated using the Kaplan-Meier methods. Relative risks were estimated by the multivariate Poisson regression analyses. Variables included in the multivariate analyses were gender, age, calendar year of SOT/start of dialysis, and origin. There were no missing data for these variables in the dataset.

Stata, version 15.1 (StataCorp, College Station, Texas, USA), was used for data analyses.

The study was approved by the Danish Patient Safety Authority I-Suite no: 03605.

3. Results

3.1. Baseline Characteristics. We included 1,989 SOT recipients and 1,305 patients who initiated chronic dialysis at Copenhagen University Hospital, Rigshospitalet, in the period 2004-2017. A total of 225 of the SOT recipients had been on chronic dialyses at Rigshospitalet prior to transplantation. Baseline characteristics are summarized in Table 1. Of the 1,989 SOT recipients, 917 (46.1%) had a kidney transplant, 530 (26.7%) a liver transplant, 365 (18.5%) a lung transplant, 158 (7.9%) a heart transplant, and 15 (0.8%) a kidney/pancreas or kidney/liver transplant. The immunosuppressive regimens used at the center in the study period are described in the supplemental material (available here).

TABLE 2: Incidence rates of tuberculosis stratified by the type of immune suppression and incidence rate ratios in analysis pooling of solid organ transplant recipients and patients on dialysis.

	Solid organ transplant recipients ($n = 1,989$) IR/100,000 PY (95% CI)	Patients on chronic dialysis ($n = 1,305$) IR/100,000 PY (95% CI)	All patients IRR (95% CI)*
All patients	41 (15-109)	262 (145-473)	
Gender			
Male	17 (2-124)	109 (35-339)	1.0 (ref.)
Female	74 (2-230)	550 (275-1,110)	4.3 (1.4-13.7)
Age			
<50 years	17 (2-119)	364 (152-877)	1.0 (ref.)
≥50 years	78 (3-243)	212 (95-473)	2.1 (0.7-6.1)
Year of study inclusion			
2004-2009	51 (16-156)	125 (40-387)	1.0 (ref.)
2010-2017	25 (4-184)	446 (223-892)	1.8 (0.6-4.9)
Origin			
Denmark	11 (2-81)	31 (4-218)	1.0 (ref.)
Greenland	0	2,579 (645-10313)	42.2 (5.8-306)
Other low TB endemic countries	0	0	NA
Other medium/high TB endemic countries	454 (147-1,408)	1,133 (567-2,266)	49.2 (10.9-222)

IR: incidence rate; IRR: incidence rate ratio; TB: tuberculosis. *All variables were included in multivariate analyses.

Most SOT recipients, 1,805 (91.0%), were from low TB endemic countries, but 184 (9.0%) originated from a medium/high TB endemic country. Of patients who initiated chronic dialysis, 1,092 (83.7%) were from low TB endemic countries and 213 (16.3%) were from a medium/high TB endemic country. A total of 43 SOT and 16 dialyses patients were second-generation immigrants from medium/high TB endemic countries.

Thirteen SOT recipients and 16 dialysis patients had been treated for active tuberculosis prior to SOT or start of chronic dialysis. None of the patients who were on chronic dialysis prior to SOT had been diagnosed with TB prior to transplantation.

3.2. Incidence of Active TB after SOT/Dialysis. SOT recipients were followed for a total of 9,785 person-years (PY) of follow-up, median 4.4 years (interquartile range (IQR) 1.7-7.4), and dialysis patients were followed for a total of 4,196 PY, median 2.4 years (IQR 1.1-4.6). Four cases of active TB were diagnosed in the SOT patient group (3 cases in kidney transplant recipients and 1 liver transplant recipient) and eleven cases among the patients on dialysis.

The incidence rates (IRs)/100,000 PY of active TB were 41 (95% confidence interval (CI) 15-109) and 262 (95% CI 145-473) for SOT and dialysis patients, respectively (Table 2), which is 8.5 and 55 times higher than in the general population, respectively. For kidney and non-kidney transplant recipients, the IRs/100,000 PY of active TB were 108 (95% CI 35-336) and 17 (95% CI 2-119), respectively. Three of the four TB cases among SOT recipients were patients from medium/high TB endemic countries and one was of Danish origin. Ten of the patients who developed active TB after initiating chronic dialyses were from TB endemic countries and one was of Danish origin. There were no cases of TB among second-generation immigrants. The IRs/100,000 PY of TB among patients from medium/high TB endemic areas were 358 (95% CI 115-1,110) and 1,266 (95% CI 681-2,354) for SOT and dialysis patients, respectively.

The Kaplan-Meier curves of time from transplantation or start of chronic dialysis to a diagnosis of active TB are shown in Figure 1. The median time to TB diagnosis was 2.6 years (IQR 0.6-5.3) and 0.9 years (IQR 0.2-1.9) among SOT and dialysis patients, respectively. No cases of TB were diagnosed within 3 months of transplantation, but two cases (50%) were diagnosed within one year of SOT, whereas three (27%) and six (34%) patients were diagnosed with active TB within three months and one year after starting chronic dialysis, respectively.

Female gender and origin from Greenland or another medium/high TB endemic area were risk factors for being diagnosed with active TB (Table 2).

3.3. TB Diagnoses. Of the fifteen patients who developed active TB, ten were diagnosed with pulmonary TB, two had TB of the spine, two had TB in lymph nodes, and one had miliary TB (Table 3). Ten cases were confirmed by culture, one by PCR, two by histology, and in two patients, it was a clinical diagnosis (based on signs and symptoms, positive interferon gamma release assay (IGRA) (QuantiFERON TB Gold), imaging, and response to TB treatment) (Table 3). Three of the patients diagnosed with TB died within the study period (129, 826, and 1,286 days after TB diagnosis, respectively).

3.4. Screening for Latent TB. We could obtain consistent data on screening for latent TB by an IGRA in the period from January 2010 and onwards. Tuberculin skin testing was not used to screen for latent TB in that period. A total of 4.4%

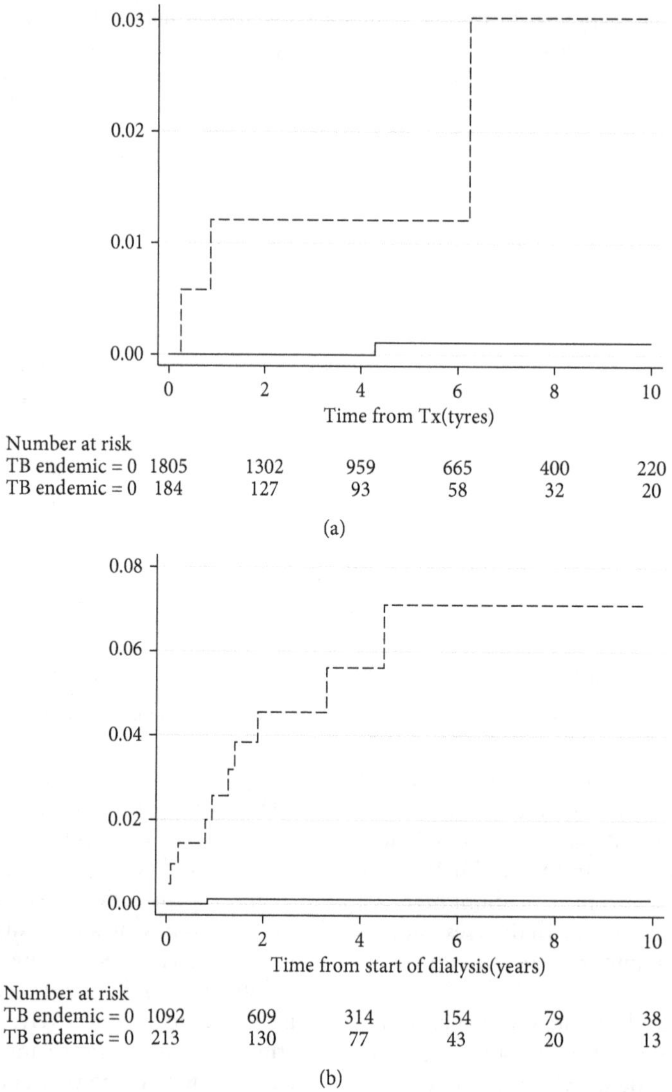

FIGURE 1: Time to diagnosis of active tuberculosis among solid organ transplant recipients (a) and dialysis patients (b) born in medium/high TB endemic countries (broken line) versus low TB endemic countries (full line).

of the SOT recipients and 3.7% of the patients on dialysis had been screened before SOT/start of chronic dialysis. Among patients from medium/high TB endemic areas, 16.5% of SOT recipients and 11.4% of dialysis patients had been screened, whereas among patients from low TB endemic countries, the corresponding proportions were 3.0% and 1.9%, respectively. Among 71 patients who were screened for latent TB prior to SOT or start of dialysis, 31 were from medium/high TB endemic areas and two of these patients (6.5%) developed active TB, whereas 5 (2.5%) of the 203 patients from medium/high TB endemic areas, who were not screened, were diagnosed with active TB after SOT or start of dialysis. Data on prophylactic treatment were not available.

4. Discussion

In this study conducted in a low TB endemic country, we found that the overall incidence of active TB among SOT and dialysis patients was 8.5 and 55 times higher than in the general population, respectively. Among study participants who were immigrants from medium/high TB endemic areas, the rates were very high, with cumulative incidences of 3-7%, whereas the incidence among patients born in countries with low TB incidence was minimal.

There are only few studies assessing the rates of active TB after SOT or dialysis in countries with low TB incidence, but our results are similar to findings from a Canadian study of SOT recipients [10], a study from the UK of patients with advanced chronic kidney disease [11], and an Australian study of dialysis patients [12]. It has previously been reported that rates of TB are 20-74 times higher in SOT recipients and patients on dialysis compared to the general population [13–15].

Patients initiating chronic dialysis tended to have a higher rate of development of active TB than patients receiving immunosuppressive therapy after SOT, but the two groups are not comparable. Dialysis patients were significantly older, and a larger proportion of dialysis patients originated from Greenland or another medium/high TB endemic country. Individuals with considerable comorbidity will not

Table 3: Characteristics of patients who developed active tuberculosis during follow-up, *n* (%).

	Solid organ transplant recipients ($n = 4$)	Patients on chronic dialysis ($n = 11$)
Male	1 (25)	3 (27)
Age < 50 years	1 (25)	5 (45)
Age ≥ 50 years	3 (75)	6 (55)
Year of study inclusion		
2004-2009	3 (75)	8 (73)
2010-2017	1 (25)	3 (27)
Origin		
Denmark	1 (25)	1 (9)
Greenland	0	2 (18)
Other non-TB endemic countries	0	0
Other TB endemic countries	3 (75)[a]	8 (73)[b]
SOT type (kidney/liver/lung/heart)	3/1/0/0	
Type of TB		
Pulmonary	4 (100)	6 (55)
Spine		2 (18)
Lymph node		2 (18)
Miliary		1 (9)
Time from SOT/dialysis to TB	2.6 years (IQR 0.6-5.3)	0.9 years (IQR 0.2-1.9)

[a]Yugoslavia: 1, Pakistan: 1, and Somalia: 1; [b]Pakistan: 2, Philippines: 2, Rumania: 1, Somalia: 1, and Turkey: 2.

undergo SOT; thus, the SOT recipients are "generally healthier" than patients on chronic dialysis. Rates of active TB were also higher among kidney transplant recipients compared to non-kidney transplant recipients, which is likely explained by the fact that a larger proportion of kidney transplant recipients originated from medium/high TB endemic countries.

The underlying pathogenic mechanisms behind the immunosuppression induced by dialysis are not well understood. However, end-stage renal disease (ESRD) is associated with functional abnormalities in a variety of immune cells including dendritic cells, B and T cells, neutrophils, monocytes, and natural killer cells, which is not reversed by dialysis [16]. Dialysis itself may also affect immune function by causing dysfunction of neutrophils, monocytes, and T cells [17–19].

Only a small proportion of patients in the present study had been screened for latent TB prior to SOT or start of chronic dialysis. The study was not powered to determine whether screening for latent TB was associated with a reduction in risk of developing active TB after start of immunosuppressive therapy, but the efficacy of treatment of latent TB to prevent progression to active disease is well documented [20].

The sensitivity of tuberculin skin tests and IGRAs is suboptimal in immunocompromised patients [21]. In studies including immunocompetent immigrants from high TB incidence countries and TB contacts, IGRAs have exhibited a rather low ability to predict development of active TB with a positive predictive value of <1-5% [22, 23]. In these groups the number needed to treat (NNT) based on results of an IGRA to guide preventive TB treatment in low TB incidence countries has been estimated to be 30-80 [23]. The NNT may be reduced to 25 if treating only those with strongly positive test results (>4.0 IU/mL) [24]. However, estimates of positive predictive value (PPV) and NNT are sensitive to the absolute risk in the population under study, and thus, the PPV may be higher and the NNT lower among SOT recipients and dialysis patients. A modelling study estimated that the NNT based on tuberculin skin test to guide preventive TB treatment was 3-7 for patients with ESRD and a renal transplant and 6-128 for patients with ESRD requiring dialysis [25].

TB and multidrug TB treatment are associated with considerable morbidity, risk of graft failure or rejection, and substantial mortality rates [26, 27], which must be taken into consideration when determining what threshold of NNT is considered acceptable. Recent studies have showed that screening for latent TB using an IGRA prior to SOT [28] or initiation of dialysis in patients from countries with high TB prevalence [29] is cost-effective. Among patients from low TB incidence countries without a history of travel-associated, occupational, or other specific TB exposure, screening with an IGRA may not be cost-effective. Indeed, in the present study, we found very low rates of active TB after immunosuppressive therapy in patients from low TB incidence countries even in the absence of screening for latent TB.

The sensitivity of IGRAs for identifying persons who will develop active TB is suboptimal, 60-70% [22]; thus, better tools for predicting the risk of active TB are needed. Future studies of biomarkers, e.g., signature cytokine profiles of patients with protective immunity in contrast to those about to lose control of the latent infection, and progress into subclinical or clinical TB may facilitate precision medicine in management of latent TB [30].

Our study had some limitations. Data on screening for latent TB were not complete in the period before 2010, and data on prophylactic treatment for latent TB and immunosuppressive therapy for the individual patient were unavailable. The numbers of patients who developed TB were low, which is why our ability to study risk factors was limited.

Strengths of the study include the large study population with long-term follow-up and access to nationwide data and registries, which made complete ascertainment of outcomes possible. The Danish Civil Registration number ensures correct linkage of data and that patients can be followed even if they transfer to other treatment centers. Further, the registers include precise data on place of birth and data on migrations. This allowed us to calculate specific incidence rates for patients originating from medium/high TB endemic countries and for those from countries with a low incidence of TB.

5. Conclusion

The risk of active TB is markedly increased among SOT recipients and patients requiring chronic dialysis compared to the general population even in a country with low TB prevalence. The incidence of active TB among immunosuppressed immigrants from TB endemic areas is high, while the absolute risk of active TB is minimal among patients from low TB incidence countries if they have no history of specific TB exposure.

Additional Points

Summary. SOT recipients and patients on dialysis had 9-55 higher rates of TB than the general population. The incidence of TB was very high in immigrants but minimal in patients from low TB endemic countries. 33% of TB cases were extrapulmonary.

Authors' Contributions

ABA fostered the idea for the study, which was designed by MH and ABA. All authors contributed to the collection and interpretation of data. MH did the data analyses and drafted the manuscript in collaboration with ABA. All authors contributed to the revisions of the draft, reviewed the manuscript, and approved the final version.

Acknowledgments

The work was supported by the Danish National Research Foundation, grant no. 126.

References

[1] J. W. Ai, Q. L. Ruan, Q. H. Liu, and W. H. Zhang, "Updates on the risk factors for latent tuberculosis reactivation and their managements," *Emerging Microbes & Infections*, vol. 5, no. 1, pp. 1–8, 2016.

[2] S. Vikrant, "Tuberculosis in dialysis: Clinical spectrum and outcome from an endemic region," *Hemodialysis International*, vol. 23, no. 1, pp. 88–92, 2018.

[3] A. M. Metry, I. al Salmi, S. al-Abri et al., "Epidemiology and outcome of tuberculosis in immunocompromised patients," *Saudi Journal of Kidney Diseases and Transplantation*, vol. 28, no. 4, pp. 806–817, 2017.

[4] H. Getahun, A. Matteelli, I. Abubakar et al., "Management of latent Mycobacterium tuberculosis infection: WHO guidelines for low tuberculosis burden countries," *The European Respiratory Journal*, vol. 46, no. 6, pp. 1563–1576, 2015.

[5] D. M. Lewinsohn, M. K. Leonard, P. A. LoBue et al., "Official American Thoracic Society/Infectious Diseases Society of America/Centers for Disease Control and Prevention Clinical Practice Guidelines: diagnosis of tuberculosis in adults and children," *Clinical Infectious Diseases*, vol. 64, no. 2, pp. 111–115, 2017.

[6] Statistics Denmark, January 2020, https://www.dst.dk/da/Statistik/emner/befolkning-og-valg#.

[7] S. S. Institut, *EPI-NYT Uge 28/33-2018*, 2018.

[8] "PERSIMUNE Data warehouse," CHIP, Department of Infectious Diseases, Rigshospitalet, January 2020, http://www.persimune.dk/How-to-get-involved/PERSIMUNE-Data-warehouse-search.

[9] M. Schmidt, S. A. Schmidt, J. L. Sandegaard, V. Ehrenstein, L. Pedersen, and H. T. Sorensen, "The Danish National Patient Registry: a review of content, data quality, and research potential," *Clinical Epidemiology*, vol. 7, pp. 449–490, 2015.

[10] Y. Natori, V. H. Ferreira, S. Nellimarla et al., "Incidence, Outcomes, and Long-term Immune Response to Tuberculosis in Organ Transplant Recipients," *Transplantation.*, vol. 103, no. 1, pp. 210–215, 2018.

[11] E. Moran, J. Baharani, M. Dedicoat et al., "Risk factors associated with the development of active tuberculosis among patients with advanced chronic kidney disease," *The Journal of Infection*, vol. 77, no. 4, pp. 291–295, 2018.

[12] C. C. Dobler, S. P. McDonald, and G. B. Marks, "Risk of tuberculosis in dialysis patients: a nationwide cohort study," *PLoS One*, vol. 6, no. 12, article e29563, 2011.

[13] D. Lopez de Castilla and N. W. Schluger, "Tuberculosis following solid organ transplantation," *Transplant Infectious Disease*, vol. 12, no. 2, pp. 106–112, 2010.

[14] A. K. Subramanian, M. I. Morris, and the AST Infectious Diseases Community of Practice, "Mycobacterium tuberculosisInfections in solid organ transplantation," *American Journal of Transplantation*, vol. 13, no. s4, Supplement 4, pp. 68–76, 2013.

[15] S. Chia, M. Karim, R. K. Elwood, and J. M. FitzGerald, "Risk of tuberculosis in dialysis patients: a population-based study," *The International Journal of Tuberculosis and Lung Disease*, vol. 2, no. 12, pp. 989–991, 1998.

[16] K. Romanowski, E. G. Clark, A. Levin, V. J. Cook, and J. C. Johnston, "Tuberculosis and chronic kidney disease: an emerging global syndemic," *Kidney International*, vol. 90, no. 1, pp. 34–40, 2016.

[17] V. Liakopoulos, A. Jeron, A. Shah, D. Bruder, P. R. Mertens, and X. Gorny, "Hemodialysis-related changes in phenotypical features of monocytes," *Scientific Reports*, vol. 8, no. 1, p. 13964, 2018.

[18] S. Lemesch, W. Ribitsch, G. Schilcher et al., "Mode of renal replacement therapy determines endotoxemia and neutrophil dysfunction in chronic kidney disease," *Scientific Reports*, vol. 6, no. 1, p. 34534, 2016.

[19] D. Ducloux, M. Legendre, J. Bamoulid et al., "ESRD-associated immune phenotype depends on dialysis modality and iron status: clinical implications," *Immunity & Ageing*, vol. 15, no. 1, p. 16, 2018.

[20] C. Pease, B. Hutton, F. Yazdi et al., "Efficacy and completion rates of rifapentine and isoniazid (3HP) compared to other treatment regimens for latent tuberculosis infection: a systematic review with network meta-analyses," *BMC Infectious Diseases*, vol. 17, no. 1, p. 265, 2017.

[21] M. Sester, F. van Leth, J. Bruchfeld et al., "Risk assessment of tuberculosis in immunocompromised patients. A TBNET study," *American Journal of Respiratory and Critical Care Medicine*, vol. 190, no. 10, pp. 1168–1176, 2014.

[22] I. Abubakar, F. Drobniewski, J. Southern et al., "Prognostic value of interferon-gamma release assays and tuberculin skin test in predicting the development of active tuberculosis (UK PREDICT TB): a prospective cohort study," *The Lancet Infectious Diseases*, vol. 18, no. 10, pp. 1077–1087, 2018.

[23] C. Lange, A. M. Mandalakas, B. Kalsdorf, C. M. Denkinger, and M. Sester, "Clinical Application of Interferon-γ Release Assays for the Prevention of Tuberculosis in Countries with Low Incidence," *Pathogens and Immunity*, vol. 1, no. 2, pp. 308–329, 2016.

[24] B. A. Winje, R. White, H. Syre et al., "Stratification by interferon-γ release assay level predicts risk of incident TB," *Thorax*, vol. 73, no. 7, pp. 652–661, 2018.

[25] D. N. Rose, "Benefits of screening for latent Mycobacterium tuberculosis infection," *Archives of Internal Medicine*, vol. 160, no. 10, pp. 1513–1521, 2000.

[26] D. Bumbacea, S. M. Arend, F. Eyuboglu et al., "The risk of tuberculosis in transplant candidates and recipients: a TBNET consensus statement," *The European Respiratory Journal*, vol. 40, no. 4, pp. 990–1013, 2012.

[27] I. S. Pradipta, N. Van't Boveneind-Vrubleuskaya, O. W. Akkerman, J. W. C. Alffenaar, and E. Hak, "Predictors for treatment outcomes among patients with drug-susceptible tuberculosis in the Netherlands: a retrospective cohort study," *Clinical Microbiology and Infection*, vol. 25, p. 761.e1, 2018.

[28] A. Kowada, "Interferon-gamma release assay for tuberculosis screening of solid-organ transplant recipients is cost-effective," *The Journal of Infection*, vol. 78, no. 1, pp. 58–65, 2018.

[29] J. R. Campbell, J. C. Johnston, L. A. Ronald et al., "Screening for Latent Tuberculosis Infection in Migrants With CKD: A Cost- effectiveness Analysis," *American Journal of Kidney Diseases*, vol. 73, no. 1, pp. 39–50, 2018.

[30] R. K. Gupta, C. T. Turner, C. Venturini et al., "Concise whole blood transcriptional signatures for incipient tuberculosis: a systematic review and patient-level pooled meta-analysis," *The Lancet Respiratory Medicine*, vol. 8, no. 4, pp. 395–406, 2020.

18

N-Acetyl Cysteine as an Adjunct in the Treatment of Tuberculosis

Dawit A. Ejigu[1] **and Solomon M. Abay**[2]

[1]*Department of Pharmacology, St Paul's Hospital Millennium Medical College, Addis Ababa, Ethiopia*
[2]*Department of Pharmacology and Clinical Pharmacy, College of Health Sciences, Addis Ababa University, Addis Ababa, Ethiopia*

Correspondence should be addressed to Dawit A. Ejigu; dawit.a.ejigu@gmail.com

Academic Editor: Vincent Jarlier

Oxidative stress is a common feature of tuberculosis (TB), and persons with reduced antioxidants are at more risk of TB. TB patients with relatively severe oxidative stress had also more advanced disease as measured by the Karnofsky performance index. Since adverse effects from anti-TB drugs are also mediated by free radicals, TB patients are prone to side effects, such as hearing loss. In previous articles, researchers appealed for clinical trials aiming at evaluating N-acetyl cysteine (NAC) in attenuating the dreaded hearing loss during multidrug-resistant TB (MDR-TB) treatment. However, before embarking on such trials, considerations of NAC's overall impact on TB treatment are crucial. Unfortunately, such a comprehensive report on NAC is missing in the literature and this manuscript reviews the broader effect of NAC on TB treatment. This paper discusses NAC's effect on mycobacterial clearance, hearing loss, drug-induced liver injury, and its interaction with anti-TB drugs. Based on the evidence accrued to date, NAC appears to have various beneficial effects on TB treatment. However, despite the favorable interaction between NAC and first-line anti-TB drugs, the interaction between the antioxidant and some of the second-line anti-TB drugs needs further investigations.

1. Introductions

Oxidative stress is a common feature of tuberculosis (TB) [1] and is evidenced by elevated lipid peroxidation products such as malondialdehyde (MDA) as well as reduced antioxidant capacity. Compared to healthy individuals, TB patients have low vitamins A, C, and E, selenium, and glutathione (GSH) amounts [2, 3]. TB patients in developing countries have even worse oxidative stress compared with their counterparts in developed nations [2]. After successful treatment with anti-TB drugs, the elevated oxidative stress in TB patients returns to normal [1]. Individuals with diminished antioxidant capacity and increased oxidative stress are also predisposed to TB [4], and TB patients with relatively advanced oxidative stress are more likely to have a severe form of the disease as measured by the Karnofsky performance index [2].

Anti-TB drugs induce several adverse effects in TB patients, and oxidative stress is implicated in mediating these adverse effects. Drug-induced liver injury (DILI) [5] and hearing loss [6] are some of these untoward effects that follow treatment with anti-TB drugs, and both adverse effects are believed to be mediated through oxidative stress. TB patients have already high oxidative stress and hence are prone to these side effects. Hence, antioxidants could potentially mitigate adverse effects induced by anti-TB drugs and facilitate recovery from TB.

Researchers previously appealed for clinical trials aiming at evaluating N-acetyl cysteine (NAC) in attenuating hearing loss in multidrug-resistant TB (MDR-TB) patients owing to the gravity of the problem [7, 8]. However, before testing NAC in TB patients for its hearing loss protective effect, considerations of how NAC would impact other aspects of TB treatment are critical. Unfortunately, there are no such comprehensive scientific reports on NAC and hence this manuscript reviews the broader effects of NAC on TB treatment. This paper discusses NAC's effect on mycobacterial clearance, hearing loss, and DILI as well as the antioxidant's interaction with anti-TB drugs. The safety of NAC itself is not covered here as it has been reviewed elsewhere [7].

2. Antimycobacterial Properties of N-Acetyl Cysteine

NAC demonstrated antimycobacterial properties in previous studies of different models [9–11]. NAC cleared mycobacteria through several mechanisms including immunomodulation [12], enhancement of GSH level [13], and direct antimycobacterial effects [14].

2.1. Antimycobacterial Mechanisms of NAC. NAC is a precursor of GSH [15], and GSH, in turn, has demonstrated direct antimycobacterial effects. NAC is deacetylated, and the resulting cysteine is used to synthesize GSH [15]. GSH has both direct and indirect antimycobacterial effects. The direct effect of GSH includes enhancing the effect of nitric oxide (NO), one of the immune effector molecules produced by the immune effector cells. Normally, NO had a short-lived antimycobacterial effect but when it is combined with GSH and forms S-nitrosoglutathione (GSSNO) [16], it was persistently released from GSSNO and this prolonged its antimycobacterial effect [17]. Additionally, GSH, being a thiol-containing molecule, might also create a redox imbalance in the mycobacteria since the bacteria use mycothiol [18, 19] as an antioxidant, eventually causing growth inhibition. Another antimycobacterial effect of GSH is through enhancing immune cell activity and cytokine production [20].

NAC also has a direct antimycobacterial effect [14] independent of GSH as well as its free radical-scavenging effects. NAC maintained similar antimycobacterial effects in the presence and absence of the nicotinamide adenine dinucleotide phosphate (NADPH) system in a study that used a knockout mouse model [14]. Had NAC exclusively depended on GSH for its antimycobacterial effect, the absence of NADPH could have diminished its antimycobacterial effect since the recycling of GSH from its oxidized form to its reduced form needs NADPH [21]. In *Escherichia coli*, intracellular cysteine-induced reactive oxygen species (ROS) leading to DNA damage [22] and a similar mechanism of cysteine were confirmed later in mycobacterium [23]. Moreover, cysteine and any other thiol-containing molecules prevented mycobacterial persistence, a state where the bacteria decrease its metabolic rate and become refractory to killing by anti-TB drugs [23]. By avoiding persistence, NAC can also facilitate sterilization by anti-TB drugs and prevent drug resistance.

Moreover, NAC modulated immunity against tuberculosis where it increased interleukin-2 (IL-2), IL-12, and interferon gamma (INF-γ) production [9, 20, 24] and these cytokines are important for suppressing mycobacterial proliferation. Additionally, NAC reduced the production of IL-10, a cytokine that favors mycobacterial proliferation [10, 11]. The antioxidant also reduced the proinflammatory cytokines such as IL-1, IL-6, and tumor necrosis factor alpha (TNF-α), cytokines known to exacerbate oxidative stress. NAC also increased the immunological activities of various cells including natural killer (NK) cells and macrophages against mycobacterium [13, 25].

2.2. Evidence from Studies Other than the In Vitro Model. NAC demonstrated antimycobacterial effects in animal studies [14, 26]. In guinea pigs infected with *Mycobacterium tuberculosis* (MTB), 60 days of oral NAC treatment partially restored red blood cell GSH concentrations and serum total antioxidant capacity. NAC also reduced spleen mycobacterial load as well as lesion burden and the severity in the lungs [26]. However, in this study, NAC did not reduce the mycobacterial load in the lungs. A different study in C57BL/6 mice NAC significantly reduced the mycobacterial load in the lungs after 7 days of treatment with the antioxidant [14].

The difference in the two studies, concerning the reduction in lung mycobacterial load, could be due to species variation, the difference in infection methodology, and the duration of infection. Guinea pigs are very susceptible to infection by MTB and clearing the mycobacteria may be difficult for them while mice are resistant to mycobacteria [27]. The study in guinea pigs also used aerosolization for infecting the animals while the mouse study used intratracheal inoculation. Moreover, the guinea pig study assessed the effect of NAC at 30 and 60 days after infection while the mice study assessed the effect only seven days postinoculation.

NAC also demonstrated several beneficial effects including facilitation of mycobacterial clearance in a clinical trial. In a double-blind, randomized clinical trial of 67 newly diagnosed TB patients, NAC as an adjunct to anti-TB drugs improved smear conversions 3 weeks after initiation of DOTs (directly observed therapies) [28]. NAC at an oral dose of 1200 mg/day resulted in a smear conversion rate of 95.8%, while the conversion rate was 58.3% in the control group. At the end of two months, smear conversion rates were 100% for the NAC group and 91.7% for the control group. Additionally, NAC improved weight gain and response to treatment as assessed by radiology. However, the attrition rate in this study was very high (28%). Two additional trials trying to assess the efficacy and safety of NAC in newly diagnosed TB patients are ongoing (NCT03281226, NCT03702738).

Despite numerous *in vitro* animal studies and a clinical trial which reported antimycobacterial effects of NAC, studies by Khameneh et al. and Vilchèze et al. did not confirm the antimycobacterial effects of the antioxidant in their experiments [23, 29] (Table 1). According to Khameneh et al., NAC did not show antimycobacterial effects against H37Rv even at a concentration of up to 40 mg/ml. However, both studies reported that NAC increased the antimycobacterial effects of anti-TB drugs. What is common in these two studies is that they used TB culture media, Middlebrook 7H9 Broth (7H9) and Lowenstein Jensen (LJ) media, in reporting the sole effect of NAC against TB. From these observations, we can estimate that for its direct anti-TB effect, NAC will probably need macrophages or other similar immune cells, and in the absence of these cells, it can only enhance the effects of other anti-TB drugs.

2.3. Interaction with Anti-TB Drugs. NAC showed additive/-synergistic antimycobacterial interaction with all first-line and some second-line anti-TB drugs [10, 24, 30]. Administration of NAC and suboptimal concentrations of isoniazid (INH) or rifampicin (RIF) to peripheral blood mononuclear

Table 1: Summary of studies on anti-TB effects of NAC against *MTB*.

Author	Year	Type of study	Anti-TB effect	Effect measurement	Type of immune cells	Type of *MTB*	Conc. of NAC	Study subjects	Remark	Reference
Venketaraman et al.	2006	Cell culture	Yes	CFU reduction, effect size not indicated	Human Øs	H37Rv	10 mM	HIV +ve and -ve		[9]
Cao et al.	2018	Cell culture	Yes	50% CFU reduction	THP-1	Erdman strain	10 mM	NA	Also showed that anti-TB drugs and NAC have synergistic effects	[10]
Venketaraman et al.	2008	Cell culture	Yes	CFU reduction, effect size not indicated	Human Øs	H37Rv	10 mM	HIV -ve	Used whole blood culture	[11]
Guerra et al.	2011	Cell culture	Yes	CFU reduction, effect size not indicated	Human NK cells	H37Rv	20 mM	HIV +ve and -ve	NK cells pretreated with NAC	[20]
Morris et al.	2013	Cell culture	Yes	CFU against control, effect size not indicated	Human Øs	H37Rv	10 mM	HIV +ve and -ve		[13]
Amaral et al.	2016	Cell culture	Yes	CFU vs. control, effect size not indicated	THP-1	H37Rv, avium, Beijing 1471, M. bovis	10 mM	HIV -ve		[14]
Guerra et al.	2011	Cell culture	Yes	CFU reduction, effect size not indicated	Human Øs	H37Rv	5, 10, 20 mM	HIV +ve and -ve		[20]
Vilchèze et al.	2017	Cell culture & 7H9	No	4-5 log CFU reduction	J774 Øs	H37Rv	5-10 mM	NA	Anti-TB effect when only combined with RIF/INH	[23]
Lamprecht et al.	2016	7H9 medium	Yes	CFU reduction, sterilized	NA	H37Rv	5 mM	NA	Combined with BDQ, Q203, and CFZ	[30]
Teskey et al.	2018	Cell culture & animal study	Yes	CFU reduction	Human PBMCs	Erdman strain	10 mM	Healthy and T2DM patients, rats		[24]
Palanisamy et al.	2011	Animal study	Yes	CFU reduction	NA	H37Rv	400 mg/kg/day for 60 days	Guinea pigs		[26]
Mahakalkar et al.	2017	Clinical trial	Yes	Sputum conversion	NA	NA	600 mg/day	Smear +ve TB patients		[28]
Khameneh et al.	2016	LJ media	No	NA	NA	H37Rv	0.04-40 mg/ml	NA	Anti-TB effect only when combined with RIF or INH	[29]

CFU: colony-forming unit; Øs: macrophages; NK cells: natural killer cells; LJ: Lowenstein Jensen; PBMC: peripheral blood mononuclear cells; T2DM: type 2 diabetes mellitus; NAC: N-acetyl cysteine; INH: isoniazid; RIF: rifampicin; BDQ: bedaquiline; CFZ: clofazimine; Q203: investigational product.

cells (PBMCs) infected with mycobacterium completely cleared mycobacterium from the culture [24]. According to this study, NAC also enhanced the antimycobacterial effect of ethambutol (EMB) in a statistically significant manner. When NAC and anti-TB drugs were also added to the cell culture of macrophages infected with *MTB*, NAC further reduced the viability of the bacteria in the macrophages [10]. In this study, the interaction of NAC with INH, RIF, EMB, and pyrazinamide (PZA) resulted in more than a fourfold further reduction of the CFU. Moreover, coadministration of NAC with clofazimine, bedaquiline, and Q203, an investigational agent, to a culture medium inoculated with *MTB* resulted in the sterilization of the culture medium [30]. According to the study, in the absence of NAC, the three drugs were not able to sterilize the culture media.

The synergistic effect of NAC with INH in clearing mycobacterium could probably be a paradox in light of previous findings on how INH works [31, 32]. INH is a prodrug requiring oxidative activation by the catalase-peroxidase hemoprotein, *KatG*, and the activation of INH by *KatG* is enhanced in the presence of a superoxide. This enhancement is evidenced by an observation that plumbagin and clofazimine, which are superoxide generators, increased the antimycobacterial effect of INH [31]. As an antioxidant, NAC reduces the free radical level, and hence, the antimycobacterial effect of INH could be expected to diminish when coadministered with NAC.

As mentioned earlier, NAC prevents a state of TB persistence, and through this mechanism, the antioxidant has the potential to reduce the duration of anti-TB treatment, reduce the rate of relapse, and prevent resistance against anti-TB drugs [23, 33, 34]. Persisters are subpopulations of the *MTB* colonies which are metabolically inactive and respond poorly to anti-TB drugs. These subpopulations are also the reason for prolonged treatment with anti-TB drugs and an important source of drug resistance. Persisters also do contribute to TB relapses [33]. According to Valchèze et al., the administration of exogenous reducing substances, such as NAC, switched persisters to metabolically active bacteria [23].

Despite synergism of NAC with the first-line anti-TB drugs and clofazimine as well as bedaquiline, assessing NAC's interactions with the remaining second-line drugs is imperative since NAC seemingly antagonized some of the antibiotics [35, 36]. Based on various reports, NAC increased the minimal inhibitory concentrations (MICs) of fluoroquinolones and aminoglycosides against various non-TB bacteria [35]. According to these reports, these effects of NAC are peculiar to the type of organisms since the antioxidant either increased or decreased the MICs depending on the type of organisms [35]. However, Rodriguez et al. explained the counterproductive effects of NAC on the antibiotics' MICs to be due to the acidic pH of the culture medium and adjustment of the medium pH to neutral avoided NAC's negative effect of the antibiotics' MICs [37]. Landini et al. also confirmed that 10 mM of NAC did not adversely affect the MIC of the antibiotics [38]. To further clear the confusion, it would be advisable to test the interaction between NAC and the remaining second-line anti-TB drugs before conducting a clinical trial of NAC in MDR-TB patients.

3. Protective Effects of NAC against Ototoxicity

Aminoglycosides are injectable anti-TB drugs used for the treatment of MDR-TB and are associated with ototoxicity [6]. The antibiotics cause loss of hair cells in the cochlea, involved in hearing, and in the vestibular apparatus, involved in maintaining balance. Early damage in the cochlea is limited to the hair cells in the basal region resulting in high-frequency losses in the inaudible range and then involves the apex affecting the low frequencies in the audible range [39]. Initially, the patient's hearing may not be affected but failure to promptly discontinue the antibiotics would diminish the patient's hearing. Ototoxicity caused by aminoglycosides is also irreversible and cumulative [40, 41].

A significant proportion of TB patients undergoing treatment with aminoglycosides develop ototoxicity [6, 42, 43]. Studies suggested that ototoxicity is more frequent in resource-limited settings than in developed nations [39]. The method of diagnosis also has an impact on the proportion of patients identified as having ototoxicity. Diagnosis with high-frequency audiometers is sensitive [44] and gives the true picture of the rates of aminoglycoside-induced ototoxicity than does clinical diagnosis, which underestimates the problem.

Several risk factors are associated with the development of aminoglycoside-induced ototoxicity. Patients with advanced age and low body mass index (BMI) are at a higher risk of ototoxicity [6]. Prolonged duration of treatment with aminoglycosides increases the probability of developing aminoglycoside-induced ototoxicity [44, 45]. Based on a systematic review, MDR-TB patients coinfected with HIV have 22% more risk of their treatment being complicated with ototoxicity [46].

The rate of ototoxicity also varies with the particular aminoglycosides used in the MDR-TB treatment. In a study comparing the rate of ototoxicity induced by capreomycin versus amikacin, the risk of ototoxicity in patients treated with amikacin was increased five times compared with those treated with capreomycin [47]. In another study, in Namibian MDR-TB patients, amikacin was associated with more risk of ototoxicity than kanamycin [48]. Moreover, according to a review on ototoxicity induced by injectable anti-MDR TB drugs, ototoxicity rates caused by streptomycin, kanamycin, and amikacin were 11.8%, 13.3%, and 19.7%, respectively [44]. However, the review seemed to overestimate the ototoxicity rate for capreomycin (25%) probably due to the enrollment in the review of only four patients treated with capreomycin.

NAC attenuated aminoglycoside-induced ototoxicity in various studies [49, 50], and its mechanism of ototoxicity attenuation could be through scavenging free radicals and inhibition of downstream molecular mechanisms of apoptosis induced by oxidative stress. Apart from its free radical-scavenging properties, NAC was shown to inhibit the activation of p38 mitogen-activated protein kinase (MAPK) [51]. The p38 MAPK and its downstream molecular mechanisms, such as activation of caspases and cytochrome c, were also shown to be responsible for aminoglycoside-induced ototoxicity [52].

Aminoglycosides cause ototoxicity through the generation of free radicals and these radicals, in turn, attack the hair cells of the vestibulocochlear nerve [53]. In this process, an iron-aminoglycoside complex is formed and unsaturated fatty acids donate electron in the process of ROS generation [54]. The free radicals cause cochlear and vestibular hair cell loss [55] through apoptosis due to the activation of the p38 MAPK system [56].

In animal studies, enhancing the antioxidant systems and/or free radical-scavenging capacity protected against aminoglycoside-induced ototoxicity. Animals overexpressing superoxide dismutase, the enzyme responsible for scavenging ROS, were resistant to kanamycin-induced ototoxicity [57]. NAC also protected gentamycin- and neomycin-induced ototoxicity in rats and zebrafish [49, 58, 59]. In a rat model which used both NAC and vitamin A for the prevention of gentamycin-induced ototoxicity, both interventions prevented ototoxicity but N-acetyl cysteine showed more protective effect [49]. However, according to an earlier study in guinea pigs by Bock et al., NAC rather worsened kanamycin-induced ototoxicity [60].

NAC protected against aminoglycoside-induced hearing loss in clinical trials of non-TB patients [50, 61, 62] (Table 2). In renal failure patients who developed peritonitis after undergoing peritoneal dialysis and were treated with aminoglycosides, NAC attenuated aminoglycoside induced-ototoxicity. In these studies, gentamycin and amikacin were administered along with NAC for four to six weeks. In a meta-analysis of these clinical trials, NAC protected 86% of the ototoxicity that might have been induced by aminoglycosides [7]. Vural et al. also confirmed that NAC protected against aminoglycoside-induced ototoxicity during a one-month treatment period with the antioxidant [63]. However, the protective effect diminished after one year. In this trial, treatments with aminoglycosides and NAC were completed at the same time. This finding probably suggests that for maximal protection with the antioxidant, we need to continue the administration of NAC for a little longer after completion of aminoglycoside administration. According to pharmacokinetic studies, aminoglycosides accumulate in the hair cells slowly and their half-life in these cells is prolonged [64, 65]. This means aminoglycosides could continue to cause hair cell damages even after they are discontinued.

4. Protective Effect of NAC against DILI

DILI is one of the major adverse effects of treatment with anti-TB drugs. Patients treated with anti-TB drugs may experience DILI ranging from simple hepatic enzyme elevations to severe clinical hepatitis. In the presence of hepatitis symptoms, such as abdominal pain, nausea, vomiting, unexplained fatigue, or jaundice, hepatotoxicity is defined as an elevation of liver enzymes, alanine (ALT) and/or aspartate (AST) transaminase, more than three times the upper limit of the normal range (ULN). But in the absence of symptoms, either of the enzymes must be elevated more than five times ULN [66, 67]. The culprits causing DILI among the first-line anti-TB drugs are INH, PZA, and RIF while from the second line drugs, the list includes fluoroquinolones, ethionamide, prothionamide, amoxicillin-clavulanate, and para-aminosalicylic acid [68]. The rate of DILI in TB patients could sometimes go up as high as 27% [69].

DILI could have serious implications on the outcome of TB patient treatment [5, 70]. Some patients with DILI may develop acute liver failure, ascites, and hepatic encephalopathy, and yet others may manifest only with simple enzyme elevations. A study in China demonstrated more than a 9-fold risk of unsuccessful treatment and more than a 2-fold increased risk of prolonged intensive phase treatment in patients with DILI compared to TB patients without DILI [70]. Anti-TB associated DILI could also result in death, and this was more common in patients who developed encephalopathy, ascites, and jaundice [5]. The mortality rate in patients who developed anti-TB-associated DILI could also be as high as 23%.

Different risk factors are associated with the development of anti-TB DILI. Various studies suggested advanced age as one of the risk factors [71, 72] even if other studies did not confirm age as a risk factor [73, 74]. Some studies also indicated HIV to be a risk factor for anti-TB-associated DILI [75, 76]. Additionally, other risk factors associated with anti-TB DILI include low BMI [77, 78], viral hepatitis [79], INH acetylation status [80], and genetic makeup of the patients [81].

NAC attenuates anti-TB DILI through scavenging free radicals formed during the metabolism of the drugs as well as through enhancing the synthesis of GSH [82]. Anti-TB drugs induce liver injury via the formation of free radicals and then the free radicals damage different cellular parts [83]. The free radicals are probably generated during the metabolism of the various anti-TB drugs [67]. Normally, these molecules are detoxified by the host's antioxidant system including GSH. However, if the antioxidant system is compromised for various reasons, the free radicals could damage different structures within the cells and perpetuate the oxidative stress through lipid peroxidation.

According to studies on genetic polymorphisms of oxidant-antioxidant systems, mutations leading to reduced antioxidant enzymes or increased prooxidant enzymes resulted in increased susceptibility to anti-TB DILI [81, 84, 85]. A loss of function mutation on *MAFK* encoding MafK (small Maf basic leucine zipper proteins) increased susceptibility to anti-TB DILI [81] (Figure 1). Normally, the binding of MafK with Nrf2 (nuclear factor erythroid 2-related factor 2) leads to the upregulation of antioxidant enzymes. Similarly, a gain of function mutations on *NOS2A*, encoding inducible nitric oxide synthase (iNOS) and *BACH1*, encoding BTB and CNC homology 1 (bach1), increased susceptibility to anti-TB DILI [81]. *NOS2A* encodes the enzyme nitric oxide synthase while *BACH1* encodes Bach1, whose binding with Nrf2 leads to the downregulation of antioxidant enzymes. Additionally, loss of function mutations on *HMOX1*, the gene encoding for heme oxygenase 1 recognized as phase II antioxidant enzyme, and *NQO1*, which encodes NAD (P)H: quinone oxidoreductase 1, were also associated with susceptibility to anti-TB DILI [84]. A meta-analysis also confirmed the association of polymorphisms

Table 2: Clinical trials conducted to investigate the otoprotective effect of 600 mg twice a day NAC against AGs in non-TB patients.

Author	Year	Effect measurement	Duration of protection	Study subjects	Sample size	Type of aminoglycoside	Country of study	Remark	Reference
Feldman et al.	2007	25% vs. 60% in favor of NAC	6 weeks	Hemodialysis patients	40	Gentamycin	Israel		[61]
Tokgoz et al.	2011	3.3% vs. 70% in favor of NAC	4 weeks	Peritoneal dialysis patients	60	Amikacin	Turkey	Amikacin combined with vancomycin	[62]
Kocyigit et al.	2015	In favor of NAC	4 weeks	Peritoneal dialysis patients	46	Amikacin	Turkey		[50]
Vural et al.	2018	In favor of NAC	4 weeks	Peritoneal dialysis patients	40	Amikacin	Turkey	Reassessment after 12 months showed reduced effects	[63]

NAC: N-acetyl cysteine; AGs: aminoglycosides.

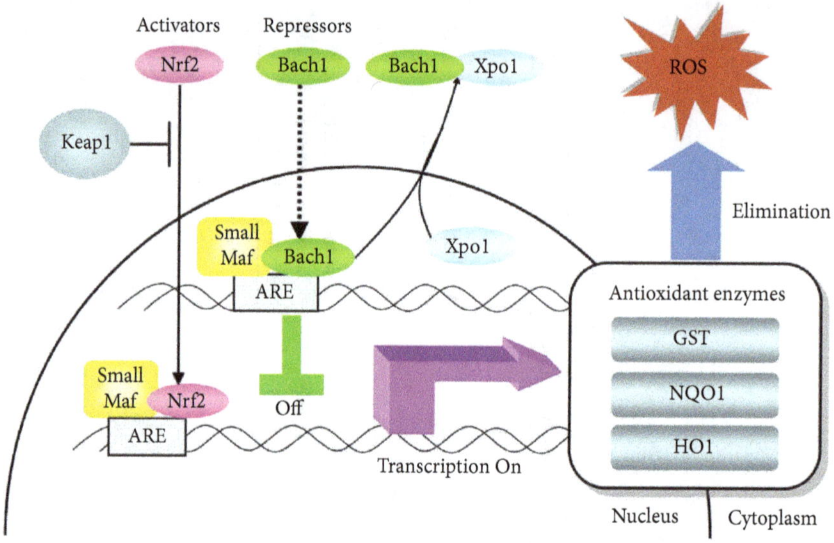

Figure 1: Activator and repressor arms in the antioxidant pathway. Schematic representation indicates the location and translocation of relevant genes involved in the activator arm (Nrf2/small Mafs/Xpo1) and repressor arm (Bach1/small Mafs/Keap1) in the antioxidant pathway as well as the transcriptional regulation of antioxidant enzymes (NQO1/HO1) against oxidative stress in hepatocytes. Nrf2: nuclear factor erythroid 2-related factor 2; Keap1: Kelch-like ECH-associated protein 1; Bach1: BTB and CNC homology 1; Xpo1: exportin 1; ARE: antioxidant-responsive element; GST: glutathione S-transferase; NQO1: NAD (P) H dehydrogenase quinone 1; HO1: heme oxygenase 1; ROS: reactive oxygen species [81].

Table 3: List of studies on the hepatoprotective effect NAC on anti-TB drugs.

Author	Year	Type of study	Types of animals or cells	Dose or concentration of NAC	Type of anti-TB	Protection by NAC	Reference
Attri et al.	2000	Animal study	Wistar rats	100 mg/kg	INH (50 mg/kg), RIF (50 mg/kg)	Yes	[83]
Rana et al.	2006	Animal study	Wistar rats	100 mg/kg	RIF (50 mg/kg)	Yes	[82]
Singh et al.	2012	*In vitro*	HepG2	10 μM	INH (100, 200 mM), RIF (50 mM), PZA (100, 200 mM)	Yes	[86]
Baniasadi et al.	2011	Clinical trial	NA	600 mg PO BID	INH, RIF, PZA, ETH	Yes	[87]

NAC: N-acetyl cysteine; INH: isoniazid; RIF: rifampicin; PZA: pyrazinamide; hepG2: human liver cancer cell line.

of GSTM1 and GSTT1, glutathione S-transferase encoding genes, with anti-TB DILI [85].

NAC prevented anti-TB drug-induced hepatotoxicity in animal studies [82, 83] (Table 3). A study in rats demonstrated that INH and RIF each at a dose of 50 mg/kg depleted GSH as well as other antioxidants and increased lipid peroxidation in the liver tissue [83]. The changes in antioxidants levels were also accompanied by histopathologic changes such as portal triaditis, lobular inflammation, and patchy necrosis. NAC at a dose of 100 mg/kg prevented all these pathologic changes and attenuated the ALT elevation from 102 IU/l to 28 IU/l and the AST elevation from 578 IU/l to 165 IU/l at 3 weeks. Another study in rats confirmed the protective effect of NAC on RIF-induced hepatotoxicity. However, the latter study did not evidence a reduction in the level of GSH after treatment with RIF alone [82]. An *in vitro* study in human liver cancer cell line (hepg2) cells also demonstrated a protective property of NAC against anti-TB-induced hepato-/cytotoxicity [86] (Table 3).

A clinical trial of NAC in newly diagnosed TB patients also showed protective effects against hepatotoxicity [87] (Table 3). Sixty patients, aged greater than 60, were recruited in this trial and followed for two weeks. The study was not blinded and controls did not receive placebo. NAC was administered orally at dose of 600 mg twice daily, and the incidence of hepatotoxicity in the control group was 37.5% and none in the NAC group. As the authors themselves acknowledged, these results need to be interpreted with caution and there is a need for well-controlled larger trials with longer follow-up.

5. Conclusions

Based on the evidence accrued to date, NAC appears to have various beneficial effects on TB treatment and its evaluation in clinical trials is justifiable. For maximal protection by NAC against anti-TB-induced hearing loss, we need to continue the administration of NAC for a little longer after completion of aminoglycoside administration. Moreover, the interaction between NAC and some of the second-line anti-TB drugs needs further investigations despite favorable interaction between NAC and first-line anti-TB drugs, bedaquiline and clofazimine.

References

[1] R. Vidhya, K. Rathnakumar, V. Balu, and K. V. Pugalendi, "Oxidative stress, antioxidant status and lipid profile in pulmonary tuberculosis patients before and after anti-tubercular therapy," *The Indian Journal of Tuberculosis*, vol. 66, no. 3, pp. 375–381, 2019.

[2] T. Madebo, B. Lindtjorn, P. Aukrust, and R. K. Berge, "Circulating antioxidants and lipid peroxidation products in untreated tuberculosis patients in Ethiopia," *The American Journal of Clinical Nutrition*, vol. 78, no. 1, pp. 117–122, 2003.

[3] B. A. Muzembo, N. C. Mbendi, N. R. Ngatu, T. Suzuki, K. Wada, and S. Ikeda, "Serum selenium levels in tuberculosis patients: a systematic review and meta-analysis," *Journal of Trace Elements in Medicine and Biology*, vol. 50, pp. 257–262, 2018.

[4] A. Z. Soh, C. B. E. Chee, Y. T. Wang, J. M. Yuan, and W. P. Koh, "Dietary intake of antioxidant vitamins and carotenoids and risk of developing active tuberculosis in a prospective population-based cohort study," *American Journal of Epidemiology*, vol. 186, no. 4, pp. 491–500, 2017.

[5] H. Devarbhavi, R. Singh, M. Patil, K. Sheth, C. K. Adarsh, and G. Balaraju, "Outcome and determinants of mortality in 269 patients with combination anti-tuberculosis drug-induced liver injury," *Journal of Gastroenterology and Hepatology*, vol. 28, no. 1, pp. 161–167, 2013.

[6] O. A. Sogebi, B. O. Adefuye, S. O. Adebola, S. M. Oladeji, and T. O. Adedeji, "Clinical predictors of aminoglycoside-induced ototoxicity in drug-resistant tuberculosis patients on intensive therapy," *Auris Nasus Larynx*, vol. 44, no. 4, pp. 404–410, 2017.

[7] K. Kranzer, W. F. Elamin, H. Cox, J. A. Seddon, N. Ford, and F. Drobniewski, "A systematic review and meta-analysis of the efficacy and safety of N-acetylcysteine in preventing aminoglycoside-induced ototoxicity: implications for the treatment of multidrug-resistant TB," *Thorax*, vol. 70, no. 11, pp. 1070–1077, 2015.

[8] A. J. Garcia-Prats, H. S. Schaaf, and A. C. Hesseling, "The safety and tolerability of the second-line injectable antituberculosis drugs in children," *Expert Opinion on Drug Safety*, vol. 15, no. 11, pp. 1491–1500, 2016.

[9] V. Venketaraman, T. Rodgers, R. Linares et al., "Glutathione and growth inhibition of Mycobacterium tuberculosis in healthy and HIV infected subjects," *AIDS Research and Therapy*, vol. 3, no. 1, p. 5, 2006.

[10] R. Cao, G. Teskey, H. Islamoglu et al., "Characterizing the effects of glutathione as an immunoadjuvant in the treatment of tuberculosis," *Antimicrobial Agents and Chemotherapy*, vol. 62, no. 11, 2018.

[11] V. Venketaraman, A. Millman, M. Salman et al., "Glutathione levels and immune responses in tuberculosis patients," *Microbial Pathogenesis*, vol. 44, no. 3, pp. 255–261, 2008.

[12] C. Guerra, K. Johal, D. Morris et al., "Control of Mycobacterium tuberculosis growth by activated natural killer cells," *Clinical and Experimental Immunology*, vol. 168, no. 1, pp. 142–152, 2012.

[13] D. Morris, C. Guerra, M. Khurasany et al., "Glutathione supplementation improves macrophage functions in HIV," *Journal of Interferon & Cytokine Research*, vol. 33, no. 5, pp. 270–279, 2013.

[14] E. P. Amaral, E. L. Conceição, D. L. Costa et al., "N-acetyl-cysteine exhibits potent anti-mycobacterial activity in addition to its known anti-oxidative functions," *BMC Microbiology*, vol. 16, no. 1, p. 251, 2016.

[15] S. Whillier, J. E. Raftos, B. Chapman, and P. W. Kuchel, "Role of N-acetylcysteine and cystine in glutathione synthesis in human erythrocytes," *Redox Report*, vol. 14, no. 3, pp. 115–124, 2009.

[16] M. Balazy, P. M. Kaminski, K. Mao, J. Tan, and M. S. Wolin, "S-Nitroglutathione, a product of the reaction between peroxynitrite and glutathione that generates nitric oxide," *The Journal of Biological Chemistry*, vol. 273, no. 48, pp. 32009–32015, 1998.

[17] V. Venketaraman, Y. K. Dayaram, M. T. Talaue, and N. D. Connell, "Glutathione and nitrosoglutathione in macrophage defense against Mycobacterium tuberculosis," *Infection and Immunity*, vol. 73, no. 3, pp. 1886–1889, 2005.

[18] S. J. Anderberg, G. L. Newton, and R. C. Fahey, "Mycothiol biosynthesis and metabolism. Cellular levels of potential intermediates in the biosynthesis and degradation of mycothiol in Mycobacterium smegmatis," *The Journal of Biological Chemistry*, vol. 273, no. 46, pp. 30391–30397, 1998.

[19] D. Morris, M. Khurasany, T. Nguyen et al., "Glutathione and infection," *Biochimica et Biophysica Acta (BBA) - General Subjects*, vol. 1830, no. 5, pp. 3329–3349, 2013.

[20] C. Guerra, D. Morris, A. Sipin et al., "Glutathione and adaptive immune responses against Mycobacterium tuberculosis infection in healthy and HIV infected individuals," *PLoS One*, vol. 6, no. 12, article e28378, 2011.

[21] S. C. Lu, "Regulation of glutathione synthesis," *Molecular Aspects of Medicine*, vol. 30, no. 1-2, pp. 42–59, 2009.

[22] S. Park and J. A. Imlay, "High levels of intracellular cysteine promote oxidative DNA damage by driving the Fenton reaction," *Journal of Bacteriology*, vol. 185, no. 6, pp. 1942–1950, 2003.

[23] C. Vilcheze, T. Hartman, B. Weinrick et al., "Enhanced respiration prevents drug tolerance and drug resistance inMycobacterium tuberculosis," *Proceedings of the National Academy of Sciences of the United States of America*, vol. 114, no. 17, pp. 4495–4500, 2017.

[24] G. Teskey, R. Cao, H. Islamoglu et al., "The synergistic effects of the glutathione precursor, NAC and first-line antibiotics in the granulomatous response against Mycobacterium tuberculosis," *Frontiers in Immunology*, vol. 9, p. 2069, 2018.

[25] M. Allen, C. Bailey, I. Cahatol et al., "Mechanisms of control of Mycobacterium tuberculosis by NK cells: role of glutathione," *Frontiers in Immunology*, vol. 6, 2015.

[26] G. S. Palanisamy, N. M. Kirk, D. F. Ackart, C. A. Shanley, I. M. Orme, and R. J. Basaraba, "Evidence for oxidative stress and defective antioxidant response in guinea pigs with tuberculosis," *PLoS One*, vol. 6, no. 10, article e26254, 2011.

[27] A. S. Dharmadhikari and E. A. Nardell, "What animal models teach humans about tuberculosis," *American Journal of*

Respiratory Cell and Molecular Biology, vol. 39, no. 5, pp. 503–508, 2008.

[28] S. M. Mahakalkar, D. Nagrale, S. Gaur, C. Urade, B. Murhar, and A. Turankar, "N-acetylcysteine as an add-on to directly observed therapy short-I therapy in fresh pulmonary tuberculosis patients: a randomized, placebo-controlled, double-blinded study," *Perspectives in Clinical Research*, vol. 8, no. 3, pp. 132–136, 2017.

[29] B. Khameneh, B. S. Fazly Bazzaz, A. Amani, J. Rostami, and N. Vahdati-Mashhadian, "Combination of anti-tuberculosis drugs with vitamin C or NAC against different Staphylococcus aureus and Mycobacterium tuberculosis strains," *Microbial Pathogenesis*, vol. 93, pp. 83–87, 2016.

[30] D. A. Lamprecht, P. M. Finin, M. A. Rahman et al., "Turning the respiratory flexibility of _Mycobacterium tuberculosis_ against itself," *Nature Communications*, vol. 7, no. 1, 2016.

[31] V. M. Bulatovic, N. L. Wengenack, J. R. Uhl et al., "Oxidative stress increases susceptibility of Mycobacterium tuberculosis to isoniazid," *Antimicrobial Agents and Chemotherapy*, vol. 46, no. 9, pp. 2765–2771, 2002.

[32] J. Y. Wang, R. M. Burger, and K. Drlica, "Role of superoxide in catalase-peroxidase-mediated isoniazid action against mycobacteria," *Antimicrobial Agents and Chemotherapy*, vol. 42, no. 3, pp. 709–711, 1998.

[33] Y. Zhang, W. W. Yew, and M. R. Barer, "Targeting persisters for tuberculosis control," *Antimicrobial Agents and Chemotherapy*, vol. 56, no. 5, pp. 2223–2230, 2012.

[34] W. W. Yew, D. P. Chan, K. C. Chang, and Y. Zhang, "Does oxidative stress contribute to antituberculosis drug resistance?," *Journal of Thoracic Disease*, vol. 11, no. 7, pp. E100–E102, 2019.

[35] F. Yang, L. H. Liu, X. P. Li et al., "Short communication: N-acetylcysteine-mediated modulation of antibiotic susceptibility of bovine mastitis pathogens," *Journal of Dairy Science*, vol. 99, no. 6, pp. 4300–4302, 2016.

[36] M. Goswami and N. Jawali, "N-acetylcysteine-mediated modulation of bacterial antibiotic susceptibility," *Antimicrobial Agents and Chemotherapy*, vol. 54, no. 8, pp. 3529-3530, 2010.

[37] J. Rodriguez-Beltran, G. Cabot, E. Y. Valencia et al., "N-acetylcysteine selectively antagonizes the activity of imipenem in Pseudomonas aeruginosa by an OprD-mediated mechanism," *Antimicrobial Agents and Chemotherapy*, vol. 59, no. 6, pp. 3246–3251, 2015.

[38] G. Landini, T. Di Maggio, F. Sergio, J. D. Docquier, G. M. Rossolini, and L. Pallecchi, "Effect of high N-acetylcysteine concentrations on antibiotic activity against a large collection of respiratory pathogens," *Antimicrobial Agents and Chemotherapy*, vol. 60, no. 12, pp. 7513–7517, 2016.

[39] Y. Chen, W. G. Huang, D. J. Zha et al., "Aspirin attenuates gentamicin ototoxicity: from the laboratory to the clinic," *Hearing Research*, vol. 226, no. 1-2, pp. 178–182, 2007.

[40] D. T. Kemp, "Otoacoustic emissions, their origin in cochlear function, and use," *British Medical Bulletin*, vol. 63, no. 1, pp. 223–241, 2002.

[41] O. W. Guthrie, "Aminoglycoside induced ototoxicity," *Toxicology*, vol. 249, no. 2-3, pp. 91–96, 2008.

[42] M. L. Aznar, A. Rando Segura, M. M. Moreno et al., "Treatment outcomes and adverse events from a standardized multidrug-resistant tuberculosis regimen in a rural setting in Angola," *The American Journal of Tropical Medicine and Hygiene*, vol. 101, no. 3, pp. 502–509, 2019.

[43] R. Prasad, A. Singh, R. Srivastava, G. B. Hosmane, R. A. S. Kushwaha, and A. Jain, "Frequency of adverse events observed with second-line drugs among patients treated for multidrug-resistant tuberculosis," *The Indian Journal of Tuberculosis*, vol. 63, no. 2, pp. 106–114, 2016.

[44] R. Sarin, D. Behera, A. Khanna, V. Singh, P. Narang, and T. S. Deepak, "Second-line injectable induced ototoxicity in drug resistant tuberculosis: a systematic review of Indian studies," *The Indian Journal of Tuberculosis*, vol. 66, no. 2, pp. 279–287, 2019.

[45] C. Modongo, J. G. Pasipanodya, N. M. Zetola, S. M. Williams, G. Sirugo, and T. Gumbo, "Amikacin concentrations predictive of ototoxicity in multidrug-resistant tuberculosis patients," *Antimicrobial Agents and Chemotherapy*, vol. 59, no. 10, pp. 6337–6343, 2015.

[46] H. Hong, C. Budhathoki, and J. E. Farley, "Increased risk of aminoglycoside-induced hearing loss in MDR-TB patients with HIV coinfection," *The International Journal of Tuberculosis and Lung Disease*, vol. 22, no. 6, pp. 667–674, 2018.

[47] A. Arnold, G. S. Cooke, O. M. Kon et al., "Adverse effects and choice between the injectable agents amikacin and capreomycin in multidrug-resistant tuberculosis," *Antimicrobial Agents and Chemotherapy*, vol. 61, no. 9, 2017.

[48] E. L. Sagwa, N. Ruswa, F. Mavhunga, T. Rennie, H. G. M. Leufkens, and A. K. Mantel-Teeuwisse, "Comparing amikacin and kanamycin-induced hearing loss in multidrug-resistant tuberculosis treatment under programmatic conditions in a Namibian retrospective cohort," *BMC Pharmacology and Toxicology*, vol. 16, no. 1, p. 36, 2015.

[49] I. Aladag, M. Guven, and M. Songu, "Prevention of gentamicin ototoxicity with N-acetylcysteine and vitamin A," *The Journal of Laryngology and Otology*, vol. 130, no. 5, pp. 440–446, 2016.

[50] I. Kocyigit, A. Vural, A. Unal et al., "Preventing amikacin related ototoxicity with N-acetylcysteine in patients undergoing peritoneal dialysis," *European Archives of Oto-Rhino-Laryngology*, vol. 272, no. 10, pp. 2611–2620, 2015.

[51] X. Gong, G. Celsi, K. Carlsson, and S. Norgren, "Protective effects of N-acetylcysteine amide (NACA) on gentamicin-induced apoptosis in LLC-PK1 cells," *Renal Failure*, vol. 34, no. 4, pp. 487–494, 2012.

[52] X. Wei, L. Zhao, J. Liu, R. C. Dodel, M. R. Farlow, and Y. Du, "Minocycline prevents gentamicin-induced ototoxicity by inhibiting p 38 MAP kinase phosphorylation and caspase 3 activation," *Neuroscience*, vol. 131, no. 2, pp. 513–521, 2005.

[53] A. Forge and J. Schacht, "Aminoglycoside antibiotics," *Audiology & Neuro-Otology*, vol. 5, no. 1, pp. 3–22, 2000.

[54] E. M. Priuska and J. Schacht, "Formation of free radicals by gentamicin and iron and evidence for an iron/gentamicin complex," *Biochemical Pharmacology*, vol. 50, no. 11, pp. 1749–1752, 1995.

[55] H. Jiang, S. H. Sha, A. Forge, and J. Schacht, "Caspase-independent pathways of hair cell death induced by kanamycin in vivo," *Cell Death and Differentiation*, vol. 13, no. 1, pp. 20–30, 2006.

[56] J. Kralova, M. Dvorak, M. Koc, and V. Kral, "p38 MAPK plays an essential role in apoptosis induced by photoactivation of a novel ethylene glycol porphyrin derivative," *Oncogene*, vol. 27, no. 21, pp. 3010–3020, 2008.

[57] S. H. Sha, G. Zajic, C. J. Epstein, and J. Schacht, "Overexpression of copper/zinc-superoxide dismutase protects from

kanamycin-induced hearing loss," *Audiology & Neuro-Otology*, vol. 6, no. 3, pp. 117–123, 2001.

[58] M. A. Somdas, F. Korkmaz, S. G. Gurgen, M. Sagit, and A. Akcadag, "N-acetylcysteine prevents gentamicin ototoxicity in a rat model," *The Journal of International Advanced Otology*, vol. 11, no. 1, pp. 12–18, 2015.

[59] C. Y. Wu, H. J. Lee, C. F. Liu, M. Korivi, H. H. Chen, and M. H. Chan, "Protective role of L-ascorbic acid, N-acetylcysteine and apocynin on neomycin-induced hair cell loss in zebrafish," *Journal of Applied Toxicology*, vol. 35, no. 3, pp. 273–279, 2015.

[60] G. R. Bock, G. K. Yates, J. J. Miller, and P. Moorjani, "Effects of N-acetylcysteine on kanamycin ototoxicity in the guinea pig," *Hearing Research*, vol. 9, no. 3, pp. 255–262, 1983.

[61] L. Feldman, S. Efrati, E. Eviatar et al., "Gentamicin-induced ototoxicity in hemodialysis patients is ameliorated by N-acetylcysteine," *Kidney International*, vol. 72, no. 3, pp. 359–363, 2007.

[62] B. Tokgoz, C. Ucar, I. Kocyigit et al., "Protective effect of N-acetylcysteine from drug-induced ototoxicity in uraemic patients with CAPD peritonitis," *Nephrology, Dialysis, Transplantation*, vol. 26, no. 12, pp. 4073–4078, 2011.

[63] A. Vural, I. Kocyigit, F. San et al., "Long-term protective effect of N-acetylcysteine against amikacin-induced ototoxicity in end-stage renal disease: a randomized trial," *Peritoneal Dialysis International*, vol. 38, no. 1, pp. 57–62, 2018.

[64] J. Aran, "Current perspectives on inner ear toxicity," *Otolaryngology and Head and Neck Surgery*, vol. 112, no. 1, pp. 133–144, 1995.

[65] K. H. Tan, M. Mulheran, A. J. Knox, and A. R. Smyth, "Aminoglycoside prescribing and surveillance in cystic fibrosis," *American Journal of Respiratory and Critical Care Medicine*, vol. 167, no. 6, pp. 819–823, 2003.

[66] A. Tostmann, M. J. Boeree, R. E. Aarnoutse, W. C. de Lange, A. J. van der Ven, and R. Dekhuijzen, "Antituberculosis drug-induced hepatotoxicity: concise up-to-date review," *Journal of Gastroenterology and Hepatology*, vol. 23, no. 2, pp. 192–202, 2008.

[67] V. Ramappa and G. P. Aithal, "Hepatotoxicity related to antituberculosis drugs: mechanisms and management," *Journal of Clinical and Experimental Hepatology*, vol. 3, no. 1, pp. 37–49, 2013.

[68] S. Keshavjee, I. Y. Gelmanova, S. S. Shin et al., "Hepatotoxicity during treatment for multidrug-resistant tuberculosis: occurrence, management and outcome," *The International Journal of Tuberculosis and Lung Disease*, vol. 16, no. 5, pp. 596–603, 2012.

[69] F. Gafar, H. Arifin, Y. D. Jurnalis et al., "Antituberculosis drug-induced liver injury in children: incidence and risk factors during the two-month intensive phase of therapy," *The Pediatric Infectious Disease Journal*, vol. 38, no. 1, pp. 50–53, 2019.

[70] P. Shang, Y. Xia, F. Liu et al., "Incidence, clinical features and impact on anti-tuberculosis treatment of anti-tuberculosis drug induced liver injury (ATLI) in China," *PLoS One*, vol. 6, no. 7, article e21836, 2011.

[71] I. Warmelink, N. H. ten Hacken, T. S. van der Werf, and R. van Altena, "Weight loss during tuberculosis treatment is an important risk factor for drug-induced hepatotoxicity," *The British Journal of Nutrition*, vol. 105, no. 3, pp. 400–408, 2011.

[72] R. Singla, S. K. Sharma, A. Mohan et al., "Evaluation of risk factors for antituberculosis treatment induced hepatotoxicity," *The Indian Journal of Medical Research*, vol. 132, pp. 81–86, 2010.

[73] S. E. Isa, A. O. Ebonyi, N. Y. Shehu et al., "Antituberculosis drugs and hepatotoxicity among hospitalized patients in Jos, Nigeria," *International Journal of Mycobacteriology*, vol. 5, no. 1, pp. 21–26, 2016.

[74] W. Abera, W. Cheneke, and G. Abebe, "Incidence of antituberculosis-drug-induced hepatotoxicity and associated risk factors among tuberculosis patients in Dawro zone, South Ethiopia: a cohort study," *International Journal of Mycobacteriology*, vol. 5, no. 1, pp. 14–20, 2016.

[75] L. G. Possuelo, J. A. Castelan, T. C. de Brito et al., "Association of slow N-acetyltransferase 2 profile and anti-TB drug-induced hepatotoxicity in patients from southern Brazil," *European Journal of Clinical Pharmacology*, vol. 64, no. 7, pp. 673–681, 2008.

[76] G. Yimer, G. Aderaye, W. Amogne et al., "Anti-tuberculosis therapy-induced hepatotoxicity among Ethiopian HIV-positive and negative patients," *PLoS One*, vol. 3, no. 3, article e1809, 2008.

[77] A. H. Ali, T. Belachew, A. Yami, and W. Y. Ayen, "Anti-tuberculosis drug induced hepatotoxicity among TB/HIV co-infected patients at Jimma University Hospital, Ethiopia: nested case-control study," *PLoS One*, vol. 8, no. 5, article e64622, 2013.

[78] H. A. Makhlouf, A. Helmy, E. Fawzy, M. El-Attar, and H. A. Rashed, "A prospective study of antituberculous drug-induced hepatotoxicity in an area endemic for liver diseases," *Hepatology International*, vol. 2, no. 3, pp. 353–360, 2008.

[79] N. Lomtadze, L. Kupreishvili, A. Salakaia et al., "Hepatitis C virus co-infection increases the risk of anti-tuberculosis drug-induced hepatotoxicity among patients with pulmonary tuberculosis," *PLoS One*, vol. 8, no. 12, article e83892, 2013.

[80] L. Ben Mahmoud, H. Ghozzi, A. Kamoun et al., "Polymorphism of the N-acetyltransferase 2 gene as a susceptibility risk factor for antituberculosis drug-induced hepatotoxicity in Tunisian patients with tuberculosis," *Pathologie Biologie*, vol. 60, no. 5, pp. 324–330, 2012.

[81] K. Nanashima, T. Mawatari, N. Tahara et al., "Genetic variants in antioxidant pathway: risk factors for hepatotoxicity in tuberculosis patients," *Tuberculosis (Edinburgh, Scotland)*, vol. 92, no. 3, pp. 253–259, 2012.

[82] S. V. Rana, S. Attri, K. Vaiphei, R. Pal, A. Attri, and K. Singh, "Role of N-acetylcysteine in rifampicin-induced hepatic injury of young rats," *World Journal of Gastroenterology*, vol. 12, no. 2, pp. 287–291, 2006.

[83] S. Attri, S. V. Rana, K. Vaiphei et al., "Isoniazid- and rifampicin-induced oxidative hepatic injury–protection by N-acetylcysteine," *Human & Experimental Toxicology*, vol. 19, no. 9, pp. 517–522, 2000.

[84] M. Yang, H. Zhang, B. Tao et al., "Possible association of HMOX1 and NQO1 polymorphisms with anti-tuberculosis drug-induced liver injury: a matched case-control study," *Journal of Clinical Pharmacy and Therapeutics*, vol. 44, no. 4, pp. 534–542, 2019.

[85] M. Zhang, S. Q. Wu, and J. Q. He, "Are genetic variations in glutathione S-transferases involved in anti-tuberculosis drug-induced liver injury? A meta-analysis," *Journal of Clinical Pharmacy and Therapeutics*, vol. 44, no. 6, pp. 844–857, 2019.

[86] M. Singh, P. Sasi, V. H. Gupta, G. Rai, D. N. Amarapurkar, and P. P. Wangikar, "Protective effect of curcumin, silymarin and N-acetylcysteine on antitubercular drug-induced hepatotoxicity assessed in an in vitro model," *Human & Experimental Toxicology*, vol. 31, no. 8, pp. 788–797, 2012.

[87] S. Baniasadi, P. Eftekhari, P. Tabarsi et al., "Protective effect of N-acetylcysteine on antituberculosis drug-induced hepatotoxicity," *European Journal of Gastroenterology & Hepatology*, vol. 22, no. 10, pp. 1235–1238, 2010.

19

Treatment Outcomes and Associated Factors in Tuberculosis Patients at Atwima Nwabiagya District, Ashanti Region, Ghana: A Ten-Year Retrospective Study

Sadick Ahmed Agyare,[1] Francis Adjei Osei,[2] Samuel Frimpong Odoom,[3] Nicholas Karikari Mensah,[3] Ernest Amanor,[2] Charles Martyn-Dickens,[3] Michael Owusu-Ansah,[2] Aliyu Mohammed,[2] and Eugene Osei Yeboah[4]

[1]*Ghana Health Service, Atwima Nwabiagya, Ghana*
[2]*Kwame Nkrumah University of Science and Technology, Kumasi, Ghana*
[3]*Komfo Anokye Teaching Hospital, Kumasi, Ghana*
[4]*Ghana Health Service, Zuarungu, Ghana*

Correspondence should be addressed to Samuel Frimpong Odoom; samfriod@gmail.com

Academic Editor: Adwoa Asante-Poku

Introduction. Tuberculosis poses a great threat to public health around the globe and affects persons mostly in their productive age, notwithstanding; everyone is susceptible to tuberculosis (TB) infection. To assess the effectiveness and performance of the tuberculosis control program activities, the percentage of cases with treatment success outcome is key. To control tuberculosis, interrupting transmission through effective treatment cannot be overemphasized. The study was conducted to determine factors associated with TB treatment outcome, in the Atwima Nwabiagya District from 2007–2017. *Method.* A Retrospective review of routine/standard TB registers was carried out in five directly observed therapy short-course (DOTS) centres at the Atwima Nwabiagya District from January 2007 to December 2017. Demographic characteristics, clinical characteristics, and treatment outcomes were assessed. Bivariate and multivariate logistic regression was conducted to determine the predictors of successful treatment outcome. *Results.* Of the 891 TB client's data that was assessed in the district, the treatment success rate was 68.46%. Patients, aged ≤ 20 years (adjusted odds ratio (aOR) = 4.74, 95%CI = 1.75 – 12.83) and 51-60 years (aOR = 1.94, 95%CI = 1.12 – 3.39), having a pretreatment weight of 35-45 kg (aOR = 2.54, 95%CI = 1.32 – 4.87), 46-55 kg (aOR = 2.75, 95%CI = 1.44 – 5.27) and 56-65 kg (aOR = 3.04, 95%CI = 1.50 – 6.14) were associated with treatment success. However, retreatment patients (aOR = 0.31, 95%CI = 0.11 – 0.84) resulted in unsuccessful treatment outcome. *Conclusion.* Successful treatment outcome among TB patients was about 20.00% and 30.00% lower compared to the national average treatment success rate and WHO target, respectively. Active monitoring, motivation, and counselling of retreatment patients and patients with advanced age are key to treatment success.

1. Background

Tuberculosis (TB) remains one of the oldest debilitating infectious diseases globally but disproportionately affect the world's poor. The clinical presentation of TB is associated with the pathogenesis of an Acid-Fast Bacilli bacterium called *Mycobacterium tuberculosis* which is transmitted through aerosols or droplets when an individual with an active infection coughs, sneezes, sings, or talks [1, 2]. Persons infected by *Mycobacterium tuberculosis* may not develop symptoms of TB (latent TB); nonetheless, infected individuals have a 5-15% lifetime risk of becoming sick within 2-5 years of getting the infection [3–5]. However, individuals who are immunocompromised such as people with HIV, diabetes, malnutrition, or heavy smokers, and older adults and children have a higher risk of developing symptoms of TB [4]. This may include a cough that produces phlegm, fever, chills, fatigue, loss of appetite, and weight loss. It is reported that a single TB patient with active infection can infect an average of 10-15 people annually if the patient is not treated [6].

Approximately 10 million cases of TB and 1.5 million deaths are recorded every year globally [7]. Out of the 30 countries with the highest burden of TB globally, 24 are in the WHO African region [8, 9]. Nearly 2.5 million people who contracted TB, 665,000 of them died from the disease in 2017 in sub-Saharan Africa [9]. Analysis of global TB data shows that the annual TB incidence has been on a downturn by an average of 1.5%, and the management of TB has significantly improved since 2000 [8]. Interestingly, about 49 million lives have been rescued as a result of early and improved TB diagnosis and appropriate treatments between 2000 and 2015 [5]. Despite the mammoth progress of global efforts, TB remains one of the leading causes of morbidity and mortality worldwide and remains a substantial public health burden in sub-Saharan Africa [10]. It is reported that the prevention, care, and control of TB has been challenging due to socioeconomic reasons [10]. Therefore, it is imperative to scale-up management efforts to meet the End TB strategy, which aims at reducing TB mortality rate by 90% by the year 2030 [11].

Successful treatment outcomes of TB vary from country to country but 83% of treatment outcomes have been attained worldwide [12]. Nonetheless, several studies have reported age, biological sex, comorbidity or underlining health conditions, pretreatment weight, and financial status or family support as factors that influence treatment outcomes of TB in sub-Saharan Africa [13, 14]. Comorbidity with HIV was found to be strongly associated with TB treatment outcomes, and apparently, treatment outcomes were best for individuals with a negative HIV status compared with those positive for HIV [12, 13, 15]. Moreover, most studies report that being male, older adults, and large family size are associated with unsuccessful treatment outcomes in sub-Saharan Africa [15, 16]. According to WHO, about 6 million adult men contracted TB and around 840,000 died from it compared with roughly 3.2 million and nearly half a million adult women who fell ill and died from TB, respectively, in 2017 [8]. However, the factors influencing treatment outcome may vary from one setting or region to another. For instance, a study reported a successful treatment outcome rate of 82.5% in the Volta region, 90.2% in the Central region, and 90.7% in the Greater Accra region of Ghana [17, 18].

In Ghana, over 46,000 new cases of active TB infection are recorded yearly, and TB mortality rate is reported at 7.5 per 1,000 infected people, indicating that TB is a burden in the country [5, 19]. Successful treatment outcomes are very crucial to mitigate the burden of TB of which several studies have reported successful outcome rates nearly similar to the national successful treatment outcome rate (87.7%) [17, 20, 21]. Furthermore, factors such as HIV comorbidity, biological sex, disease category, patient category, financial status, the distance of patient from the treatment centre, among others were found to be associated with treatment outcomes [20, 21]. Successful treatment outcomes were associated with females, HIV-negative status, high financial index, and the proximity of patients to treatment centres. However, pretreatment weight varied [17, 18, 20, 22].

Evaluating the treatment outcome of TB cases and its determinants is important to inform health authorities and policymakers on the management of the disease. However, studies exploring TB treatment outcomes and the associated factors are limited in Ghana and lacking in many districts in the Ashanti Region of Ghana. Given the paucity of evaluation data on TB treatment outcome in the Ashanti Region, it is essential to conduct this study to contribute to the body of knowledge and provide health managers and policy makers with evidence necessary to improve the current situation.

Therefore, this study is aimed at assessing treatment outcomes of TB and the factors that influence the observed treatment outcomes in TB patients at the Atwima Nwabiagya District, Ashanti Region, Ghana.

2. Materials and Methods

2.1. Study Area. The study was conducted in the Atwima Nwabiagya district in the Ashanti Region of Ghana. The district is perched approximately on latitude 6°32′N and 6°75′N and longitude 1°45′W and 2°00′W. It covers an estimated area of 294.84 square km with a population of 176,171 and is situated in the western part of the Ashanti Region. The five DOTS centres in the Districts that were selected are Nkawie-Toase Hospital, Abuakwa Health Centre, Akropong Health Centre, Asuofua Health Centre, and Barekese Health Centre.

2.2. Study Design. A retrospective review of standard TB registers was conducted from January 2007 to December 2017 to determine successful TB treatment outcome and associated factors among TB patients.

2.3. Study Population. All patients diagnosed with and treated with TB and had treatment outcomes in the TB registers were included in the study whereas patients who were referred or entries with incomplete information on treatment outcomes were excluded.

2.4. Sample Size Determination and Sampling Technique. The sample size was determined by using a single population prevalence formula.

$$n = \frac{(Z_\alpha + Z_\beta)^2 p(1-p)}{d^2}, \quad (1)$$

where n is the minimum required sample size. Z_α is the desired level of statistical significance: 95% confidence level which translate to 1.96 to a standard normal deviate of 1.96. Z_β is the desired power of the test: 80% which translates to 0.84 standard normal deviate. p is the prevalence of successful treatment outcome of TB patients from previous study: 82.5% [22]. d is the margin of error: 4%.

Substituting the above values into the formula;

$$n = \frac{(1.96 + 0.84)^2 0.825(1 - 0.825)}{0.04^2}, \quad (2)$$

$$n = 707.43, \quad (3)$$

$$n \approx 707. \quad (4)$$

After accounting for a 20% nonresponse rate of missing data, the minimum sample size was 848.

Study participants who met the inclusion criteria were selected from the standard TB registers through convenient sampling technique at the 5 DOTS centres.

2.5. Data Collection, Data Quality, and Data Analysis. Data were collected from the standard TB registers (the TB registers are used to capture information of all TB patients been treated at all DOTS centres in the districts) using a pilot-tested data abstraction sheet. The abstraction sheet was designed electronically using Open Data Kit (ODK). The sheet was pilot tested at Komfo Anokye Teaching Hospital's (KATH), TB Clinic, which provides similar services to TB patients as the study site. The data were collected by trained research assistants. The data were reviewed by a data manager for completeness and discrepancies. Information such as demographic characteristics, clinical characteristics, and treatment outcomes were collected from the TB registers.

The data were exported from the ODK to Microsoft Excel, cleaned, and exported to Stata/SE 14.0 statistical software (Stata Corp 4905 Lakeway Drive College Station, Texas 77845, USA) for analysis. Descriptive statistical analysis such as mean, standard deviation, and frequencies (percentages) was used to describe the study population. Bivariate and multivariate logistic regression analysis was done with 95% confidence interval (CI) to calculate the crude odds ratio (OR) and adjusted odds ratio (aOR) to measure the strength of the association between the outcome (treatment outcome) and predictor variables (age, gender, pretreatment weight, HIV status, diseases classification, type of patient, availability of treatment supporter, and adverse drug reaction).

2.6. Operational Definitions and Treatment Regimen. Table 1 displays the operational terms used in this study. The operation was based on the standard definitions adopted from the World Health Organization guideline [7].

The recommended DOTS treatment regimens are guidelines for each category of TB in Ghana by the National TB Control Program and the National AIDS Control Program [23] (Table 2).

2.7. Ethical Considerations. Ethical approval for the conduct of the study was obtained from the ethical review board of the Ghana Health Service Research and Development Division (Ref. No. GHS-ERC: 76/12/18). Permission was also sought from the Ashanti Regional Health Directorate, Atwima Nwabiagya District Health Directorate, and the five DOTS centres. The information obtained from the TB registers was used for only research purposes and is kept confidential in accordance with the declaration of Helsinki (1964). No identification information such as names was extracted or captured from the records.

3. Results

3.1. Background Characteristics of the TB Patients. A total of 1,032 TB patients were registered at the 5 DOT centres at the Atwima Nwabiagya District during the period (2007-2017) of review. Of these, 891 (86.34%) patients had complete data and were therefore included in the study (Figure 1). More than half 599 (67.23%) of the patients were females. The age distribution of the patients ranged from 12–95 years, with a mean and standard deviation of 46.63 and 16.24 years, respectively. Nearly one-quarter 217 (24.35%) were within the ages of 31-40 years. Before the initiation of the regimen, 260 (29.18%) of the patients weighed 36-45 kg with a mean and standard deviation of weight as 49.64 kg and 9.42 kg, respectively. HIV/TB coinfection was observed in 82 (9.20%) of the patients. More than half, 535 (60.04%), of the patients were classified as extrapulmonary TB and more than three quarters of 793 (89.00%) were newly diagnosed with TB. Few 4 (0.45%) of the patients had adverse reactions to the TB regimen (Table 3).

3.2. Treatment Outcomes of TB Patients. The proportion of death among the TB patients was 10.21%. A total of 366 (37.71%) and 274 (30.75%) of the patients completed their treatment and were cured, respectively, giving a successful treatment rate of 68.46% ($n = 610$). Treatment failure was observed among 10 cases (1.12%) and a default rate of 20.2% ($n = 180$). Unsuccessful treatment was observed in 281 (31.54%) of them (Table 4).

3.3. Factors Associated with Treatment Outcome. Unadjusted logistics regression analysis revealed that the odds of achieving a successful treatment outcome was 5.57 ($95\%CI = 2.08 - 14.90$, $p \leq 0.001$) and 2.06 ($95\%CI = 1.20 - 3.53, p = 0.009$) higher among patients aged at less or equal to 20 years and 51-60 years compared to their age counterparts. Patients with weights between 36-45, 46-55, and 56-65 kg were 2.54, 2.50, and 2.79 times more likely to develop treatment success compared to patients with weight greater than 65 kg, respectively (($OR = 2.54$, $CI = 1.36 - 4.74$, $p = 0.004$), ($OR = 2.50$, $CI = 1.36 - 4.59$, $p = 0.003$), ($OR = 2.79$, $CI = 1.44 - 5.40$, $p = 0.002$)) (Table 5)

Adjusted logistic regression revealed that patients aged less or equal to 20 years and 51-60 years were 4.74 and 1.94 times more likely to develop treatment success as compared to other age groups (($aOR = 4.74$, $CI = 1.75 - 12.83$, $p \leq 0.002$), ($aOR = 1.94$, $CI = 1.12 - 3.39$, $p = 0.019$)). Patients weight between 36-45, 46-55, and 56-65 kg were 2.43, 2.49, and 2.75 times more likely to develop treatment success as compared to patients with weight greater than 65 kg (($aOR = 2.54$, 1.32-4.87, $p = 0.005$), ($aOR = 2.75$, $CI = 1.14 - 5.27$, $p = 0.002$), ($aOR = 3.04$, $CI = 1.50 - 6.14$, $p = 0.002$)). Retreatment patients were 69.0% less likely to develop treatment success ($OR = 0.31$, $CI = 0.11 - 0.84$, $p = 0.021$) (Table 5).

4. Discussion

Improved diagnosis and successful treatment of TB have been instrumental in mitigating and averting millions of TB

Table 1: Operational definitions used in this study.

Term	Definition
Cured	A pulmonary positive TB patient who has completed a full course of treatment and has tested negative to smear or culture-negative in the last month of treatment and at least one previous occasion.
Treatment completed	A TB patient who completed treatment without failure of treatment and with no evidence to show that sputum smear or culture results in the last month of treatment and on at least one previous occasion were negative, either because tests were not done or because results are unavailable.
Treatment failure	A TB patient who remains sputum smear or culture positive at month five or later during treatment regardless of adherence to the prescribed treatment protocols
Died	A TB patient who dies for any reason before starting or during treatment.
Default	A patient who interrupted treatment consecutively for two weeks or more after initiation of treatment
Transferred in	A patient who has been transferred from another TB register to continue treatment transferred to another reporting and recording unit for continuation of treatment, for whom treatment outcome is unknown.
HIV infection	Being infected with the human immune deficiency virus (HIV) that is confirmed by first and second line serologic tests
HIV/TB coinfection	The presence of both HIV and TB infection in a patient.
Successful treatment	A combination of cure and treatment completed.
Unsuccessful treatment	A combination of death, default, and treatment failure
New patient	A patient who has never had treatment for TB or who has taken anti-TB drugs for less than 1 month
Relapse	A patient previously treated for TB declared cured or treatment completed and who is diagnosed bacteriological (+) TB (smear or culture).
Failure	A patient who is restarted on a TB treatment after having failed previous treatment
Treatment supporter	A person who assists the patient in following treatment schedule throughout treatment. It can be a relative or a health professional

Table 2: TB treatment regimen.

Patient category	Definition	Initial phase treatment* Daily (28 doses/month)	Continuous phase treatment Daily (28 doses/month)
All new clients	New smear-positive New smear-negative pulmonary TB Concomitant HIV disease Extrapulmonary TB	2 (HRZE)[¥] = 56 doses of HRZE	4 (HR) = 112 doses of HR
Previously treated sputum smear-positive pulmonary TB	Relapse Treatment after interruption Treatment failure	2 (HRZE)S + 1(HRZE) = 84 doses of HRZE + 56 doses of S	5 (HRE) = 140 doses of HRE
Children[a]	Children below 12 years	2 (HRZ) = 56 doses of HRZ	4 (HR) = 112 doses of HR

*Direct observation of treatment intake is required and always in regimen including rifampicin. [¥]Streptomycin may be used instead of ethambutol. In meningitis, ethambutol should be replaced by streptomycin. [a]In children with meningitis, add streptomycin in the initial phase. Codes for Tb drugs: H: isoniazid; R: rifampicin; Z: pyrazinamide; S: streptomycin; E: ethambutol. Fixed drug combinations (FDC) codes: (HR): isoniazid + rifampicin; (HRZ): isoniazid + rifampicin + pyrazinamide; (HRZE): isoniazid + rifampicin + pyrazinamide + ethambutol.

deaths annually. However, TB treatment programs in sub-Saharan Africa are faced with several challenges that make these programs not as highly effective as expected, and thus, these factors result in unsuccessful treatment outcomes. We evaluated the TB treatment outcomes and the predictors of successful and unsuccessful treatment outcomes which is very key to the performance of a National TB control program. The findings of this study show that most TB clients were either cured or completed treatment; hence, the rate of successful treatment outcome in the study areas was

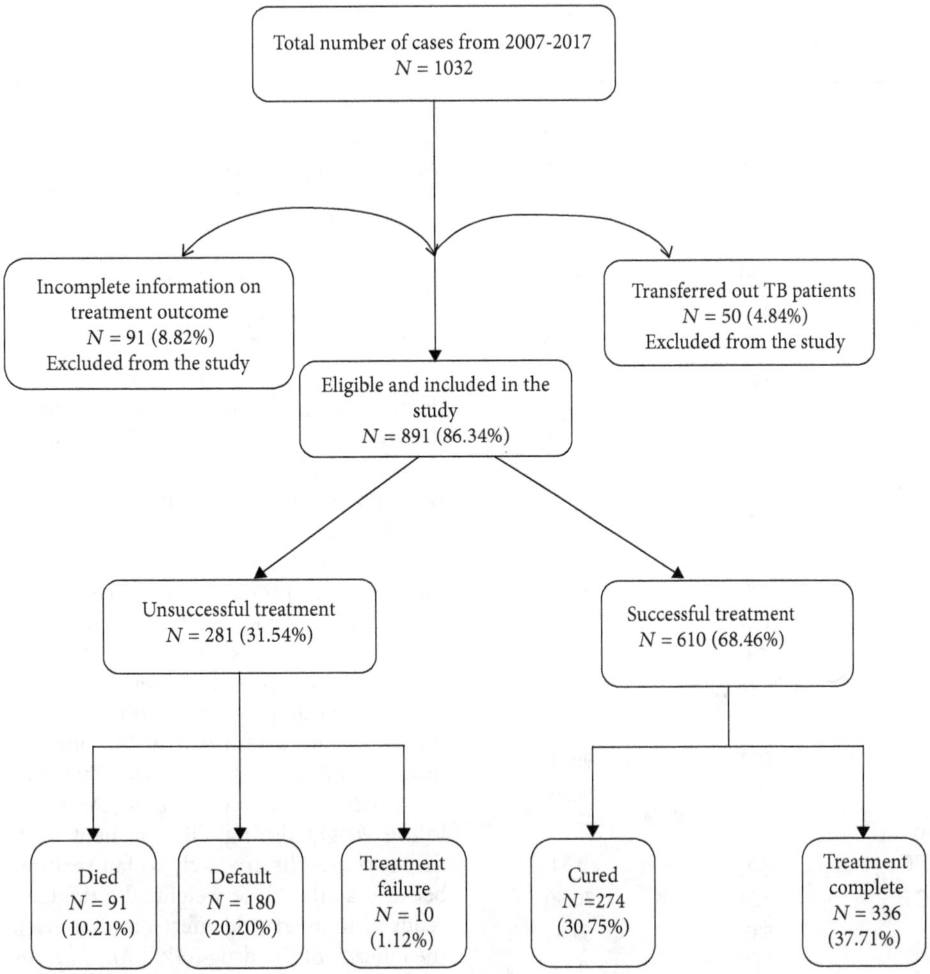

FIGURE 1: Flowchart of TB treatment outcome in Atwima Nwabiagya District, Ashanti Region, Ghana from 2007-2017.

68.46%. Though majority of the patients responded to the treatment, the rate of treatment success was below the national treatment success rate of 87.7% [16, 20] and rates recorded in other parts of the country [17, 18, 22] as well as rates in other countries like Ethiopia (Southwest 85.9%, Eastern 92.5%) [12, 24], Kenya (82.4%) [25], and Iran (91.7%) [26]. However, our finding is similar to the rate of treatment success reported by a study in South Africa (70%) [14].

The difference in treatment success observed in this study compared to other previous studies could be due to variations of the study duration, which was usually 5 years for most studies, and sample size, which was relatively low given the duration of this study [12, 24, 25]. The unsatisfactory treatment outcome can also be explained by the high number of defaulters, few participants who died, and the very few who failed treatment which was higher in the study compared to other previous studies [12, 24, 25]. This probably implies patient follow-up or treatment supervision has been poor in the district or patient delay in seeking TB care as a result of stigma or inadequate community involvement in TB care. Furthermore, patients who failed treatment might have developed resistance to anti-TB medication. Therefore, it is important to ensure rigorous treatment supervision and to engage all stakeholders in patient care through the community TB care, an intervention that recognizes social capital and connectedness as a tool to effective TB treatment and control.

Globally, TB morbidity and mortality are significantly higher among men than women, and it is reported that the ratio of male to female TB mortality and/or morbidity is about 2 : 1 in low-and middle-income countries [27, 28]. Though the cause of this observation is not clearly understood, it is believed that epidemiological factors could be the impetus driving this trend [29]. Studies have revealed that men are less likely to have a timely TB diagnosis due to the fear of stigmatization, and, within the context of HIV, men are likely to default their treatment and experience worse outcomes [28, 30]. On the other hand, women are more likely to seek timely diagnosis but due to socioeconomic constraints and stigmatization, many resort to orthodox or home treatment [26, 31]. Contrary to previous studies, our findings revealed that most of the reported TB cases were females compared to males, and the rate of treatment success was nearly the same for both genders. Nonetheless, there was no significant association between gender and treatment outcomes. This may suggest that women access diagnostic and screening services more than men or men are at a disadvantage in seeking and accessing TB care.

TABLE 3: Background characteristics of TB patients.

Variable	Frequency ($n = 891$)	Percentage (%)
Gender		
Female	599	67.23
Male	292	32.77
Age (years)		
≤20	48	5.39
21-30	150	16.84
31-40	217	24.35
41-50	214	24.02
51-60	117	13.13
>60	145	16.27
Mean (SD)	43.63 (±16.24)	
Pretreatment weight (kg)		
≤35	48	5.39
36-45	260	29.18
46-55	366	41.08
56-65	164	18.41
>66	53	5.95
Mean (SD)	49.64 (9.42)	
HIV status		
Negative	809	90.80
Positive	82	9.20
Disease classification		
Smear positive PTB	85	9.54
Smear negative PTB	270	30.30
Extra-PTB	535	60.04
MDR-TB	1	0.11
Patient category		
New	793	89.00
Relapse	53	5.95
Transfer in	8	0.90
Failure	18	2.02
Retreatment	19	2.13
Treatment support		
No	89	9.99
Yes	802	90.01
Adverse drug reaction		
No	887	99.55
Yes	4	0.45

TABLE 4: Distribution of treatment outcomes of the TB patients.

Variable	Frequency ($n = 891$)	Percentage (%)
Successful	610	68.46
(i) Cured	274	30.75
(ii) Treatment complete	336	37.71
Unsuccessful	281	31.54
(i) Died	91	10.21
(ii) Defaulted	180	20.20
(iii) Treatment failure	10	1.12

The majority of the respondents are between the ages range 31-40 years and 41-50 years, and this was consistent with a few studies in Ghana [17, 22, 32]. This suggests that individuals of the productive age group are mostly infected by TB in the district. However, the odds of successful treatment outcomes were better for respondents at age less or equal to 20 years (5.57) and 51-60 years (2.06). Based on this evidence, the economy could be burdened because the majority of the TB patients fall within the age group who might not be able to work and support the nonworking force due to the disease. Given that TB mostly affects individuals of the productive age group but less likely to have treatment success demands that community TB care must be pursued vigorously in the district. According to our findings, pretreatment weight between 36-45 kg, 46-55 kg, and 56-65 kg were significantly associated with successful treatment outcome compared to those less than 35 kg and greater than 65 kg. Furthermore, pretreatment weight between 36-45 kg, 46-55 kg, and 56-65 kg were more likely to record successful treatment outcomes. Although the effect of pretreatment weight differences on treatment outcome varies between settings, our finding is similar to the outcomes of a study conducted in the eastern part of Ethiopia [12]. TB is a wasting disease, and it has been shown that bodyweight variations can predict TB treatment outcome [33]. Thus, TB patients losing weight during TB treatment particularly within the first two months are likely to fail treatment [33, 34]. This is because as they lose weight, the dosage of drugs has to be reduced to avert side effects, and as result, this may reduce the efficacy of the drug to kill *M. tuberculosis*.

Unlike several studies that reported a strong association between HIV comorbidity and treatment outcome [21, 27, 35], this study recorded an insignificant association between treatment outcome and HIV comorbidity. Likewise, the majority of the patients reviewed were negative for HIV which contradicts the status quo of high preponderance of HIV among TB patients [36, 37]. These differences might be a result of the poor reading of HIV test results or insensitive HIV test kits; however, this could not be validated since the study was based on the retrospective review of patients' documents. In this study, majority of the TB patients were extra-PTB and smear-negative PTB compared to smear-positive and MDR-TB which was consistent with several studies in other parts of Ghana and other countries. However, extra-PTB and smear-negative PTB were not associated with treatment outcome which contravenes with several other studies. The high proportion of extra-PTB and smear-negative PTB cases recorded might be due to overdiagnosis or misdiagnosis or misclassification bias since these disease categories are diagnosed only based on the clinical condition of the patient. Moreover, it is assumed some suspected TB cases might have been diagnosed first in one health facility and transferred to another health facility; hence, the clinicians might overlook the sputum test and might rush to diagnose the patient as extra-PTB or smear-negative PTB. This in effect could affect treatment outcomes; therefore, we suggest sputum test plus clinical condition as in

TABLE 5: Bivariate and multivariate analysis of factors associated with successful treatment.

Variable	OR (95% CI)	p value	aOR (95% CI)	p value
Age (years)				
(i) ≤20	5.57 (2.08-14.90)	<0.001	4.74 (1.75-12.83)	0.002
(ii) 21-30	1.19 (0.74-1.90)	0.480	1.22 (0.74-2.00)	0.428
(iii) 31-40	1.48 (0.95-2.30)	0.081	1.47 (0.92-2.35)	0.103
(iv) 41-50	1.28 (0.82-1.99)	0.273	1.31 (0.83-2.07)	0.251
(v) 51-60	2.06 (1.20-3.53)	0.009	1.94 (1.12-3.39)	0.019
(vi) >60	Ref		Ref	
Gender				
(i) Male	Ref		Ref	
(ii) Female	0.86 (0.64-1.17)	0.350	0.76 (0.55-1.06)	0.111
Pretreatment weight (kg)				
(i) ≤35	Ref		Ref	
(ii) 36-45	2.54 (1.36-4.74)	0.004	2.54 (1.32-4.87)	0.005
(iii) 46-55	2.50 (1.36-4.59)	0.003	2.75 (1.44-5.27)	0.002
(iv) 56-65	2.79 (1.44-5.40)	0.002	3.04 (1.50-6.14)	0.002
(v) >65	1.66 (0.75-3.65)	0.210	1.78 (0.78-4.04)	0.170
HIV status				
(i) Negative	Ref		Ref	
(ii) Positive	0.69 (0.44-1.11)	0.127	0.68 (0.41-1.11)	0.119
Disease classification				
(i) Smear positive PTB	Ref		Ref	
(ii) Smear negative PTB	0.86 (0.51-1.47)	0.583	0.83 (0.48-1.45)	0.518
(iii) Extra-PTB	0.91 (0.55-1.50)	0.713	0.89 (0.53-1.50)	0.668
(iv) MDR-TB	—	—	—	—
Patient category				
(i) New	Ref		Ref	
(ii) Relapse	0.63 (0.35-1.11)	0.110	0.60 (0.34-1.08)	0.090
(iii) Transfer in	3.13 (0.38-25.57)	0.287	3.00 (0.34-26.54)	0.322
(iv) Failure	2.24 (0.64-7.79)	0.207	1.90 (0.52-6.90)	0.329
(v) Retreatment	0.40 (0.16-1.00)	0.051	0.31 (0.11-0.84)	0.021*
Treatment support				
(i) No	Ref		Ref	
(ii) Yes	1.05 (0.66-1.68)	0.823	0.92 (0.56-1.51)	0.740

the case of smear-positive PTB for all disease categories during monitoring of treatment outcome.

Most of the TB cases were new cases, and most of the patient categories were likely to be successful with treatment. Nevertheless, patients on retreatment were less likely to be successful with treatment. Similar findings from other studies in Ghana [38, 39], South Africa [40, 41], Ethiopia [42, 43], and Kenya [29] also reported that retreatment was significantly associated with unsuccessful treatment outcome. The reasons for these observations might be that as the patients were continually exposed to the anti-TB medication, suboptimal therapy and drug resistance might have occurred.

5. Conclusion

This study found an overall treatment success rate of 68.46%, which was lower compared to the national average treatment success rate of 87.0% and 90.0% target for WHO. It was deduced that the contributing factors to successful treatment outcome were age, pretreatment weight, and patient category including those who relapse, transfer in, failure of treatment, and retreatment. Based on the findings of this study, we recommend active monitoring, motivation, and counselling of TB patients during treatment to avoid defaulting of treatment procedures especially in those advanced in age.

5.1. Limitation of This Study. The major limitation to our study is the use of retrospective secondary data. Variables such as comorbidities (diabetes, hypertension, etc.), distance to health facility, income level, treatment- and disease-related factors (drug resistance and adherence), behavioural factors (knowledge and attitude about TB), and smoking and alcohol history were not routinely captured in the TB registers.

Also, incomplete data and transferred out patients might have had an impact on treatment outcome or the results of the study.

Authors' Contributions

SAA and FAO conceptualized and designed the study. MO-A, CM-D, SFO, NKM, and EOY designed and managed the tools for data collection. SFO and NKM analyzed and interpreted the data. FAO, SFO, AM, and EA drafted the initial manuscript and was subsequently reviewed by all authors. All authors approved the final manuscript and agreed to be accountable for all aspects of the work before it was finally submitted.

Acknowledgments

The authors are grateful to the staffs at the TB clinics at the five DOTS centres for their cooperation and help in retrieving the TB registers.

References

[1] E. A. Tanue, D. S. Nsagha, T. N. Njamen, and N. J. C. Assob, "Tuberculosis treatment outcome and its associated factors among people living with HIV and AIDS in Fako Division of Cameroon," *PLoS One*, vol. 14, no. 7, pp. 1–14, 2019.

[2] B. A. Talip, R. D. Sleator, C. J. Lowery, J. S. G. Dooley, and W. J. Snelling, "An update on global tuberculosis (TB)," *Infectious Diseases: Research and Treatment*, vol. 6, pp. 39–50, 2013.

[3] H. Esmail, C. E. Barry 3rd, D. B. Young, and R. J. Wilkinson, "The ongoing challenge of latent tuberculosis," *Philosophical Transactions of the Royal Society of London. Series B, Biological Sciences*, vol. 369, no. 1645, p. 20130437, 2014.

[4] P. Narasimhan, J. Wood, C. R. Macintyre, and D. Mathai, "Risk factors for tuberculosis," *Pulmonary Medicine*, vol. 2013, Article ID 828939, 11 pages, 2013.

[5] G. Aryee, E. Kwarteng, R. Essuman et al., "Estimating the incidence of tuberculosis cases reported at a tertiary hospital in Ghana: a time series model approach," *BMC Public Health*, vol. 18, no. 1, p. 1292, 2018.

[6] P. L. Lin and J. L. Flynn, "Understanding latent tuberculosis: a moving target," *Journal of Immunology*, vol. 185, no. 1, pp. 15–22, 2010.

[7] World Health Organization, *Treatment of tuberculosis guidelines*, 4th edition, , 2019https://www.who.int/tb/publications/global_report/en/.

[8] WHO, *Global Tuberculosis Report*, WHO, Geneva, 2019.

[9] B. Z. Katale, P. M. Mbelele, N. A. Lema et al., "Whole genome sequencing of mycobacterium tuberculosis isolates and clinical outcomes of patients treated for multidrug-resistant tuberculosis in Tanzania," *BMC Genomics*, vol. 21, no. 1, p. 174, 2020.

[10] A. Zumla, E. Petersen, T. Nyirenda, and J. Chakaya, "Tackling the tuberculosis epidemic in sub-Saharan Africa - unique opportunities arising from the second European Developing Countries Clinical Trials Partnership (EDCTP) programme 2015-2024," *International Journal of Infectious Diseases*, vol. 32, pp. 46–49, 2015.

[11] K. Floyd, P. Glaziou, R. M. G. J. Houben, T. Sumner, R. G. White, and M. Raviglione, "Global tuberculosis targets and milestones set for 2016-2035: definition and rationale," *The International Journal of Tuberculosis and Lung Disease*, vol. 22, no. 7, pp. 723–730, 2018.

[12] A. Tola, K. M. Minshore, Y. Ayele, and A. N. Mekuria, "Tuberculosis treatment outcomes and associated factors among TB patients attending public hospitals in Harar town, Eastern Ethiopia: a five-year retrospective study," *Tuberculosis Research and Treatment*, vol. 2019, Article ID 1503219, 11 pages, 2019.

[13] G. Abebe, Z. Bonsa, and W. Kebede, "Treatment outcomes and associated factors in tuberculosis patients at Jimma University Medical Center: a 5-year retrospective study," *International Journal of Mycobacteriology*, vol. 8, no. 1, pp. 35–41, 2019.

[14] K. Peltzer and J. Louw, "Prevalence and associated factors of tuberculosis treatment outcome among hazardous or harmful alcohol users in public primary health care in South Africa," *African Health Sciences*, vol. 14, no. 1, p. 157, 2014.

[15] K. Peltzer and J. S. Louw, "Prevalence and factors associated with tuberculosis treatment outcome among hazardous or harmful alcohol users in public primary health care in South Africa," *African Health Sciences*, vol. 14, no. 1, pp. 157–166, 2014.

[16] G. Aliyu, S. S. el-Kamary, A.'. Abimiku, W. Blattner, and M. Charurat, "Demography and the dual epidemics of tuberculosis and HIV: analysis of cross-sectional data from sub-Saharan Africa," *PLoS One*, vol. 13, no. 9, p. e0191387, 2018.

[17] A. K. Tetteh, E. Agyarko, J. Otchere, L. Bimi, and I. Ayi, "An evaluation of treatment outcomes in a cohort of clients on the DOTS strategy, 2012–2016," *Tuberculosis Research and Treatment*, vol. 2018, 7 pages, 2018.

[18] S. A. Ohene, S. Fordah, and P. dela Boni, "Childhood tuberculosis and treatment outcomes in Accra: a retrospective analysis," *BMC Infectious Diseases*, vol. 19, no. 1, p. 749, 2019.

[19] R. P. Frimpong-Mansoh, B. N. Calys-Tagoe, E. T. Coffie, and K. O. Antwi-Agyei, "Evaluation of the tuberculosis surveillance system in the Ashaiman Municipality of the Greater Accra Region," *Pan African Medical Journal Conference Proceedings*, vol. 1, 2018.

[20] J. Amo-Adjei and K. Awusabo-Asare, "Reflections on tuberculosis diagnosis and treatment outcomes in Ghana," *Archives of Public Health*, vol. 71, no. 1, 2013.

[21] G. A. Ansa, J. D. Walley, K. Siddiqi, and X. Wei, "Assessing the impact of TB/HIV services integration on TB treatment outcomes and their relevance in TB/HIV monitoring in Ghana," *Infectious Diseases of Poverty*, vol. 1, no. 1, 2012.

[22] E. Osei, S. Oppong, D. Adanfo et al., "Reflecting on tuberculosis case notification and treatment outcomes in the Volta region of Ghana: a retrospective pool analysis of a multicentre cohort from 2013 to 2017," *Global Health Research and Policy* vol. 4, no. 1, 2019.

[23] WHO and USAID, *Guidelines for the clinical management of TB and HIV co-infection in Ghana*, Ghana Health Service, 2007.

[24] T. Abebe and M. T. Angamo, "Treatment outcomes and associated factors among tuberculosis patients in Southwest Ethiopia," *Gulhane Medical Journal*, vol. 57, no. 4, pp. 397–407, 2015.

[25] D. J. Mibei, J. W. Kiarie, A. Wairia, M. Kamene, and M. E. Okumu, "Treatment outcomes of drug-resistant tuberculosis patients in Kenya," *The International Journal of Tuberculosis and Lung Disease*, vol. 20, no. 11, pp. 1477–1482, 2016.

[26] S. M. Alavi, S. Salmanzadeh, P. Bakhtiyariniya, A. Albagi, F. Hemmatnia, and L. Alavi, "Prevalence and treatment outcome of pulmonary and extrapulmonary pediatric tuberculosis in southwestern Iran," *Caspian Journal of Internal Medicine*, vol. 6, no. 4, pp. 213–219, 2015.

[27] World Health Organization, *Global tuberculosis report 2018*, WHO Press, 2021.

[28] K. C. Horton, P. MacPherson, R. M. G. J. Houben, R. G. White, and E. L. Corbett, "Sex differences in tuberculosis burden and notifications in low- and middle-income countries: a systematic review and meta-analysis," *PLoS Medicine*, vol. 13, no. 9, pp. e1002119–e1002119, 2016.

[29] B. N. Muture, M. N. Keraka, P. K. Kimuu, E. W. Kabiru, V. O. Ombeka, and F. Oguya, "Factors associated with default from treatment among tuberculosis patients in nairobi province, Kenya: A case control study," *BMC Public Health*, vol. 11, no. 1, 2011.

[30] N. A. Ifebunandu and K. N. Ukwaja, "Tuberculosis treatment default in a large tertiary care hospital in urban Nigeria: prevalence, trend, timing and predictors," *Journal of Infection and Public Health*, vol. 5, no. 5, pp. 340–345, 2012.

[31] J. Samal, "Health seeking behaviour among tuberculosis patients in India: a systematic review," *Journal of Clinical and Diagnostic Research*, vol. 10, no. 10, pp. 1–6, 2016.

[32] S. Boateng, T. Kodama, T. Tachibana, and N. Hyoi, "Factors contributing to tuberculosis (TB) defaulter rate in New Juaben Municipality in the Eastern Region of Ghana," *Journal of the National Institute of Public Health*, vol. 59, no. 3, pp. 291–297, 2010.

[33] A. Bernabe-Ortiz, C. P. Carcamo, J. F. Sanchez, and J. Rios, "Weight variation over time and its association with tuberculosis treatment outcome: a longitudinal analysis," *PLoS One*, vol. 6, no. 4, p. e18474, 2011.

[34] M. T. Gler, R. Guilatco, J. C. Caoili, J. Ershova, P. Cegielski, and J. L. Johnson, "Weight gain and response to treatment for multidrug-resistant tuberculosis," *The American Journal of Tropical Medicine and Hygiene*, vol. 89, no. 5, pp. 943–949, 2013.

[35] M. Biruk, B. Yimam, and H. Abrha, "SB-A in P, 2016 undefined," *Treatment outcomes of tuberculosis and associated factors in an Ethiopian University Hospital*, 2021, https://www.hindawi.com/journals/aph/2016/8504629/.

[36] E. Ibrahim and A. Baess, "Diseases MAM-EJ of C, 2017 undefined," in *Pattern of prevalence, risk factors and treatment outcomes among Egyptian patients with multidrug resistant tuberculosis*, Elsevier, 2021.

[37] M. Bates, B. J. Marais, and A. Zumla, "Tuberculosis comorbidity with communicable and noncommunicable diseases," *Cold Spring Harbor Perspectives in Medicine*, vol. 5, no. 11, p. a017889, 2015.

[38] T. C. Bouton, A. Forson, S. Kudzawu et al., "High mortality during tuberculosis retreatment at a Ghanaian tertiary center: a retrospective cohort study," *Pan African Medical Journal*, vol. 33, 2019.

[39] A. Forson, A. Kwara, S. Kudzawu et al., "A cross-sectional study of tuberculosis drug resistance among previously treated patients in a tertiary hospital in Accra, Ghana: public health implications of standardized regimens," *BMC Infectious Diseases*, vol. 18, no. 1, p. 149, 2018.

[40] K. Middelkoop, L.-G. Bekker, E. Shashkina, B. Kreiswirth, and R. Wood, "Retreatment tuberculosis in a South African community: the role of re-infection, HIV and antiretroviral treatment," *The International Journal of Tuberculosis and Lung Disease*, vol. 16, no. 11, pp. 1510–1516, 2012.

[41] G. Kigozi, C. Heunis, P. Chikobvu, S. Botha, and D. van Rensburg, "Factors influencing treatment default among tuberculosis patients in a high burden province of South Africa," *International Journal of Infectious Diseases*, vol. 54, pp. 95–102, 2017.

[42] J. L. Lenjisa, "Assessment of tuberculosis retreatment case rate and its treatment outcomes at Adama Hospital Medical College, East Showa, Ethiopia," *Journal of Steroids & Hormonal Science*, vol. 6, no. 1, pp. 1–6, 2015.

[43] A. Melese and B. Zeleke, "Factors associated with poor treatment outcome of tuberculosis in Debre Tabor, Northwest Ethiopia," *BMC Research Notes*, vol. 11, no. 1, p. 25, 2018.

20

Evaluation of TB/HIV Collaborative Activities: The Case of South Tongu District, Ghana

Vasco Ayere Avoka[1] **and Eric Osei**[2]

[1]Department of Epidemiology and Biostatistics, School of Public Health, University of Health and Allied Sciences, Ho, Ghana
[2]Department of Population and Behavioural Sciences, School of Public Health, University of Health and Allied Sciences, Ho, Ghana

Correspondence should be addressed to Vasco Ayere Avoka; vavokaphdc14@uhas.edu.gh

Academic Editor: Vincent Jarlier

Background. There is a complex interaction between infection with human immunodeficiency virus (HIV) and tuberculosis (TB) infection that results in a synergistic increase in their prevalence, morbidity, and mortality. In Ghana, 32% of TB cases were estimated to be coinfected with the human immunodeficiency virus and acquired immune deficiency syndrome (HIV/AIDS) epidemic HIV, with the highest number of coinfections in the Volta Region. This study assessed the extent of linkage between the TB and HIV collaborative activities in the South Tongu District of Ghana. *Method.* The study employed both qualitative and quantitative methods to assess the coverage of activities to reduce the burden of TB in people living with HIV and the coverage of activities to reduce the burden of HIV in TB patients and explored the barriers to collaborative activities from the providers' perspective. *Results.* The study showed that 344 (94.8%) HIV-positive clients were screened for TB, of which 10 (8.5%) were bacteriologically confirmed. Among those positive for TB, 6 (60%) received cotrimoxazole preventive therapy (CPT) and antiretroviral therapy. Sixty-seven (93.1%) TB patients were screened for HIV. Of these, 28 (38.9%) were retropositive, among whom 14 (50%) received anti-TB treatment. However, there were no records of isoniazid preventive therapy (IPT) for these patients. Inadequately trained personnel leading to work overload, manual record-keeping, lack of staff motivation, and absence of "enablers" packages for patients were identified as barriers to TB/HIV collaboration. *Conclusion.* Overall, there was a moderate linkage between TB and HIV collaborative activities in the study setting. Notwithstanding, there exist some barriers that mitigate against the successful implementation of the collaborative process from the providers' perspective, hence we recommend for measures to ensure effective, efficient, and sustained integrated TB/HIV activities by addressing these barriers.

1. Background

There is a complex interaction between infection with human immunodeficiency virus (HIV) and tuberculosis (TB) infection that results in a synergistic increase in their prevalence, morbidity, and mortality [1]. The coexistence of TB and HIV is a great public health problem looming as a potential pandemic in Ghana and other African countries [2]. In recognition of the dual burden and impact of these two diseases, the World Health Organization (WHO) in 2004 initiated the TB/HIV collaborative activities as an integral part of national and international responses to the joint TB/HIV treatment at all levels of service delivery [1]. As part of the policy, TB patients are to be screened for HIV and positive cases are provided with cotrimoxazole preventive therapy (CPT) and antiretroviral therapy (ART) where indicated. HIV patients are also to be regularly screened for TB and managed appropriately [2].

Despite the proven efficacy of TB/HIV treatment and prevention, studies in Ghana have found that the prevalence of HIV in TB patients is approximately 25-30% and that as many as 50% of patients with a chronic cough could be HIV positive [2]. Cultural and system-wide differences between HIV and TB care providers present operational difficulties for providing effective and appropriate interventions which have contributed to a lack of progress in expanding collaborative TB/HIV activities [3].

Since the national launch of TB/HIV collaborative activities in Ghana in 2007 and operation in 2009, not many studies have focused on the operational effectiveness of the integrative process, especially in the Volta Region. This study, therefore, assessed the TB/HIV collaborative activities in a district hospital in the Volta Region of Ghana.

2. Materials and Methods

2.1. Study Setting. South Tongu is one of the 26 administrative districts of the Volta Region. The population of South Tongu District, according to the 2010 Population and Housing Census, is 87,950 representing 4.1% of the region's total population. Males constitute 45.5% and females represent 54.5%. About eighty-seven (87.1%) of the population resides in rural localities with a sex ratio (number of males to 100 females) of 83.5%.

2.2. Study Design and Population. The study employed both qualitative and quantitative methods to assess the coverage of activities to reduce the burden of TB in PLHIV and the coverage of activities to reduce the burden of HIV in TB patients and explored the barriers to collaborative activities from the providers' point of view. The quantitative tool was used to measure the linkage of the TB and HIV collaborative activities. Data were extracted from the TB and HIV registers at the Voluntary Counselling and Testing (VCT) unit and Chest Clinic from 1st January 2014 to 31st December 2016 in the district hospital. All cases of TB and HIV registered at the hospitals during the period were included for the analysis. The qualitative method allowed for the identification of barriers to collaboration from the healthcare providers' perspective. The TB and HIV coordinators from the district hospital were interviewed to establish the barriers to collaboration.

2.3. Data Analysis. Quantitative data were exported to IBM SPSS for analysis. Data cleaning and validation were done to ensure data quality before analysis was carried out. Descriptive statistics such as proportions, frequencies, mean, and standard deviation were used to describe the population. Qualitative data were analysed thematically, and pattern building was done using a priori themes that were used to design the study as well as emergent ones. Interviews were recorded directly in words using pen and paper. Data was then organized manually into easily retrievable sections assigned with unique codes, or by breaking up field notes into sections identified by date, or by context using both sentences and paragraphs as the units of analysis. These codes (salient themes, recurring ideas, patterns of beliefs, etc.) were then refined or combined to form themes or categories of issues.

2.4. Ethical Issues. This study was approved by the Ghana Health Service Ethical Review Committee with reference no. GHS-ERC 57/05/17. Participation was completely voluntary, and participants could choose not to participate or leave the study at any time during data collection.

3. Results

3.1. Characteristics of HIV and TB Cases. There were 363 HIV cases registered during the study period. Of these, females accounted for nearly three-quarters (272, 74.7%). The majority (215, 59.2%) belong to the economically active age group (20-39 years). The minimum and maximum ages were 12 and 77 years, respectively, with the median age of 36 years (Table 1).

Of the 72 TB cases registered during the study period, the majority 37 (51.4%) were males. The majority (57, 79.2%) were in the age group 20-59 years. The minimum and maximum ages were 3 and 87 years, respectively, with a median age of 40 years (iqr = 18). Forty-three (59.7%) of them were pulmonary positive and 1 (1.4%) was an extrapulmonary case (Table 2).

3.2. TB and HIV Collaborative Activities. Of the 363 HIV cases, 344 (94.8%) of them were screened for TB, of whom 10 (8.5%) were bacteriologically confirmed TB; six (60%) of the HIV-positive TB patients had access to cotrimoxazole preventive therapy (CPT) and antiretroviral therapy (Figure 1).

Among the 72 TB cases, 67 (93.1%) were screened for HIV, of whom 28 (38.9%) were positive for HIV. Of the 28 HIV-positive TB patients, 14 (50%) were put on antituberculosis treatment (Figure 2). There were no records of isoniazid preventive therapy (IPT) for TB/HIV patients.

3.3. Barriers to Collaboration. Several barriers that mitigate against the successful implementation of TB and HIV control collaborative activities were enumerated by key health personnel involved in TB and HIV control at the hospital. Prominent among the barriers mentioned were inadequate staff leading to work overload. This was what the TB facility coordinators had to say:

"*I am the only qualified staff here (the DOTS centre) so I am not able to go out to the field (to follow up cases) and leave my patients in the ward. This has affected service delivery because I am not able to trace defaulters.*" (facility TB coordinator)

The Voluntary Counselling and Testing unit was located on a different block of the hospital and was being overseen by a senior nurse. When the in-charge was asked about the challenges of the unit, she also reiterated the lack of qualified personnel.

"*We are three in this unit but the other two are not regular staff because of that the workload on me is too much hence I am not able to visit some clients because the clinic runs every day and I have to be here at all times. This makes me very tired so am not able to work effectively.*" (facility VCT coordinator)

Manual data capture and records keeping was also mentioned as one of the barriers to successful TB/HIV collaborative activities at the hospital. At the DOTS centre, patients' information was recorded in folders and papers and stored in a cupboard. According to the nurse-in-charge, the process makes retrieval of folders and some records very cumbersome and time wasting.

Table 1: Age and sex distribution of HIV cases registered (2014-2016).

Period Variable	2014 ($n = 134$) n	 %	2015 ($n = 112$) n	 %	2016 ($n = 117$) n	 %	All years ($n = 363$) n	 %
Sex								
Female	103	76.9	82	73.2	87	74.4	272	74.7
Male	32	23.1	30	26.8	30	25.6	92	25.3
Age range (years)								
≤19	4	3.0	1	0.9	3	2.6	8	2.2
20-39	78	58.2	65	58.0	72	61.5	215	59.2
40-59	43	32.1	42	37.5	37	31.6	122	33.6
≥60	9	6.7	4	3.6	5	4.3	18	5.0

Table 2: Characteristics of tuberculosis cases registered from 2014 to 2016.

Variable	2014 $n = 26$	 %	2015 $n = 23$	 %	2016 $n = 23$	 %	All years $n = 72$	 %
Sex								
Female	16	61.5	12	52.2	7	34.4	35	48.6
Male	10	38.5	11	47.8	16	69.6	37	51.4
Age (years)								
≤19	1	3.9	0	0.00	1	4.6	2	2.8
20-59	18	69.2	22	95.6	17	73.9	57	79.2
≥60	7	26.9	1	4.4	5	21.7	13	18.0
Disease type								
PP	14	53.9	15	65.2	14	60.9	43	59.7
PN	12	46.1	8	34.8	8	34.8	28	38.9
EP	0	00.0	0	00.0	1	4.4	1	1.4
Treatment outcome								
Completed	9	34.62	4	18.2	4	17.4	17	23.9
Cured	12	46.15	13	59.1	13	56.5	38	53.5
Died	5	19.23	5	22.7	4	17.4	14	19.7
LTF	0	0.00	0	00.0	2	8.7	2	2.8

PP: pulmonary positive; PN: pulmonary negative; EP: extrapulmonary; LTF: lost to follow-up.

"Because the records are kept manually, it is difficult to retrieve some folders sometimes when they (patients) come for follow up visits. Some of the folders can get missing or destroyed when they are packed together. It is also difficult to monitor to see whether a referred patient to VCT unit go to the unit or not because the records are kept in folders which cannot be seen and used by more than one person at a time." (facility TB coordinator)

To ensure that TB/HIV clients adhere to their treatment regimens, food was added as a package which as described by service providers as an "enablers" package. However, this package was scrapped in 2015 after funds dwindled, which posed a major challenge to the TB/HIV collaborative activities.

"The enabling package should be re-introduced so that patients would adhere to their treatment since this serves as a motivation for them. Most patients do not visit the clinic as scheduled and when they come and if we ask them, they say they the drugs make them a week to travel to the clinic." (TB coordinator)

As confirmed by Mbilinyi et al. [4], health worker motivation plays a critical role in the quality of service rendered by healthcare providers. The lack of motivation for staff working in TB/HIV units adversely affect the quality of the service rendered according to the hospital DOTS centre in-charge.

"The lack of motivation may not affect me as a person but other staff like the OPD nurses, or the laboratory personnel. If they are not given some motivation, they would not help us with the detection of cases. This can affect our case detection rate." (facility TB coordinator)

4. Discussion

TB screening among people living with HIV almost reached universal in this study site, similar to what Lima et al. [5] found in their study in Johannesburg, South Africa, where more than 9 in 10 TB patients received an HIV test. The high screening rates as observed in this study mean that the healthcare providers adhere to the WHO recommendation

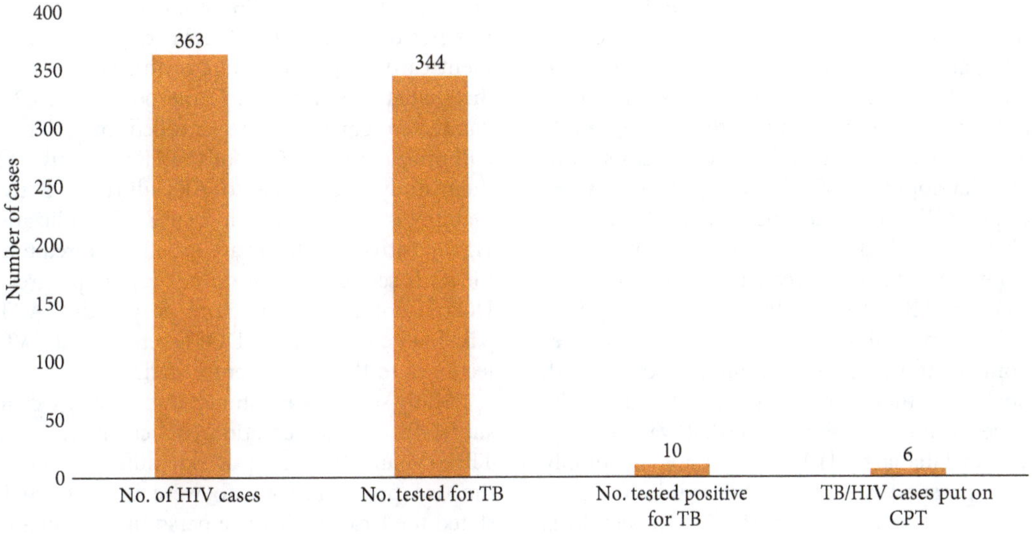

FIGURE 1: TB collaborative activities among HIV patients.

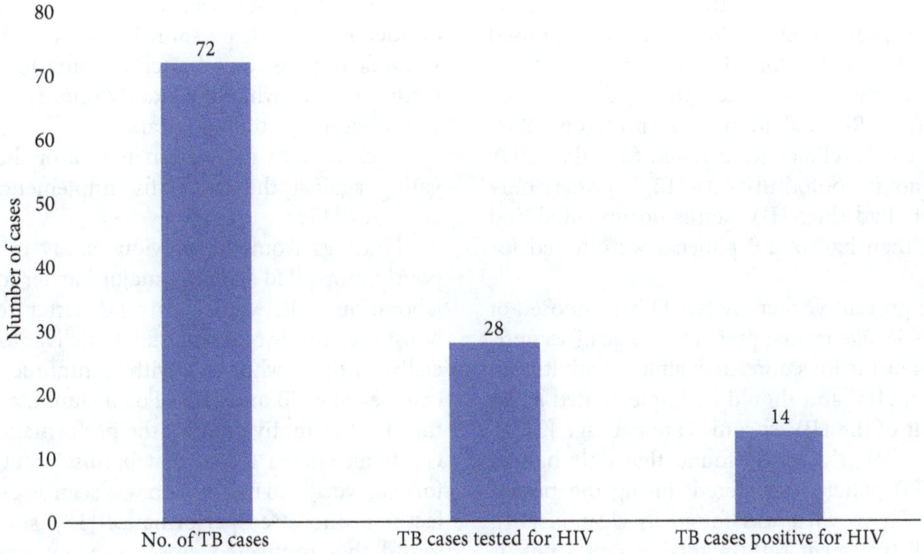

FIGURE 2: HIV collaborative activities among TB patients.

that all TB patients must be screened for HIV. This implies that treatment outcomes in TB patients would be improved and also transmission to contact persons would be reduced. Early detection of TB among people living with HIV, followed by prompt initiation of treatment, can improve patient treatment outcomes and reduce transmission in communities and healthcare settings [6]. TB screening is also essential in evaluating PLHIV infection or AIDS for isoniazid preventive therapy (IPT) eligibility in order to avoid the risk of isoniazid monotherapy resistance [6]. WHO emphasizes the relevance of screening for TB in PLHIV to reduce the impact of TB among people living with HIV (PLHIV).

In order to lessen the burden of TB in HIV patients, new HIV-positive TB patients should receive a TB regimen containing 6 months of rifampicin and should be put on ART regardless of CD4 count as soon as possible within the first 8 weeks of antituberculosis treatment [3]. In this study, 6 in 10 of all eligible HIV-positive TB patients received TB treatment. This implies that the other 4 cases go untreated for TB, and they would continue to infect others from the healthy population who they come into contact with.

Studies have proven that IPT is as efficacious but safer than rifampicin- and pyrazinamide-containing regimens used for the prevention of latent TB infection and effective in reducing the incidence of TB and death from TB in HIV-infected patients with a positive tuberculin skin test result [3]. Although WHO recommend IPT as part of the standard care for HIV patients without active TB, IPT uptake could not be measured in this study as it was not indicated in the registers whether patients receive IPT or not. This study result is similar to a study in Ethiopia which found that IPT intake could not be measured due to an incomplete TB register [7]. While this study could not measure the level of IPT uptake, in Ethiopia, it was found that 19.4% of TB and HIV/AIDS patients received IPT [8]. IPT has been proven to reduce the incidence of TB cases among HIV patients. A study in Ethiopia to compare the incidence rate of TB and TB-free survival time and identify factors associated with the development of TB among HIV-infected individuals on pre-ART follow-up found that IPT use was associated with a 50% reduction in new cases of tuberculosis, and implementing the widespread use of IPT had the potential to reduce TB rates substantially among HIV-infected individuals in addition to other tuberculosis prevention and control efforts in resource-limited settings [9].

In this study, more than 9 in 10 TB patients during the period were screened for HIV, similar to what was found in an earlier study in Ghana by [10]. This result favourably compares with a prospective observational study to determine the burden and treatment of HIV in tuberculosis patients in Papua Province, Indonesia, which established that 85.2% of all TB patients were tested for HIV [11]. A quantitative assessment at 3 clinics in Johannesburg, South Africa, to evaluate TB/HIV integration at the primary care level established that the proportion of clients newly diagnosed with HIV who were screened for TB symptoms could not be determined, because it was not systematically documented [12]. Correspondingly, Rie et al. found that in Ethiopia 85% of TB patients at DOTS clinics were tested for HIV/AIDS [13]. Our result is not in conformity with [12, 13] where only 75% of TB patients had their HIV status documented and only a little more than half of TB patients were tested for HIV, respectively.

Cotrimoxazole preventive therapy (CPT) is composed of multiple antimicrobial agents that prevent a range of secondary bacterial and parasitic infections in eligible TB adults and children living with HIV and should be implemented as an integral component of the HIV chronic care package [3]. In terms of access to CPT, this study found that only half of all HIV-positive TB patients registered during the period received CPT, similar to what was found in Uganda [14]. However, the CPT treatment rate in this current study is lower than what was found in Ethiopia where 8 in 10 HIV-positive TB patients received CPT [11, 14] and in India where more than 9 in 10 HIV-positive TB patients were given CPT [7]. The rest of the eligible HIV-positive TB patients who did not receive CPT would be more prone to secondary and parasitic infections, and this may affect their treatment outcomes [7].

HIV is a predictor for active TB both in people with new infection or with latent *Mycobacterium tuberculosis* infection. Improving access to TB prevention, treatment, care, and support services for health-care workers, as well as of workers in congregate settings, is, therefore, crucial [3].

Antiretroviral therapy (ART) greatly improves the survival and the quality of life of TB patients living with HIV and prevents HIV transmission and reduces mortality risk between 54% and 95% [3]. In this study, of the 72 TB cases registered, ART service could not be established because there was no documented record on ART in the TB register. Pontororing et al. found that in South Africa ART coverage among patients with TB could not be ascertained as ART was not documented in the TB register or on the TB treatment card [12]. The results of this study, however, contradicts what was found in Cameroon where 82% of TB/HIV coinfected patients were enrolled on ART [15, 16]; the authors found that 52% of the HIV-positive TB patients in their study had access to ART during TB treatment. The inability of this study to measure ART utilization is because HIV-positive TB clients are usually referred to the VCT unit for such services which do not report progress back to the DOTS centre. It is therefore proper that ART for eligible patients be given at the DOTS centre or the VCT staff gives feedback to the DOTS centre staff.

Many studies have shown that there are challenges to the successful implementation of collaborative activities of TB/HIV and this study is not different. Focal persons for the two programmes who were interviewed in this study stated the lack of adequate personnel, leading to high workload as a major challenge to successful TB/HIV collaboration. In sub-Saharan Africa, many patients were attended to by a few providers at the DOTS centres [16]. Retirement from active service by service providers could account for the lack of adequate health personnel in this study. It is likely that some facility personnel after working for some time go for further studies while the elderly ones retire from active service when they attain 60 years.

Lack of staff motivation is one of the challenges mitigating against the successful implementation of TB/HIV activities [17].

Findings from the previous study in Ghana also cited poorly motivated staff as a major barrier to the TB/HIV collaboration [10]. Motivation and better remunerations can boost the morale of health staff to deliver to their fullest especially for those who work with communicable and infectious diseases like TB and HIV. For instance, a study to establish the effect of motivation on the performance of employees at GT Bank Ghana found that bonuses motivate staff to perform at work and motivation was seen as a silent contributing factor to increased performance [18], similar to Jasmi who found that motivated employees not only influence their work performance but also the whole organization's performance and business productivity [19].

Manual record-keeping was also found to be a challenge to the TB/HIV collaborative activities in the facility. Due to the nature of manual records, it was not easily accessed by more than one person at a time and usually difficult to transport [20].

The inability to be accessed by more than one person at a time makes it impossible or difficult for staff at the unit to monitor clients who have been referred to the other unit for other services. Again, navigation through manual records is cumbersome and highly time-consuming and this may delay the delivery of health services, supported by [21] who concluded that experts and policymakers believe that electronic health records are beneficial to the patient and society if they are used in a meaningful way.

"The termination of 'enabling' packages as a motivation and support found to be a challenge to the successful collaboration of TB/HIV collaborative activities. Due to the burden

of the TB pills, the program initiated a package in the form of food to motivate and help them adhere to and complete their treatment in time. However, this 'enabling' package of late has been irregular in supply to the TB patients." (TB coordinator)

This may lead to high default rates and nonadherence and also affect negatively TB patients' participation in HIV services, as evidenced by Ciobanu et al. in 2014 who observed that provision of enablers such as cash and food to TB patients significantly improves the treatment success rate and should be continued [21]. Also, lack of food was among the other factors identified as a barrier to adherence to TB treatment in patients on concomitant TB and HIV treatment.

5. Conclusion

Though some aspects of the collaborative activities are commendable, more effort is needed to ensure the linkage of all activities between TB and HIV/AIDS programmes and to address the exiting factors that mitigate against the implementation of these collaborative activities to reduce the burden of HIV on TB patients and vice visa. If more pragmatic measures are not put in place, the 90-90-90 target cannot be achieved.

Abbreviation

AIDS: Acquired immune deficiency syndrome
ART: Antiretroviral therapy
CHPS: Community-based health planning and services
CPT: Cotrimoxazole prophylaxis therapy
DOTS: Directly observed therapy short course
GHS: Ghana Health Service
HIV: Human immunodeficiency virus
IPT: Isoniazid preventive therapy
IRIS: Idiopathic immune reconstitution syndrome
NACP: National AIDS Control Program
NTP: National Tuberculosis Program
PLHIV: People living with human immunodeficiency virus
SSA: South-Saharan Africa
TB: Tuberculosis
VRHD: Volta Regional Health Directorate
VCT: Voluntary counselling and testing
WHO: World Health Organization

Consent

Participation in this study was completely voluntary and participants could choose not to participate or leave the study at any time during data collection without any penalty or lose any existing benefits of accessing health within the catchment area of the study site and elsewhere.

Disclosure

This research article was submitted to and published by the 13th INTEREST Conference 2019 in Accra (*Abstracts Book, page 215*).

Authors' Contributions

EO conceived the study. VAA reviewed the literature and collected and analysed the data. EO and VAA wrote the first draft. Both authors read and approved the final draft.

Acknowledgments

The South Tongu District Health Directorate staff deserve special recognition for their selfless support during the period of this study. We say "Ayekoo" to them.

References

[1] Ghana Health Service, *Guidelines for the Clinical Management of TB and HIV Co-infection in Ghana*, Ghana Ministry of Health, 2007.

[2] World Health Organization, *Tuberculosis*, WHO, 2016.

[3] World Health Organization, *WHO Policy on Collaborative TB/HIV Activities. Guidelines for National Programmes and Other Stakeholders*, World Health Organization, 2012, WHO/HTM/TB: 1–34.

[4] D. Mbilinyi, M. L. Daniel, and G. T. Lie, "Health worker motivation in the context of HIV care and treatment challenges in Mbeya Region, Tanzania: a qualitative study," *BMC Health Services Research*, vol. 11, no. 1, p. 266, 2011.

[5] Y. V. De Lima, D. Evans, L. Page-Shipp et al., "Linkage to care and treatment for TB and HIV among people newly diagnosed with TB or HIV-associated TB at a large, Inner City South African Hospital," *PLoS One*, vol. 8, no. 1, pp. 1–8, 2013.

[6] World Health Organization, *A Guide to Monitoring and Evaluation for Collaborative TB/HIV*, World Health Organization, 2009.

[7] A. Kassa, D. Jerene, Y. Assefa, A. Teka, A. Aseffa, and A. Deribew, "Evaluation of collaborative TB/HIV activities in a general hospital in Addis Ababa, Ethiopia," *BMC Research Notes*, vol. 5, no. 1, p. 67, 2012.

[8] H. T. Ayele, M. S. M. van Mourik, and M. J. M. Bonten, "Effect of isoniazid preventive therapy on tuberculosis or death in persons with HIV: a retrospective cohort study," *BMC Infectious Diseases*, vol. 15, no. 1, article 334, 2015.

[9] L. F. Assebe, H. L. Reda, A. D. Wubeneh, W. T. Lerebo, and S. M. Lambert, "The effect of isoniazid preventive therapy on incidence of tuberculosis among HIV-infected clients under pre-ART care, Jimma, Ethiopia: a retrospective cohort study," *BMC Public Health*, vol. 15, no. 1, article 346, 2015.

[10] J. Amo-Adjei, "Views of health service providers on obstacles to tuberculosis control in Ghana," *Infectious Diseases of Poverty*, vol. 2, no. 1, article 9, 2013.

[11] G. A. Ansa, J. D. Walley, K. Siddiqi, and X. Wei, "Health system barriers and facilitators influencing TB/HIV integration in Ghana," *International Journal of TROPICAL DISEASE & Health*, vol. 9, no. 2, 2015.

[12] G. J. Pontororing, E. Kenangalem, D. B. Lolong et al., "The burden and treatment of HIV in tuberculosis patients in Papua Province, Indonesia: a prospective observational study," *BMC Infectious Diseases*, vol. 10, no. 1, article 362, 2010.

[13] L. Page-Shipp, Y. V. de Lima, K. Clouse et al., "TB/HIV integration at primary care level: A quantitative assessment at 3

clinics in Johannesburg, South Africa," *Southern African Journal of HIV Medicine*, vol. 13, no. 3, pp. 138–143, 2012.

[14] M. H. Assfaw, *The Prevalence of HIV among Registered TB Patients in Public DOTS*, University of Bergen, 2011.

[15] N. Raizada, L. S. Chauhan, B. S. Babu et al., "Linking HIV-infected TB patients to cotrimoxazole prophylaxis and antiretroviral treatment in India," *PLoS One*, vol. 4, no. 6, article e5999, 2009.

[16] H. A. Yumo, C. Kuaban, and F. Neuhann, "WHO recommended collaborative TB/HIV activities: evaluation of implementation and performance in a rural district hospital in Cameroon," *The Pan African Medical Journal*, vol. 10, p. 30, 2011.

[17] A. A. Howard and W. M. El-Sadr, "Integration of tuberculosis and HIV services in sub-Saharan Africa: lessons learned," *Clinical Infectious Diseases*, vol. 50, no. s3, pp. S238–S244, 2010.

[18] W. Van Eerde, *Motivation and Reward Systems*, Wiley Online Library, 2017.

[19] M. Nduro, *The effect of motivation on the performance of employees at GT Bank Ghana by A Thesis submitted to the Institute Of Distance Learning, Kwame Nkrumah University of Science and Technology, in partial fulfilment of the requirements for the degree of COMMO*, European Centre for Research Training and Development UK, 2012.

[20] S. Al Jasmi, *A Study on Employees Work Motivation and its Effect on their Performance and Business Productivity, By Student Name: Samira Al Jasmi, Student ID number: 90040, Dissertati*, The British University in Dubai (BUiD), 2012.

[21] A. Ciobanu, L. Domente, V. Soltan et al., "Do incentives improve tuberculosis treatment outcomes in the Republic of Moldova?," *Public Health Action*, vol. 4, Supplement 2, pp. S59–S63, 2014.

21

Mobile Health Technologies May be Acceptable Tools for Providing Social Support to Tuberculosis Patients in Rural Uganda: A Parallel Mixed-Method Study

Angella Musiimenta,[1,2] Wilson Tumuhimbise,[1] Esther C. Atukunda,[1] Aaron T. Mugaba,[1,2] Conrad Muzoora,[1] Mari Armstrong-Hough,[3,4,5,6] David Bangsberg,[7] J. Lucian Davis,[3,4,5] and Jessica E. Haberer[8,9]

[1]*Mbarara University of Science and Technology, Mbarara, Uganda*
[2]*Angels Compassion Research and Innovations Centre, Mbarara, Uganda*
[3]*Uganda Tuberculosis Implementation Research Consortium, Makerere University, Kampala, Uganda*
[4]*Department of Epidemiology of Microbial Diseases, Yale School of Public Health, New Haven, Connecticut, USA*
[5]*Pulmonary, Critical Care and Sleep Medicine, Yale School of Medicine, New Haven, Connecticut, USA*
[6]*New York University College of Global Public Health, New York, New York, USA*
[7]*Oregon Health & Science University-Portland State University School of Public Health, USA*
[8]*Harvard Medical School, Boston, MA, USA*
[9]*Massachusetts General Hospital Center for Global Health, Boston, MA, USA*

Correspondence should be addressed to Angella Musiimenta; amusiimenta@must.ac.ug

Academic Editor: José R. Lapa e Silva

Background. Social support has been shown to mitigate social barriers to medication adherence and improve tuberculosis (TB) treatment success rates. The use of mobile technology to activate social support systems among TB patients, however, has not been well explored. Moreover, studies that tie supportive SMS (Short Message Service) texts to electronic monitoring of TB medication adherence are lacking. *Objective.* To explore TB patients' current access to social support and perceptions of utilizing real-time adherence monitoring interventions to support medication adherence. *Methods.* We purposively selected TB patients who owned phones, had been taking TB medications for ≥1 month, were receiving their treatment from Mbarara Regional Referral Hospital, and reported having ≥1 social supporter. We interviewed these patients and their social supporters about their access to and perceptions of social support. We used STATA 13 to describe participants' sociodemographic and social support characteristics. Qualitative data were analyzed using content analysis to derive categories describing accessibility and perceptions. *Results.* TB patients report requesting and receiving a variety of different forms of social support, including instrumental (e.g., money for transport and other needs and medication reminders), emotional (e.g., adherence counselling), and informational (e.g., medication side effects) support through mobile phones. Participants felt that SMS notifications may motivate medication adherence by creating a personal sense of obligation to take medications regularly. Participants anticipated that limited financial resources and relationship dynamics could constrain the provision of social support especially when patients and social supporters are not oriented about their expectations. *Conclusion.* Mobile telephones could provide alternative approaches to providing social support for TB medication adherence especially where patients do not stay close to their social supporters. Further efforts should focus on optimized designs of mobile phone-based applications for providing social support to TB patients and training of TB patients and social supporters to match their expectations.

1. Introduction

Globally, Uganda ranks among the 30 countries with the highest burden of TB (tuberculosis), with a prevalence rate of 253/100,000 people and an incidence rate of 201/100,000 people [1]. Although treatment is freely available in Uganda, significant treatment adherence challenges remain, constraining TB treatment success and increasing its transmission. The implementation of DOTS (Direct Observed Treatment Short Course) has been limited in Uganda. This is because DOTS demands significant time and financial burden from patients as they travel to the clinic; it also demands time commitment from health workers and treatment supporters who have to supervise patients taking their medication [2]. Social factors such as poverty, stigma, and limited knowledge of tuberculosis (TB) can constrain adherence to tuberculosis medications [3–8]. Provision of social support, defined as instrumental, emotional, and informational assistance from one's social network, can enhance TB medication adherence by mitigating the social barriers to medication adherence. For instance, money can facilitate transport to the clinic for pill refills, while encouragement or positive feedback makes people feel cared for and empowered to cope with stigma and social discrimination [9, 10]. Importantly, social support has been shown to improve clinical outcomes, such as the treatment success rate [11].

Traditional approaches to providing social support (such as face-to-face counselling interventions) may be limited by geographical boundaries and are often expensive due to the time and transport costs involved. Given the widespread adoption of wireless technologies, such as mobile phones in sub-Saharan Africa (76% ownership in 2015; [12]), these technologies can provide accessible and potentially affordable means of providing social support. In a recent study carried out in central Uganda, 75% of TB patients reported owning mobile phones and being willing to receive TB-related communication via their phones [13]. Mobile phones are thus a promising alternative approach for providing social support to TB patients.

Prior studies have utilized mobile technology to support adherence to TB medications, including randomized, controlled trials of SMS reminders in Pakistan [14], daily mobile phone calls in Thailand [15], and video directly observed therapy (VDOT) in California and Mexico [16]. These approaches have generally been found feasible and acceptable [16] and have also shown improvements in clinical outcomes, including treatment completion and sputum conversion rates in some studies (e.g., [15]) but not all (e.g., [17]). Overall, mobile technology is becoming widely used to support TB adherence, although the majority of studies have focused on reminders and DOT (directly observed therapy). Moreover, the use of mobile technologies to activate social support systems has not been well explored. Moreover, there is lack of studies that tie supportive SMS texts to electronic monitoring (which may be an attractive alternative to DOT) although limited evidence in HIV is promising [18–20].

In this study, we used a parallel mixed-method design to explore the types of social support that adults with presumed drug-sensitive TB in rural Uganda receive during TB treatment and to assess how patients utilize mobile phones to obtain social support. We also explored how these adults would perceive social support for a possible future TB adherence intervention that we were planning. This intervention includes (1) real-time audits of adherence using a digital monitoring device, (2) SMS reminders to patients, and (3) SMS notifications to patients' social supporters. WHO [21] guidelines recommend directly observed therapy (DOT) using a community-based model in which a family member or close friend is designated as an adherence supporter, which includes the responsibility to watch the patient take his or her medications every day. In this study, we define social supporters as friends or family who have previously helped TB patients with medication or other needs (such as transport to clinic, food, child care, and/or guidance).

2. Materials and Methods

2.1. Study Design and Setting. This formative study employed a parallel mixed-method study design that utilized semistructured interviews and surveys. TB patients were recruited from the TB clinic within Mbarara Regional Referral Hospital (MRRH) in rural, southwestern Uganda. Uganda ranks among the 30 countries with the highest burden of TB/HIV in the world in 2017 [22]. The treatment completion rate stands at 75% in Uganda [23]. The Mbarara TB unit provides care to approximately 600 TB patients annually. TB treatment to newly diagnosed patients is provided according to WHO guidelines [21] with a daily short course regimen delivered in fixed-dose combination tablets containing isoniazid, rifampin, pyrazinamide, and ethambutol for two months. At the two-month visit, sputum is examined, and those who convert the smear examinations to negative continue with isoniazid and rifampin only for four months in the continuation phase. The period of treatment can be extended up to eight months to cater for missed medication pick-ups. All patients with new cases of TB self-administer their medications. The clinic does not employ directly observed therapy due to inadequate staff time and excessive travel costs for patients to attend the clinic.

2.2. Selection of Study Participants. Between June 2017 and June 2018, authors AMT and WT purposively selected patients receiving TB treatment in Mbarara. We aimed to achieve balanced representation by gender and HIV status to elicit diverse perspectives. Inclusion criteria for TB patient participants were as follows: (a) having documented drug-sensitive TB, (b) receiving treatment with a first-line 6-month course of anti-TB regimen as described above for at least one month, (c) having a personal mobile phone, (d) able to send and receive SMS, (e) being 18 years or older, (f) residing in Mbarara district, (g) being willing and able to give consent, (h) being willing and able to name one social supporter, and (i) being able to speak the local language (Runyankole) or English.

We asked patients to identify social supporters at enrollment on the basis of an ongoing relationship, social supporter knowledge of the patient's TB status, and previous or current provision of social support (e.g., assistance to travel to the clinic and/or medication adherence advice) to the study participant. Inclusion criteria for the social supporter participants were as follows: (a) owning a personal mobile phone, (b) being able to send and received SMS, (c) being 18 years or older, (d) residing in Mbarara district, (e) knowing the study participant's TB/HIV status (ascertained through patients' self-reports), and (f) willing and able to provide consent.

2.3. Study Procedures

2.3.1. Intervention Demonstration. At enrollment, and before conducting each interview, we oriented each participant about the planned interventions to support adherence to TB medication. First, we explained that a real-time adherence monitor (Wisepill device; Wisepill Technologies, Cape Town, South Africa; Figure 1) is a pill bottle that records a date-and-time stamp when opened. We demonstrated how the adherence monitor works, including how to open it and put tablets in and how to close it after taking tablets. We indicated that the device monitors openings as proxies of medication ingestion and sends alerts to researchers if it is not opened by the expected time. We demonstrated how the monitor holds up to 28 tablets of TB medication. Participants were then given the monitor and asked to explain what it does and to practically demonstrate how it works to the researcher. We then explained to participants how we will send SMS reminders on a scheduled (e.g., daily) or triggered (e.g., triggered by a delayed/missed dose as detected through the monitor) basis to TB patients to help them take their medications. We further explained that the device could send SMS notifications of nonadherence to the patients' social supporters to encourage provision of assistance to the patient.

2.3.2. Data Collection. Immediately after orienting participants about the intervention (at enrolment), authors WT and AMT administered surveys eliciting information about sociodemographics, health status, social support, and general preferences for the planned wireless intervention. Within two weeks of enrolment, WT, AM, and AMT carried out semistructured in-depth interviews with TB patients (following reorientation about the intervention); both authors are bilingual in English and Runyankole and trained in qualitative research and research ethics. All questions in the interview guide were translated into Runyankole and back-translated to English by a different translator. Interviews were conducted in Runyankole, digitally recorded, transcribed, and translated to English. Interviews were conducted in a private space at the research office near the MRRH. Each interview lasted between 30 and 60 minutes. We elicited information about any current social support obtained by TB patients and how they feel about the social support they obtain, as well as their expectations of the wireless adherence monitoring intervention vis-à-vis social support. In interviews with social supporters, we also solicited information about the challenges they faced in providing medication adherence-related social support to TB patients

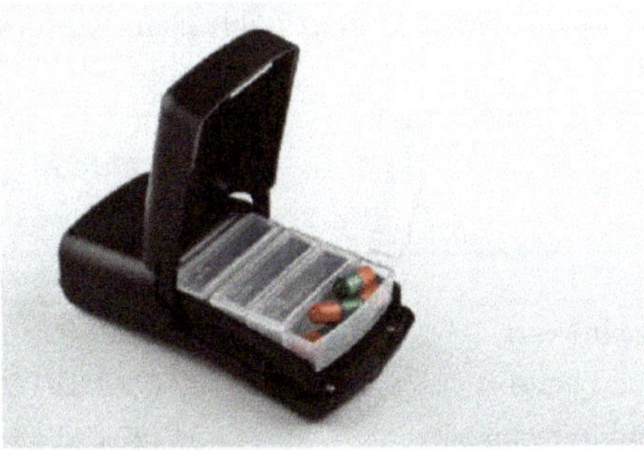

FIGURE 1: The Wisepill device.

and how the intervention might influence these challenges. Interviews were conducted until thematic saturation was achieved. Following each interview, author AM, with support from JEH and JLD, reviewed the transcripts for quality, clarity, and detail.

2.3.3. Analysis. Participants' sociodemographic details and preferences were summarized descriptively using STATA 13 by ATM and TW. We used inductive content analysis [24] to derive qualitative categories describing how participants currently use their phones to support TB-related treatment and how they perceived the planned wireless adherence monitoring intervention. Initially, AM, WT, and ATM reviewed and discussed 20% of transcripts for content relevant to current social support and expectations of the intervention. AM and WT then assembled a codebook from the identified concepts, using an iterative process, which included developing codes to represent content, writing operational definitions, and selecting illustrative quotes. JEH, JLD, and DB also reviewed and discussed the codebook. Differences in coding were harmonized through discussion. Following completion of the codebook, interviews were coded by AM and WT using NVIVO 11.

2.3.4. Ethical Approval. Ethical approvals were obtained from the Research Ethics Committee of Mbarara University of Science and Technology, the Uganda National Council for Science and Technology, and the Partners Human Research Committee for Massachusetts General Hospital.

3. Results and Discussion

3.1. Participant Characteristics. Of 53 screened TB patients, 18 (34%) were excluded for the following reasons (individuals could have >1 criterion): having no cellphone ($n = 6$; 11.3%), inability to use SMS text messages ($n = 5$; 9.4%), unwillingness or inability to name at least one social supporter ($n = 3$; 5.7%), being <18 years old ($n = 2$; 3.8%), having drug-resistant TB ($n = 1$; 1.9%), and/or inability to provide informed consent ($n = 1$; 1.9%). A total of 35 TB patients, of whom 15 (42.8%) were persons living with HIV/AIDS, enrolled in the study between February 2017 and April 2018.

Of 24 screened social supporters, 15 (62.5%) were enrolled in the study. Nine social supporters were excluded for the following reasons (individuals could have >1 criterion): having no cellphone ($n = 3$; 12.5%), living beyond

Table 1: Sociodemographic and health characteristics of study participants.

Characteristic	TB patients ($n = 35$)	Social supporters ($n = 15$)
Female	15 (42.9%)	9 (60.0%)
Median age in years	32.0	37.0
Able to read English	27 (77.1%)	10 (66.7%)
Able to read Runyankole	34 (97.1%)	14 (93.3%)
Had regular income	18 (51.4%)	8 (53.3%)
Worried about food security	20 (57.1%)	8 (53.3%)
Living with HIV	15 (42.9%)	1 (6.7%)
Mean (standard deviation) of TB treatment period completed (months)	3.3 (1.5)	—

Table 2: Survey results from patients.

Current social support received by patients*	
Reminders/encouragement to take medication	24 (69%)
Transport to clinic	21 (60%)
Food and drinks	20 (57%)
Help with chores	20 (57%)
Assistance with child care	10 (29%)
Counselling (e.g., encouragement to be positive about having TB)	5 (14%)
Money for other needs	3 (9%)
Adequacy of the social support received	
Social support enough	14 (40%)
Social support not enough	21 (60%)
Preference of notifications of social supporter	
Preferred notifications that instruct how the social supporter should help	15 (43%)
Preferred notifications that do not instruct how the social supporter should help	20 (57%)

*Participants could select multiple responses.

Mbarara district ($n = 2$; 8.33%), not knowing the study participant's TB/HIV status ($n = 2$; 8.3%), being <18 years of age ($n = 1$; 4.2%), and inability to provide informed consent ($n = 1$; 4.2%).

The sociodemographics, self-reported HIV status, and TB treatment progress of the study participants are indicated in Table 1. Just over half of the TB patients were male and the median age was 32 years. The mean period of TB treatment completed at the time of interview was 3.3 months. Most social supporters were female with a median age of 37 years. The majority of social supporters were TB patients' biological relatives ($n = 8$, 53%), 4 (27%) were spouses, and 3 (20%) were friends.

3.2. Survey Results. The most frequently reported type of social support was being reminded/encouraged to take medication—24 (69%) (Table 2). The majority of patients also reported that they were currently not receiving enough social support—21 (60%). Patients preferred SMS notifications that do not instruct how social supporters should help—20 (57.2%), compared to notifications that do offer such guidance.

3.3. Interview Results. TB patient participants reported utilizing mobile phones to obtain social support related to TB medication and treatment by (1) requesting and receiving instrumental support from social supporters, (2) requesting and receiving emotional support from social supporters, and (3) receiving informational support from healthcare providers. In reference to the anticipated intervention, social supporters and TB patients reported that SMS notifications may motivate medication adherence. Social supporters reported being concerned that they would at times be unable to provide the required support. TB patients reported the possibility of strain on relationships as a result of sending notifications linked to missed doses to social supporters. TB patients highlighted the need for the clinic/researchers to orient social supporters and patients about their expectations after receiving SMS notifications of nonadherence.

3.4. Use of Mobile Phones for Social Support

3.4.1. Requesting and Receiving Instrumental Support. TB patients described having used mobile phones to call their social supporters to request and obtain financial assistance in the form of mobile money (i.e., money sent and received using mobile phones). Patients reported using the obtained financial assistance to transport themselves to the clinic to obtain TB medication, buy food and drinks to ease pill taking, and pay bills both related and unrelated to TB (e.g., clinic bills, children's school fees, and housing bills).

> *Interviewer (I): What challenges do you face in picking your TB medication from the hospital? For example, how do you normally come to the hospital to pick your TB medication?*
> *Respondent (R): When I got sick, I moved to stayed with my sister so that she can assist me with washing, cooking, and generally taking care of me when I am too weak. So, I do not stay with my mother who provides money for transport to the clinic for my medication. I always have to use my mobile phone to call my mother to send me transport using mobile money. (Female, 39 yrs, TB patient living with HIV)*

This support was particularly helpful for patients without a regular source of income.

3.4.2. Requesting and Receiving Emotional Support. TB patients reported using mobile phones to call their social supporters, who in turn provided them with multiple forms of emotional social support. Common modes of emotional support included encouraging patients to take medication, encouraging them to live positively, and accompanying them to the TB clinic.

> *I: Please tell me about a time when someone used a mobile phone to help you with anything related to your TB?*
> *R: I used my phone to call my sister, and she escorted me to the hospital, and took me to the theatre. She would encourage me to take medicine, and ensured that I was taken good care of myself.*
> *I: How did you feel about the support that she gave to you?*
> *R: I felt good and cared for because she is the one that was always with me.*
> *I: So why do you think she helped you the way she helped you?*
> *R: She helped because she cares about my life. (Female, 28 yrs, TB patient)*

Patients described feeling good and cared for when their social supporters checked on them during telephone and SMS interactions.

3.4.3. Informational Support from Healthcare Providers. In addition to their social networks, TB patients also reported using their mobile phones to call healthcare providers and inquire about side effects, such as feeling dizzy or experiencing a change of urine color after taking the medication. These calls helped patients get useful medication-related advice, such as the need to eat and drink before taking medication.

> *I: First, I would like to know a little about how you use your cell phone. Do you ever use your phone for anything related to your health?*
> *R: Yes. Sometimes when I take my medication and become dizzy I call the nurse nearby our trading center called X and she tells me what to do.*
> *I: Please tell me more about that.*
> *R: When I call her, she tells me that it's the side effect of the TB pills and that to reduce it, I need to drink a lot and ensure that I do not take medicine on an empty stomach. (Female, 37 yrs, TB patient)*

TB patients, especially those who stayed far from the clinic, reported calling healthcare providers to make inquiries about the availability of drugs and clinic opening times. This information saved patients the expense of having to buy medicine from private pharmacies when they are freely available at the public clinic or traveling to the clinic outside operating hours.

> *I: Have you ever gotten assistance in taking your TB medication through your mobile phone?*
> *R: Yes I have ever called a doctor because I wanted to find out about the availability of the drugs at the TB treatment unit. The doctor told me that the drugs are always available and advised me to always come and pick the medication. He also discouraged me from buying medication from the pharmacy in case of failure to come to the hospital because they are expensive in terms of costs. (Male 39 yrs, TB patient)*

Instrumental and emotional support from friends and family, as well as informational support from clinicians, are important resources that can be accessed using mobile phones and used to facilitate completion of TB treatment.

3.5. Perceptions about the Planned Intervention

3.5.1. SMS Notifications to Social Supporters May Motivate TB Medication Adherence. Regarding the planned wireless adherence monitoring technology, social supporters and TB patients reported that receiving SMS texts when patients miss taking medication may "force" TB patients "not to forget taking medicine on time." This "force" was described positively, because it is motivated by the shared desire for the patient to get well.

> *I: How do you think [study participant] will feel when he knows that you receive his SMS when he misses taking his medication?*
> *R: He will like it very well and knowing that I will receive his SMS text when he misses taking his medication will force him not to forget taking his medicine on time.*
> *I: Why would he be forced not to forget?*
> *R: He knows me as a very strict person who has cared about his sickness since testing up to now. I agreed with him to always tell me, how he picks his medication and whenever he does medical checkup since it's me who gives him transport as my son. (Male, 65 years, social supporter)*

> *I: How do you feel about sending SMS notification to your social supporter when you miss taking your pills in time?*
> *R: It is a good thing because it will help me get cured quickly.*
> *I: Please tell me more about that.*
> *R: It forces me to take my drugs on time to get well, and also make him happy by seeing that he did not waste his efforts in supporting me. (Male, 45 years, patient)*

Social supporters felt that access to updates about patients' adherence would create a personal sense of obligation to take medication on time among patients.

3.5.2. Economic Constraints Could Limit Resources to Provide Support. Despite the anticipated motivation, participants had some concerns about implementing the planned intervention. First, although social supporters reported a desire and willingness to assist TB patients, those without a regular source of income reported being worried about the possibility of not being able to provide support for the TB patients even after receiving the SMS notification from the planned intervention.

> *It is not easy for me now, and it would not be easy for me when you send me a notification. I have to provide him all the support he needs to take his medicine well. Yet, I am also a poor woman struggling to live. (Female, 63, social supporter)*

This inability to provide support when needed created feelings of disappointment and embarrassment for both the social supporters and TB patients.

3.5.3. Receipt of the Planned SMS Notifications Could Strain Relations. Second, in addition to stress arising from limited resources, some TB patients and social supporters expressed concern that adherence-related messages could introduce conflict into their relationships. For example, patients noted that receiving notifications of missed doses could strain their relationship with social supporters.

> *"Once she knows that I have missed taking my medication and she has received an SMS notification from you. I am sure she will quarrel with me. Most of the times when she finds that I have forgotten taking my TB medication, she quarrels." (Male, 50 yrs, TB patient)*

This strain could potentially negatively affect the relationships between TB patients and their social supporters.

3.5.4. Orienting Social Supporters and TB Patients May Improve the Impact of SMS Notifications. In response to these challenges, TB patients and social supporters described the need to be oriented about the planned SMS notifications. This orientation could be done by the clinic or researchers and should highlight times and/or scenarios when SMS notifications can be sent and multiple ways how social supporters can help. During these orientations, patients can be helped to understand that social supporters may at times be unable to provide instrumental support due to inadequate resources.

> *I: So do you want the SMS notifications to inform your social supporter that you forgot to swallow your TB medication in order for her to help you well in taking you are TB medication?*
> *R: The best thing is to tell me to come with her here and you teach both of us so that each of us knows what to do after receiving the SMS. (Male, 50 yrs, TB patient)*

Providing orientation may be helpful in matching expectations of TB patients and their social supporters.

4. Discussion

In this mixed-method study of social support for adherence to TB treatment, TB patients described requesting and receiving instrumental, emotional, and informational social support using their mobile phones. Reminders and encouragement were the most common type of support received, followed by transport to the clinic, food and drinks, and help with chores. Participants felt that SMS notifications may motivate medication adherence by creating a personal sense of obligation to take medication on time. However, TB patients and social supporters reported that limited resources and relationship dynamics may constrain the provision of social support. Participants expressed the need to be oriented about the use of SMS notifications before they start receiving them in order to match expectations of patients and those of social supporters.

Traditional approaches to providing social support (such as counselling support, family and community support, and health education) have been shown to positively impact TB treatment success [9, 10]. A systematic review by van Hoorn and colleagues (which includes studies from low income countries of Nepal, Burkina Faso, and Haiti) reports that social support in the form of counseling, food supplements, home visits, and economic support improves TB treatment completion [25]. Other studies [26, 27] report the positive influence of instrumental support (in the form of monetary incentives and food packages) on TB treatment success and TB medication adherence in Asia and Russia. A randomized, controlled trial carried out by Tola and colleagues reports decreased nonadherence to TB medication adherence as a result of a social support intervention composed of counselling and health education in Ethiopia [28]. Despite the benefits, traditional approaches for providing social support may involve transport and time burdens, especially among patients who do not stay close to their social supporters. Delivering social support using mobile phones may be an inexpensive, accessible, and convenient approach that can potentially overcome geographical barriers to the provision of social support.

In this study, TB patients and their supporters largely agreed that SMS reminders linked to adherence monitoring technology could improve adherence. Such interventions have been shown to increase adherence to HIV antiretroviral therapy. In China, mobile phone-based SMS reminders are reported to be acceptable and useful in establishing antiretroviral adherence routines [29]. In South Africa, adherence measured by a real-time monitoring technology emerged as one of the best predictors of antiretroviral drug resistance and virological failure [30]. In the same setting in Uganda, a mobile adherence monitoring intervention composed of real-time adherence technology and SMS reminders was reported to be acceptable [19] and to improve adherence to antiretroviral therapy [18]. Similar or related interventions need to be tested in supporting TB medication adherence.

Our findings emphasize the need for researchers and intervention designers to consider social support in light of complex interpersonal relationships. Sending SMS notifications to social supporters when patients miss their TB medications may motivate patients to consistently take their medication on time to avoid letting down the efforts of social supporters who are caring for their health. Social supporters' frequent receipt of SMS notifications may, however, be perceived as patients' lack of commitment to medication adherence. This scenario may potentially result in misunderstandings which may affect the quality of support provided and the relationship itself, as noted by our participants. Additionally, the anticipated conflict as a result of unmatched or unmet expectations between patients and their social supporters was indeed reported in the antiretroviral adherence intervention in the same setting [31] and no definitive benefit of social support was seen [18].

Since findings indicate that potential strain on relationships and resources could limit the feasibility/acceptability of social support interventions, managing such strains is likely critical to the successful implementation of these interventions. Mobile phone-based support has a great potential, but the complexities of resource scarcity and interpersonal relationships necessitate careful human management of the process. Additional interventions for boosting the economic status (e.g., [32]) of social supporters or identifying alternative sources of support when possible (e.g., other members of the patient's social network) may improve the feasibility of the social support intervention. Providing orientation and counseling to patients and social supporters could also help in clarifying their roles, managing and harmonizing expectations, and highlighting the negative effect of persistent nonadherence on relationships.

This study has some limitations. Since we used purposive sampling, the proportions may not accurately summarize the characteristics or opinions of the overall TB patient and supporter populations from which we selected. It is based on a single setting—results may be different in different settings where culture, use of technology, resources, interpersonal dynamics, and other factors vary. The study only included patients who possess mobile phones and know how to use SMS texts; patients without phones or/and without knowledge of using SMS texts may have different views. This study is also based on self-reported responses about sensitive topics, which may be vulnerable to social desirability bias. Importantly, several of our findings reflect views of an anticipated intervention without the benefit of experience of the intervention. Experiences with the intervention will be assessed in an upcoming trial (NCT03800888). This study also has a number of strengths. First, the achievement of theme saturation suggests the sample was adequate. The study highlights potential ways in which mobile phones could be used to promote TB medication. Our findings are important for understanding the potential acceptability of the use of SMS texts combined with electronic monitoring to support TB medication adherence, which may potentially be an attractive alternative to DOT. Additionally, these findings can inform ideal study design for future mobile health-based and other related interventions.

5. Conclusions

Mobile telephones could provide alternative approaches to providing social support for TB medication adherence especially where patients do not stay close to their social supporters. This could relieve transport and time burdens associated with traditional face-to-face delivery of support. This advantage may be particularly useful in resource-limited settings where mobile phones are widely adopted and other support is difficult to obtain. Further efforts should focus on optimized designs of mobile phone-based applications for providing social support to TB patients and training of TB patients and social supporters to match their expectations.

Acknowledgments

The study was funded by a grant from the Fogarty International Center of the National Institutes of Health (K43TW010388). Author JEH is also supported through K24MH114732. The study was registered with ClinicalTrials.gov (NCT03800888). The authors would like to acknowledge the contributions of Anne Katahoire and the project directors and principal investigators of the PART project, which facilitated a Mixed Methods Fellowship in Makerere University. This fellowship provided technical guidance on writing mixed-method manuscripts.

References

[1] MOH and National Tuberculosis and Leprosy Control Programme, *Revised national strategic plan 2015/16-2019/20*, Ministry of Health (MOH), 2017.

[2] A. Wynne, S. Richter, L. Banura, and W. Kipp, "Challenges in tuberculosis care in Western Uganda: health care worker and patient perspectives," *International Journal of Africa Nursing Sciences*, vol. 1, pp. 6–10, 2014.

[3] S. H. Chang and J. K. Cataldo, "A systematic review of global cultural variations in knowledge, attitudes and health responses to tuberculosis stigma," *The International Journal of Tuberculosis and Lung Disease*, vol. 18, no. 2, pp. 168–173, 2014.

[4] G. M. Craiga and A. Zumlab, "The social context of tuberculosis treatment in urban risk groups in the United Kingdom: a qualitative interview study," *International Journal of Infectious Diseases*, vol. 32, pp. 105–110, 2015.

[5] A. L. Cremers, M. M. de Laat, N. Kapata, R. Gerrets, K. Klipstein-Grobusch, and M. P. Grobusch, "Assessing the consequences of stigma for tuberculosis patients in urban Zambia," *PLoS One*, vol. 10, no. 3, article e0119861, 2015.

[6] R. C. de Abreu Temoteo, F. D. Tavares de Luna, S. N. Batista Lacerda et al., "Accession to tuberculosis treatment: individual and social vulnerability elements," *International Archives of Medicine*, vol. 8, no. 206, 2015.

[7] G. Sulis, A. Roggi, A. Matteelli, and M. C. Raviglione, "Tuberculosis: epidemiology and control," *Mediterranean Journal of Hematology and Infectious Diseases*, vol. 6, no. 1, article e2014070, 2014.

[8] R. D. da Silva, F. D. T. de Luna, A. J. de Araújo et al., "Patients' perception regarding the influence of individual and social vulnerabilities on the adherence to tuberculosis treatment: a qualitative study," *BMC Public Health*, vol. 17, no. 1, p. 725, 2017.

[9] R. D. Deshmukh, D. J. Dhande, K. S. Sachdeva, A. N. Sreenivas, A. M. V. Kumar, and M. Parmar, "Social support a key factor for adherence to multidrug-resistant tuberculosis treatment," *Indian Journal of Tuberculosis*, vol. 65, no. 1, pp. 41–47, 2018.

[10] X. Li, B. Wang, D. Tan et al., "Effectiveness of comprehensive social support interventions among elderly patients with

tuberculosis in communities in China: a community-based trial," *Journal of Epidemiology and Community Health*, vol. 72, no. 5, pp. 369–375, 2018.

[11] J. Yin, X. Wang, L. Zhou, and X. Wei, "The relationship between social support, treatment interruption and treatment outcome in patients with multidrug-resistant tuberculosis in China: a mixed-methods study," *Tropical Medicine & International Health*, vol. 23, no. 6, pp. 668–677, 2018.

[12] International Telecommunication Union, "Key global telecom indicators for the world telecommunication service sector," 2016, October 2017, http://www.itu.int/en/ITU-D/Statistics/Documents/statistics/2016/ITU_Key_2005-2016_ICT_data.xls.

[13] J. M. Ggita, C. Ojok, A. J. Meyer et al., "Patterns of usage and preferences of users for tuberculosis-related text messages and voice calls in Uganda," *The International Journal of Tuberculosis and Lung Disease*, vol. 22, no. 5, pp. 530–536, 2018.

[14] S. Mohammed, R. Glennerster, and A. J. Khan, "Impact of a daily SMS medication reminder system on tuberculosis treatment outcomes: a randomized controlled trial," *PLoS One*, vol. 11, no. 11, article e0162944, 2016.

[15] P. Kunawararak, S. Pongpanich, S. Chantawong et al., "Tuberculosis treatment with mobile-phone medication reminders in northern Thailand," *The Southeast Asian Journal of Tropical Medicine and Public Health*, vol. 42, no. 6, pp. 1444–1451, 2011.

[16] R. S. Garfein, K. Collins, F. Muñoz et al., "Feasibility of tuberculosis treatment monitoring by video directly observed therapy: a binational pilot study," *The International Journal of Tuberculosis and Lung Disease*, vol. 19, no. 9, pp. 1057–1064, 2015.

[17] S. Mohammed, O. Siddiqi, O. Ali et al., "User engagement with and attitudes towards an interactive SMS reminder system for patients with tuberculosis," *Journal of Telemedicine and Telecare*, vol. 18, no. 7, pp. 404–408, 2012.

[18] J. E. Haberer, A. Musiimenta, E. C. Atukunda et al., "Short message service (SMS) reminders and real-time adherence monitoring improve antiretroviral therapy adherence in rural Uganda," *AIDS*, vol. 30, no. 8, pp. 1295–1299, 2016.

[19] A. Musiimenta, E. C. Atukunda, W. Tumuhimbise et al., "Acceptability and feasibility of real-time antiretroviral therapy adherence interventions in rural Uganda: mixed-method pilot randomized controlled trial," *JMIR mHealth and uHealth*, vol. 6, no. 5, article e122, 2018.

[20] C. Orrell, K. Cohen, K. Mauff, D. R. Bangsberg, G. Maartens, and R. Wood, "A randomized controlled trial of real-time electronic adherence monitoring with text message dosing reminders in people starting first-line antiretroviral therapy," *JAIDS Journal of Acquired Immune Deficiency Syndromes*, vol. 70, no. 5, pp. 495–502, 2015.

[21] WHO, "Guidelines on tuberculosis infection prevention and control, 2019 update," 2019, June 2019, https://www.who.int/tb/publications/2019/guidelines-tuberculosis-infection-prevention-2019/en/.

[22] WHO, "2017 global tuberculosis report," 2017, May 2019, https://www.who.int/tb/publications/global_report/gtbr2017_main_text.pdf.

[23] WHO, "Tuberculosis country profiles," 2018, June 2019, https://www.who.int/tb/country/data/profiles/en/.

[24] H. F. Hsieh and S. E. Shannon, "Three approaches to qualitative content analysis," *Qualitative Health Research*, vol. 15, no. 9, pp. 1277–1288, 2005.

[25] R. van Hoorn, E. Jaramillo, D. Collins, A. Gebhard, and S. van den Hof, "The effects of psycho-emotional and socio-economic support for tuberculosis patients on treatment adherence and treatment outcomes – a systematic review and meta-analysis," *PLoS One*, vol. 11, no. 4, article e0154095, 2016.

[26] K. Davtyan, S. Aghabekyan, H. Davtyan et al., *Social support programme for tuberculosis patients in Armenia: perceptions of patients and doctors*, Public Health Panorama, 2015, http://hdl.handle.net/10144/618901.

[27] B. Garden, A. Samarina, I. Stavchanskaya et al., "Food incentives improve adherence to tuberculosis drug treatment among homeless patients in Russia," *Scandinavian Journal of Caring Sciences*, vol. 27, no. 1, pp. 117–122, 2013.

[28] H. H. Tola, D. Shojaeizadeh, A. Tol et al., "Psychological and educational intervention to improve tuberculosis treatment adherence in Ethiopia based on health belief model: a cluster randomized control trial," *PLoS One*, vol. 11, no. 5, article e0155147, 2016.

[29] L. L. Sabin, L. Mansfield, M. B. DeSilva et al., "Why it worked: participants' insights into an mHealth antiretroviral therapy adherence intervention in China," *The Open AIDS Journal*, vol. 12, pp. 20–37, 2018.

[30] C. Orrell, K. Cohen, R. Leisegang, D. R. Bangsberg, R. Wood, and G. Maartens, "Comparison of six methods to estimate adherence in an ART-naïve cohort in a resource-poor setting: which best predicts virological and resistance outcomes?," *AIDS Research and Therapy*, vol. 14, no. 1, p. 20, 2017.

[31] E. C. Atukunda, A. Musiimenta, N. Musinguzi et al., "Understanding patterns of social support and their relationship to an ART adherence intervention among adults in rural southwestern Uganda," *AIDS and Behavior*, vol. 21, no. 2, pp. 428–440, 2017.

[32] S. D. Weiser, E. A. Bukusi, R. L. Steinfeld et al., "*Shamba Maisha*: randomized controlled trial of an agricultural and finance intervention to improve HIV health outcomes," *AIDS*, vol. 29, no. 14, pp. 1889–1894, 2015.

22

Engaging Informal Private Health Care Providers for TB Case Detection: Experiences from RIPEND Project in India

Santosha Kelamane,[1] Srinath Satyanarayana,[2] Sharath Burugina Nagaraja,[3] Vikas Panibatla,[1] Ramesh Dasari,[1] Rajeesham,[4] Amera Khan,[5] and Vishnuvardhan Kamineni[5,6]

[1]*TB Alert India, Hyderabad, India*
[2]*Independent Public Health Consultant, New Delhi, India*
[3]*ESIC Medical College and PGIMSR, Bengaluru, India*
[4]*State TB Office, Telangana State, Hyderabad, India*
[5]*Stop TB Partnership, Geneva, Switzerland*
[6]*Senior Advisor, Public Health, Bengaluru, India*

Correspondence should be addressed to Sharath Burugina Nagaraja; sharathbn@yahoo.com

Academic Editor: Karl Drlica

Background. Informal (unqualified) health care providers are an important source of medical care for persons with presumptive TB (PPTB) in India. A project (titled RIPEND) was implemented to engage informal providers for the identification of PPTBs and TB patients in 4 districts of Telangana State, India, during October 2018-December 2019 project period. Engagement involved sensitizing the informal providers about TB, providing them financial incentives to identify PPTBs, and linking these PPTBs to diagnostic and treatment services provided by the Government of India's National TB Elimination Programme. *Objectives.* To describe (a) the characteristics of the informal providers, along with their self-reported practices on TB diagnosis, treatment, and challenges encountered by the RIPEND project staff in engaging them in the project and (b) the outputs and outcomes of this engagement. *Methods.* We used a combination of one-on-one interviews with informal providers, group interviews with RIPEND project staff, and secondary analysis of data available within the project's recording and reporting systems. *Results.* A total of 555 informal providers were actively engaged under the project. The majority (87%) had a nonmedicine-related graduate degree and had been providing medical care for more than 10 years. Most (95%) were aware that a cough for 2 weeks or more is a symptom of pulmonary TB and that such patients should be referred for sputum-smear microscopy at a government health facility. Challenges in engaging the informal providers included motivating them to participate in the study, suboptimal mobile usage for referral services, and delays in providing financial incentives to them for referring PPTBs. During the project period (October 2018-December 2019), 8342 PPTBs were identified of which 1003 TB patients were detected and linked to TB treatment services. *Conclusion.* This project showed that engaging informal providers is feasible and that a large number of PPTB and TB patients can be identified through this effort. The Government of India should consider engaging informal providers for the early diagnosis of TB to reduce the missing TB cases in the country.

1. Introduction

India accounts for nearly 27% of the global tuberculosis (TB) burden [1]. Despite the efforts of the Government of India's Revised National TB Control Programme (RNTCP) over the past couple of decades, TB continues to be a major public health problem. The country has now renamed RNTCP to National TB Elimination Programme (NTEP) with a goal of reducing the TB burden drastically by 2025, five years ahead of the United Nations' Sustainable Development Goals

(SDG). The road map for TB elimination is outlined in National Strategic Plan (2017-2025) [2].

For eliminating TB, it is essential to diagnose and treat all TB cases occurring in the community [3]. In countries like India, involvement of private health care providers is one of the quintessential processes to achieve TB elimination [4]. The private health sector comprises both formal and informal health care providers in almost equal proportions [5]. The formal private sector is relatively expensive, particularly for the economically poor and vulnerable groups. Therefore, they avail medical services from the informal private sector, which is more affordable and easily accessible [6]. In India, nearly 70% of the persons with presumptive TB (PPTB), especially those from low and middle-income communities, first approach a nearby private health care provider who is usually an informal provider [7–9]. It is sometimes thought that the quality of care is compromised by informal care providers and that this often leads to delayed diagnosis and inappropriate treatment [10]. However, it is important for a national health programme to have a greater accessibility and deeper penetrability in the community.

The Government of India's NTEP has made several efforts to engage the formal private health care providers [11, 12], but the efforts made to engage the informal providers have not been commensurate to the need. The main reason for hesitancy to engage informal providers is that these providers are technically unqualified and therefore illegal practitioners of medical care. Any effort to engage them is seen as a sign of acknowledging and legitimising their presence [13]. However, it is now being increasingly recognised that it is essential to engage informal providers for reaching out to all TB patients because of their widespread presence in all parts of the country and their deep connection with the lower socioeconomic strata of the population who are disproportionately affected by TB disease [2, 14]. There is sparse evidence in the country on successful models to engage these providers [12, 15].

TB Alert India, an international nongovernment organisation, is implementing a project called RIPEND (Roping Informal Private Providers for Enhanced TB case Detection) with funding support from the Stop TB Partnership's TB REACH Wave 6 grant [16] in the state of Telangana, India. The first phase of this project was implemented in rural and semiurban areas of 8 TB Units (covering a population of ~2.2 million people) with an aim of training and engaging informal private health care providers in early detection of TB among patients and referring them for health/medical care. Under this project, we mapped all the informal providers in the TB units, if they met certain eligibility criteria (the criteria are described in Methods). The engaged informal provider underwent a one-day training on the identification of PPTB, the referral of PPTB to undergo TB diagnostic evaluation as per the NTEP diagnostic algorithm, and the linkage of diagnosed TB patients to treatment services. The presumptive TB patients are subjected to sputum-smear examination and chest radiography for TB diagnosis. If the smear results are negative and chest X-ray suggestive of TB or not, the presumptive TB patient shall be subjected to cartridge-based nucleic acid amplification test (CB-NAAT) for the detection of *Mycobacterium tuberculosis* and rifampicin resistance. The patients who get the CBNAAT test (1) are smear positive and have chest X-ray suggestive of TB, (2) are smear positive but have chest X-ray not suggestive of TB, (3) are smear negative but have chest X-ray suggestive of TB, and (4) have high clinical suspicion (smear negative or unavailable and chest X-ray not suggestive of TB or unavailable).

As part of the RIPENED project, we examined (a) the sociodemographic characteristics of the informal providers, along with their self-reported practices on TB diagnosis and treatment, and the challenges encountered by the RIPEND project staff in engaging them in the project and (b) the outcomes of this engagement in terms of the number of PPTB identified, the numbers assessed for TB with various TB diagnostic tests, and the numbers of TB patients diagnosed and linked to TB treatment services under the NTEP.

2. Methods

2.1. Study Design. Under objective 1, we adopted a cross-sectional study design for assessing the sociodemographic characteristics of the informal providers, along with their self-reported practices on TB diagnosis and treatment. For assessing the challenges encountered in engaging informal providers, we conducted qualitative interviews with TB Alert program staff who were responsible for engagement activities. *Under objective 2*, for describing the outcomes of the engagement, we analysed the data collected on the persons with PPTB identified by the informal providers under the project.

2.2. Study Setting. TB Alert India implemented the RIPEND project in eight tuberculosis units (TUs) of four districts, Karimnagar, Jangaon, Jagtial, and Warangal in the State of Telangana. This project was implemented in close partnership with the District/State TB programme managers.

In all eight TUs, the field coordinators of the project ($n = 16$) had line listed all informal health care providers. Providers who met the following eligibility criteria mentioned were involved under the project: (a) provide consultations to at least 10 patients per day, (b) willing to participate in the project, and (c) have an android smart phone and are willing to use it for recording and reporting patient details. All the engaged providers were trained about the programme and the project, including usage of a mobile application (an application for usage in the smart android mobile phones) for presumptive TB patient referrals by the trained RIPENED project staff. A nominal financial incentive (INR 40 for PPTB identification and referral for testing under the project and an additional INR 250 if PPTB were to be diagnosed as TB) was provided to the providers for identifying the presumptive pulmonary TB patient (PPTB) during their routine outpatient consultations and entering the PTC into the project's IT platform via their smartphones.

2.3. Study Period. The study was conducted between October 2018 and December 2019.

2.4. Study Population, Sampling, and Sample Size. For the quantitative component of the first study objective, all the informal providers willing to be part of the project were enrolled for the study; for the qualitative component, we conducted group interviews with the staff of the RIPEND project (~20). For the second study objective, we included all persons with PPTB identified by the informal providers during the project period without any exclusion.

2.5. Recording and Reporting Systems under the Project. Project RIPEND has established a paper-based and a mobile (both Android and iOS applications) web-based IT platform for documenting the information on the informal providers enrolled in the project. For each PPTB enrolled into the project, the following was documented: (a) general characteristics of the patients and their presentation such as name, age, sex, address, symptoms, and their duration; (b) type of diagnostic tests and their results, such as sputum smear microscopy, chest radiography, and CB-NAAT such as Xpert MTB/Rif® tests; and (c) the basis of diagnosis for treatment initiation and the type of sector under which treatment was initiated. The data from this information technology platform was exported to Microsoft Excel and analysed. This database was used to generate the quarterly reports that were shared with the local TB programme managers and the funders. The validity/accuracy of the data contained in the recording and reporting system was periodically assessed by RIPEND project managers during routine supervisory visits and external TB REACH monitoring and evaluation visits. If any discrepancy was noted in the data, it was rectified immediately.

2.6. Data Variables, Data Collection, and Sources of the Data. For objective 1, we used a structured questionnaire to capture the following information from the informal providers: age, sex, qualification, number of years in the field, type of clinic, other facilities with clinic (pharmacy or laboratory), location (crowded place/isolated), building (rented/own), average consultation fees per patient, average time spent on each patient, whether the provider conducts home visits and does the provider conduct a mobile clinic, TB diagnostic practices (referral for sputum/chest X-ray/both/others), diagnosis of TB made by self/other qualified professionals and diagnostic tests used, TB treatment practices (NTEP drugs/private drugs from pharmacies) anti-TB drugs/others-additional/-both/self-made preparation, willingness to update his knowledge/undergo training on TB (yes/no), time desirable to spend on knowledge improvement (1 hr/4 hr/7 hr), preferred day in a week (week days/weekends), mode of knowledge improvement (pamphlet/mobile messages/one-to-one discussion/class room teaching/others), and frequency of knowledge improvement (monthly/quarterly).

We used an interview guide to conduct group interviews with our project staff to collect the information on the challenges encountered in engaging informal care providers (like training, enrolment, and continuous engagement of informal providers and sustainability). The key informant interviews were conducted by trained researchers in the local language (Telugu) at a place and time convenient to them. Interviews were audio recorded. The transcripts were translated into English and used for analysis. We ensured the accuracy of translation through the translation-back translation method.

For objective 2, from the project's mobile app-based recording and reporting system, we obtained the following data for each PPTB: their demographic characteristics include age, sex, type, and duration of symptoms with a specific focus on cough, type of diagnostic tests, and test results (sputum smear, chest radiography, and CB-NAAT); if TB were diagnosed, type of TB (new smear-positive, new smear-negative, retreatment smear-positive, and rifampicin-resistant TB), source of TB treatment (public/private), and the TB notification status to NTEP were recorded.

2.7. Data Analysis. For objective 1, the quantitative data were entered in a standard data entry software (EpiData, Odense, Denmark) and were analysed using EpiData analysis software. For the qualitative component of the data, the content analysis of the transcripts was done. The two study investigators (SS and SBN) independently identified all codes and generated themes. Then, the codes and themes were compared, and the differences were sorted out through consensus and detailed discussions. The verbatim quotes to support the codes and themes were used to describe the results of the qualitative study.

For objective 2, we imported the data from Microsoft Excel and analysed the data in Stata Statistical Software (version 15, Stata Corp, College Station, Texas, US). We have summarized the various patient characteristics by numbers and proportions.

2.8. Ethics Approval. Ethics approval for the study was obtained by the Institutional Ethics Committee of National TB Institute, Bengaluru, Karnataka. We obtained informed consent from all study participations under objective 1. We got a waiver from obtaining informed consent from the study participants under objective 2. We have maintained the confidentiality of the data throughout the study.

3. Results

3.1. Sociodemographic Characteristics. Under objective 1, a total of 555 informal providers were enrolled in the study. The sociodemographic characteristics of the practitioners are shown in Table 1. The majority of them were in the age group of more than 40 years (60%) and were males (99%). The highest number of providers was enrolled from the Jagtial TU (21%), followed by Warangal DTC TU (20%) and Karimnagar DTC TU (18%). The majority (82%) of the providers had completed graduate-level education in a nonmedicine-related field and had more than 10 years of experience; 50% of them had clinics in rented buildings. Most of the clinics operated during both the mornings and evening hours; the majority catered to about 10-20 out-patient attendees per day. They charged the patients anywhere between 0.5 and 1 USD per consultation.

3.2. Tuberculosis Management Practices. The TB management practices of the providers at the baseline are shown in Table 2. They revealed that the majority (95%) of the providers were aware that a cough of two weeks or more is the predominant symptom of TB disease, and for persons with such symptoms, most are prescribed sputum smear

TABLE 1: Sociodemographic characteristics of informal providers involved in RIPENED project, Telangana State, India, 2018-19 ($N = 555$).

S. no	Variables		Number (%)
1	Age group (years)	<40	216 (39)
		40-50	204 (37)
		51-60	100 (18)
		>60	35 (6)
2	Sex	Male	551 (99.5)
		Female	4 (0.5)
3	Tuberculosis unit	Mulkanoor	69 (12)
		Station Ghanpur	71 (13)
		Warangal DTC	111 (20)
		Choppadandi	44 (8)
		Karimnagar DTC	99 (18)
		Jangaon	46 (8)
		Jagtial	115 (21)
4	Area of clinic	Urban	486 (87)
		Rural	69 (13)
5	Qualification	High school	26 (5)
		10th standard	36 (6)
		12th standard	8 (1)
		Diploma degree	196 (35)
		Degree science	187 (34)
		Degree others	102 (18)
6	Health facility	Rented	277 (50)
		Own building	267 (48)
		Not recorded	11 (2)
7	Clinic timings	Morning	1 (0)
		Morning and evening	546 (97)
		Evening	6 (3)
8	Experience in medical practice (in years)	<10	101 (18)
		10-20	240 (43)
		20-30	152 (28)
		>30	62 (1)
9	No. of daily consultations	<10	4 (0)
		10-20	469 (85)
		20-30	80 (14)
		>30	4 (1)
10	Consultation charges (INR)	50	21 (4)
		50-75	524 (94)
		>75	10 (2)

examination at a government health facility. None of them preferred to order chest radiography or blood tests as the first choice of investigation for TB disease. Nearly 84% of them were sensitized on TB by the project's personnel. Few of the providers (4%) were also treatment supporters or DOT providers under NTEP.

About 40% of the practitioners were using the mobile application for enrolling PPTBs under the project. The remaining were using a logbook (provided by the project) to maintain the PPTB details from which data were subsequently entered into the mobile application. After six months of initiating the project, 85% of the providers mentioned that they were receiving the incentives on time for referring the presumptive cases or TB patients. Most of the providers were willing to undergo at least four hours of updated training.

3.3. Challenges to Engage Informal Care Providers: Perspectives of Project Staff. During group interviews, the

TABLE 2: TB management practices of Informal providers at the time of involvement under RIPENED project, Telangana State, India, during 2018-19 ($N = 555$).

S. no	Variables		Number (%)
1	Symptoms of presumptive TB	Cough ≥ 2 weeks	528 (95)
		Not recorded	27 (5)
2	Action taken when encountered presumptive TB	Referred	1 (0.5)
		Order TB test	553 (99)
		Not recorded	1 (0.5)
3	Where do you refer?	Government	555 (100)
		Private	0
4	Do you ask for chest radiography?	Yes	0
		No	552 (99)
		Not recorded	3 (1)
5	Do you ask for sputum smear microscopy?	Yes	553 (100)
		No	0
		Not recorded	2 (0)
6	Do you ask for blood test?	Yes	0
		No	554 (99)
		Not recorded	1 (1)
7	Are you sensitized on TB by project staff?	Yes	466 (84)
		No	87 (16)
		Not recorded	2 (0)
8	Where were you sensitized?	Government	454 (82)
		Private	7 (3)
		Not recorded	94 (17)
9	Are you a DOT provider?	Yes	25 (4)
		No	518 (94)
		Not recorded	12 (2)
10	Do you use project mobile application routinely?	Yes	218 (40)
		No	330 (60)
		Not applicable	2 (0)
		Not recorded	5 (1)
11	Have you received incentives from project for referrals? (Initial 3 months)	Yes	86 (15)
		No	466 (85)
		Not recorded	3 (0)
12	Are you willing to undergo programmatic sensitization?	Yes	528 (95)
		No	16 (3)
		Not applicable	3 (1)
		Not recorded	8 (1)
13	How many hours can you devote for sensitization?	4 hours	537 (97)
		1 day	1 (0)
		Not recorded	17 (3)

challenges faced by the staff in engaging with the informal providers are listed in Table 3. The challenges were predominantly related to sensitization, referral activities, and financial incentives. Most of the project staff opined that it is essential to engage the informal health care providers under the national TB programme, as they provide medical care to a significant proportion of the population.

"*...it is difficult to mobilise them [informal providers] for sensitization, though they are interested, they don't want to lose their livelihood...*" Male, 33 years, Karimnagar DTC TU.

TABLE 3: Key challenges encountered by the RIPENED project staff.

During sensitization
(i) Availability of informal providers in a timely manner for group sensitization programs
(ii) Incompatible smart phones of informal providers to support the project mobile application
During referral activities
(i) Inefficient usage of mobile application for referral activities
(ii) Frequently deleting the mobile application from their phones
(iii) Referring the symptomatic to private hospitals
(iv) Referring of symptomatic with less than one-week cough to sputum smear microscopy
(v) Inadequate emphasis of chest x-ray on patients when smear results are negative and symptoms are present
Financial incentives
(i) The providers perceived the incentive provided as low
(ii) Delays in disbursement of funds to the providers bank accounts

"*...some [informal providers] don't have smart phones and those who have it use it for basic services like phone calls and whatsapp!...we have to be behind them every day to make them refer patients through mobile application...very difficult!*" Male 28 years, Station Ghanpur TU.

"*...though incentive is not of great attraction to them [informal providers]...at times...they complain about not receiving it!...they expect it to happen immediately...how is it possible?...*" Male, 42 years, Mulkanoor TU.

3.4. Clinical-Demographic Features of Referred Presumptive TB Patients. During the project period, approximately 8342 PPTBs were identified and referred for testing. Their demographic and clinical characteristics are presented in Table 4. Nearly 44% of the patients were in the age group of 18-45 years, 63% were males, and 92% had cough as the presenting symptom with 85% having cough for 2 to 3-week duration. Of all the presumptive TB cases screened, 54% of them knew their HIV status and 0.6% of them were found to be HIV positive. Nearly 3.5% of the persons had a past history of TB.

3.5. Diagnostic Tests Undergone by the Presumptive Cases. The diagnostic tests undergone by the 8342 persons with presumptive pulmonary TB are given in Table 5. Approximately 10% of the persons with presumptive pulmonary TB had undergone X-ray, of which 32% had X-ray findings suggestive of TB. Approximately two-thirds of the persons with presumptive TB had undergone sputum smear examination, of which 6.5% had sputum smear-positive results. Approximately a third of the persons with presumptive TB had undergone CB-NAAT tests, and of these who had taken this test, 23% had a positive result, indicating the presence of TB bacilli.

3.6. Notification to the Public Health System. Of the total 8342 persons with presumptive TB patients, 1003 cases of TB were diagnosed, data that were communicated to the public health systems. The testing pattern of TB diagnostic tests performed, the number of patients who underwent tests, and those diagnosed with TB are shown in Table 6. The number and proportion of patients subjected to only a single diagnostic test were (a) microscopy (4785, 57%), (b) CB-NAAT (1984, 24%), and (c) chest X-ray (235, 3%), while the number and proportion of patients who underwent two diagnostic tests are (d) microscopy and chest X-ray (235, 3%), (e) microscopy and CB-NAAT (431, 5%), and (f) chest X-ray and CB-NAAT (223, 3%). The patients who underwent (g) microscopy and chest X-ray and CB-NAAT were 98 (1%).

TABLE 4: Characteristics of persons with presumptive TB enrolled under RIPENED project, Telangana State, India, during 2018-19 ($N = 8342$).

S. no	Characteristics	Number	(Percent)
1	Age group		
	<18	378	(4)
	18-45	3604	(44)
	>45 to 60	2636	(32)
	>60	1724	(20)
2	Gender		
	Female	3079	(37)
	Male	5260	(63)
	Transgender	3	(0)
3	Cough		
	Yes	7688	(92)
	Unknown	573	(7)
	No	81	(1)
4	Cough (duration), weeks		
	<2	207	(3)
	2-3	6627	(85)
	≥4	935	(12)
5	HIV status		
	Positive	53	(0)
	Negative	4464	(54)
	Unknown	3252	(39)
	Not recorded	573	(7)
6	Previous history of TB		
	Yes	289	(3)
	No	7480	(90)
	Unknown/not recorded	573	(7)

Similarly, the number and proportion of TB patients who were diagnosed based on single diagnostic tests were (a) microscopy (201, 20%), (b) CB-NAAT (29, 3%), and (c) chest X-ray (417, 42%). The number and proportion of patients who underwent two diagnostic tests were (d) microscopy and chest X-ray (44, 4%), (e) microscopy and CB-NAAT (150, 15%), and (f) chest X-ray and CB-NAAT (104, 10%). The patients who underwent (g) microscopy and chest X-ray and CB-NAAT were (58, 6%).

3.7. Clinical-Demographic Features of Diagnosed TB Cases. The TB detection rate among persons with presumptive TB disaggregated by their demographic and clinical status is

TABLE 5: Results of different TB diagnostic tests of Presumptive TB patients enrolled under RIPENED project, Telangana State, India, during 2018-19 ($N = 8342$).

S. no	Characteristics	Number	(%)
	Sputum microscopy		
1	Not done	2793	(33)
	Done	5549	(67)
	Microscopy results (if done)		
2	Negative	5186	(93)
	Positive	363	(7)
	Chest X-ray result		
3	Not done	7551	(90)
	X-ray done	791	(10)
	X-ray result (if done)		
4	Not suggestive of TB	537	(68)
	Suggestive of TB	254	(32)
	CB-NAAT test		
	CB-NAAT test not done	5606	(67)
	CB-NAAT test done	2736	(33)
	CB-NAAT result (if done)		
5	MTB not detected	2073	(76)
	CB-NAAT result not available	33	(1)
	MTB detected-RIF sensitive	512	(19)
	MTB detected-RIF resistant	115	(4)

given in Table 7. Within different age groups, TB detection ranged from 10% in those aged less than 18 years to 15% in those aged 18-45 years. In males, 14% were detected with TB when compared to 9% among females. 13% of those who had a cough were diagnosed with TB. In those that were HIV positive, 32% were detected with TB when compared to 12% of those whose HIV status was unknown. The previous history of TB was detected among 33% of patients when compared to 12% among those without a past history of TB.

4. Discussion

The study describes the process, challenges, outputs, and outcomes of a project that was aimed towards engaging the informal providers. Through this project, ~555 informal providers were engaged, and through them, 8342 PPTBs were identified and subjected to diagnostic tests, of which 1003 persons were diagnosed with TB and all the patients were initiated on treatment according to programme guidelines. Sputum smear microscopy was the major diagnostic test for TB case detection.

The study findings suggest that the majority of the informal health care providers are educated, have knowledge of TB management practices, and can be engaged in the detection of TB patients in the community. The major challenges faced by the project staff were motivating the rural practitioners to participate in the study, suboptimal mobile usage for referral services, and delayed financial incentives for the referred presumptive TB patients.

The study has the following programmatic implications. First, informal providers can be successfully engaged, and sustained efforts will result in increasing presumptive identification and promote early TB diagnosis, particularly improving TB care among the vulnerable groups. Despite being technically unqualified to provide health care services, they had been providing the basic services in their locality for many years; hence, the NTEP should seriously consider engaging the informal providers (through training, incentives) for early identification of PPTBs by building their capacity and to accept referrals to government health services for TB management. [2, 14, 17]. A similar finding was observed in a study conducted at Jharkhand by Project Axshya [18]

Second, the informal providers were given nominal financial incentives under the project to encourage them to identify and refer PPTB for testing. We strongly believe that this incentive played a role in their engagement. Although there were instances of delayed disbursement of incentives for the providers under the project, it did not deter the identification and referral of PPTBs from the providers. The NTEP has provisions for providing incentives to the private health care providers for diagnosis of TB [12]. This should be extended for identification and referral of PPTBs as well.

Third, engagement of informal providers resulted in the identification of large numbers of PPTB, roughly constituting 7-8% of the TB patients detected in these TB Units [19]. The yield in the absolute number of PPTBs and TB cases was higher than a similar project conducted in Odisha State of India [20]. In the absence of this project, the 8342 PPTBs identified under this project either would have not been subjected to TB diagnostic evaluation or would have been subjected to diagnostic evaluation at a later stage. This would

TABLE 6: The testing patterns of TB diagnostic tests performed, number of patients who underwent tests and those diagnosed with TB under RIPENED project, Telangana State, India, during 2018-19 ($N = 8342$).

Testing patterns of TB diagnostic tests	Number of patients who underwent the test ($N = 8342$) n (%)	Number diagnosed with TB ($N = 1003$) n (%)
(a) Microscopy only	4785 (57)	201 (20)
(b) Chest X-ray only	235 (3)	29 (3)
(c) CB-NAAT only	1984 (24)	417 (42)
(d) Microscopy+chest X-ray only	235 (3)	44 (4)
(e) Microscopy+CB-NAAT only	431 (5)	150 (15)
(f) Chest X-ray+CB-NAAT only	223 (3)	104 (10)
(g) Microscopy+chest X-ray+CB-NAAT	98 (1)	58 (6)
(h) No tests done	351 (4)	0 (0)

TABLE 7: Proportion of TB cases detected among different characteristics of presumptive TB patients under RIPENED project, Telangana State, India, during 2018-19 ($N = 8342$).

S. no	Characteristics	Presumptive TB patients	TB patients	(%)
1	Age group			
	<18	378	38	(10)
	18-45	3604	499	(15)
	>45 to 60	2636	306	(13)
	>60	1724	160	(12)
2	Gender			
	Female	3079	287	(9)
	Male	5260	716	(14)
	Transgender	3	0	(0)
3	Cough			
	Yes	7688	959	(13)
	Unknown	573	32	(6)
	No	81	12	(15)
4	Cough (duration), weeks			
	<2	207	18	(8)
	2-3	6627	667	(10)
	≥4	935	266	(28)
5	HIV status			
	Positive	53	17	(32)
	Negative	4464	586	(13)
	Unknown	3252	368	(11)
	Not recorded	573	32	(6)
6	Previous history of TB			
	Yes	289	94	(33)
	No	7480	877	(2)
	Unknown/not recorded	573	32	(6)

have resulted in missed diagnosis or delayed diagnosis [21]. This would have increased the morbidity, mortality among these individuals, and the transmission of TB in the community, which was perhaps mitigated by the implementation of this project [20].

Fourth, based on anecdotal information obtained by the project's field coordinators, we feel that 8342 persons with TB symptoms identified under the project do not represent all cases of presumptive TB, and therefore, the number of persons with TB symptoms identified under this project is a gross underestimate of the actual number of presumptive TB patients seeking care from them. In our project, we tried to enhance the identification of presumptive TB patients by interacting with the informal providers at regular intervals through field coordinators and also provided a token financial incentive for identification and referral of presumptive TB cases through mobile application. But it appeared to be insufficient, and several other steps may have to be undertaken to enhance the completeness of referrals by informal health care providers, probably because the field coordinators felt that the informal providers still weighed the economic condition of the PPTBs and referred them to private health care facilities that perhaps gave them higher kick-backs. Lesser technical skills of informal providers to elicit proper history and to identify atypical presentations of PPTB [22] are a limitation. Identifying other strategies is an area for future operational research.

Fifth, there were several gaps in diagnostic tests undergone by PPTBs enrolled under the project, especially with respect to X-ray testing, sputum smear microscopy, and CB-NAAT testing. The reasons for these gaps appear to be nonavailability of these tests at the local level and difficulties in accessing these tests at the site of their availability. The project tried to mitigate these problems by establishing sputum collection and transportation systems (for sputum smear microscopy and CB-NAAT tests), identifying X-ray facilities, and linking patients to these facilities. Despite these measures, the gaps remained.

Sixth, the TB detection rate was 12% among all the presumptive TB patients enrolled in this project. This is comparable to the TB positivity under the NTEP [19]. Though this is a significant proportion, we feel that it is an underestimate, given that all persons with presumptive TB did not undergo a full diagnostic evaluation as per the NTEP diagnostic algorithm. Therefore, the true magnitude of TB cases among these PPTB is unknown. Also, as expected, the TB detection rates were higher in certain high-risk groups (persons who were HIV positive, persons with a past history of TB, and those who had a cough of longer duration) as shown in Table 7.

Lastly, anecdotal evidence suggests that there is a lack of trust in the public health system, preference for treatment under the care of private health care providers (despite incurring out-of-pocket expenditure), and the fear that accessing treatment from the public health facilities may affect the confidentiality of the disease similar to what has been reported in other studies [8, 9]. More work needs to be done for addressing these concerns and to help patients access treatment from public health facilities.

The major strength of study is that it was conducted under programmatic settings and reflects reality in the field. The major limitation of this study is the fact that the referral of TB cases by the informal care providers was incentivized and the sustainability of the referrals after the project period is unknown.

To conclude, this project demonstrated that engaging informal health care providers is feasible. Keeping informal providers updated about availability and accessibility of TB services in their areas is of paramount importance, and having robust mechanisms to monitor informal providers will lead to better TB case detection. However, this study also showed that there are several challenges that need to be addressed; the most prominent ones are ensuring completeness in the identification of persons with presumptive TB; ensuring that all persons with presumptive TB undergo complete diagnostic tests as per the NTEP's algorithm; and finally ensuring that all TB patients are treated under the public health system.

Authors' Contributions

SK,SS, SBN, VP, and RD are responsible for the conception of the study. SK, SS and SBN drafted the study protocol. SK, SS, SBN, VP, and RD performed the data collection. SS, SBN, and SK did the data analysis and interpretation. SS, SBN, and SK prepared and finalized the manuscript. SS, SBN, SK, VP, RD, AK, RJ, and VK approved the final manuscript. SBN, SK and SS addressed the reviewers' comments.

Acknowledgments

We would like to acknowledge all the informal providers and patients who were part of this project. We would like to thank all the NTEP programme managers and staff at the state and the districts for their coordination and support. We appreciate the efforts of RIPENED project staff for their dedication and commitment for the implementation of the project.

References

[1] World Health Organization, *Global Tuberculosis Report*, World Health Organization, Switzerland, 2019.

[2] Central TB Division, "National Strategic Plan for Tuberculosis Elimination 2017-2025," in *Directorate General of Health Services, Ministry of Health and Family Welfare*, Government of India, New Delhi, 2017.

[3] World Health Organisation, *The End TB Strategy*, WHO, Geneva, Switzerland, 2015.

[4] S. Deo, P. Jindal, D. Gupta et al., "What would it cost to scale-up private sector engagement efforts for tuberculosis care? Evidence from three pilot programs in India," *PLOS ONE*, vol. 14, no. 6, p. e0214928, 2019.

[5] M. Sudhinaraset, M. Ingram, H. K. Lofthouse, and D. Montagu, "What is the role of informal healthcare providers in developing countries? A systematic review," *PLoS ONE*, vol. 8, no. 2, p. e54978, 2013.

[6] M. Gautham, K. M. Shyamprasad, R. Singh, A. Zachariah, R. Singh, and G. Bloom, "Informal rural healthcare providers in North and South India," *Health Policy and Planning.*, vol. 29, suppl 1, pp. i20–i29, 2014.

[7] S. K. Kapoor, A. V. Raman, K. S. Sachdeva, and S. Satyanarayana, "How Did the TB Patients Reach DOTS Services in Delhi? A Study of Patient Treatment Seeking Behavior," *PLoS ONE*, vol. 7, no. 8, article e42458, 2012.

[8] N. Mistry, S. Rangan, Y. Dholakia, E. Lobo, S. Shah, and A. Patil, "Durations and Delays in Care Seeking, Diagnosis and Treatment Initiation in Uncomplicated Pulmonary Tuberculosis Patients in Mumbai, India," *PLOS ONE*, vol. 11, no. 3, p. e0152287, 2016.

[9] N. Mistry, E. Lobo, S. Shah, S. Rangan, and Y. Dholakia, "Pulmonary tuberculosis in Patna, India: durations, delays, and health care seeking behaviour among patients identified through household surveys," *Journal of epidemiology and global health.*, vol. 7, no. 4, pp. 241–248, 2017.

[10] J. Das, A. Holla, V. Das, M. Mohanan, D. Tabak, and B. Chan, "In urban and rural India, a standardized patient study showed low levels of provider training and huge quality gaps," *Health Affairs.*, vol. 31, no. 12, pp. 2774–2784, 2012.

[11] T. Anand, R. Babu, A. G. Jacob, K. Sagili, and S. S. Chadha, "Enhancing the role of private practitioners in tuberculosis prevention and care activities in India," *Lung India*, vol. 34, no. 6, p. 538, 2017.

[12] Central TB Division M, *Guidance Document on Partnerships*, Central TB Division, Ministry of Health and Family Welfare, Government of India, New Delhi, 2019.

[13] G. Bloom, B. Kanjilal, and D. H. Peters, "Regulating health care markets in China and India," *Health Affairs.*, vol. 27, no. 4, pp. 952–963, 2008.

[14] B. Kaboru, M. Uplekar, and K. Lönnroth, "Engaging informal providers in TB control: what is the potential in the implementation of the WHO stop TB strategy? A discussion paper," *World Health & Population*, vol. 12, no. 4, pp. 5–13, 2011.

[15] P. K. Dewan, S. S. Lal, K. Lonnroth et al., "Improving tuberculosis control through public-private collaboration in India: literature review," *BMJ*, vol. 332, no. 7541, pp. 574–578, 2006.

[16] T. B. Stop, "Partnership TB REACH - Wave 6," June 2020, http://www.stoptb.org/assets/documents/global/awards/tbreach/Wave%206%20Selected%20Projects.pdf.

[17] J. Das, A. Chowdhury, R. Hussam, and A. V. Banerjee, "The impact of training informal health care providers in India: a randomized controlled trial," *Science*, vol. 354, no. 6308, pp. -aaf7384–aaf7384, 2016.

[18] B. M. Prasad, S. S. Chadha, P. Thekkur, S. Nayak, V. S. Rajput, and R. Ranjan, "Is there a difference in treatment outcome of tuberculosis patients: rural healthcare providers versus com-

munity health workers?," *Journal of Family Medicine and Primary Care*, vol. 9, no. 1, pp. 259–263, 2020.

[19] Central TB Division M, *India TB Report*, Central TB Division, Ministry of Health and Family Welfare, Government of India, New Delhi, 2019.

[20] A. Dutta, S. Pattanaik, R. Choudhury et al., "Impact of involvement of non-formal health providers on TB case notification among migrant slum-dwelling populations in Odisha, India," *PLOS ONE*, vol. 13, no. 5, p. e0196067, 2018.

[21] C. T. Sreeramareddy, Z. Z. Qin, S. Satyanarayana, R. Subbaraman, and M. Pai, "Delays in diagnosis and treatment of pulmonary tuberculosis in India: a systematic review," *The International Journal of Tuberculosis and Lung Disease.*, vol. 18, no. 3, pp. 255–266, 2014.

[22] A. Kwan, B. Daniels, V. Saria et al., "Variations in the quality of tuberculosis care in urban India: A cross-sectional, standardized patient study in two cities," *PLoS medicine*, vol. 15, no. 9, p. e1002653, 2018.

23

Tuberculosis Drug Susceptibility, Treatment and Outcomes for Belarusian HIV-Positive Patients with Tuberculosis: Results from a National and International Laboratory

Daria N. Podlekareva,[1] Dorte Bek Folkvardsen,[2] Alena Skrahina,[3] Anna Vassilenko,[4] Aliaksandr Skrahin,[3,4] Henadz Hurevich,[3] Dzmitry Klimuk,[3] Igor Karpov,[4] Jens D. Lundgren,[1] Ole Kirk,[1,5] and Troels Lillebaek[2,6]

[1] *CHIP, Rigshospitalet, University of Copenhagen, Denmark*
[2] *International Reference Laboratory of Mycobacteriology, Statens Serum Institut, Copenhagen, Denmark*
[3] *Republican Scientific and Practical Center for Pulmonology and TB, Minsk, Belarus*
[4] *Belarusian State Medical University, Minsk, Belarus*
[5] *Department of Infectious Diseases, Rigshospitalet, University of Copenhagen, Denmark*
[6] *Global Health Section, Department of Public Health, University of Copenhagen, Denmark*

Correspondence should be addressed to Daria N. Podlekareva; daria.podlekareva@regionh.dk

Academic Editor: Karl Drlica

Background. To cure drug-resistant (DR) tuberculosis (TB), the antituberculous treatment should be guided by *Mycobacterium tuberculosis* drug-susceptibility testing (DST). In this study, we compared conventional DST performed in Minsk, Belarus, a TB DR high-burden country, with extensive geno- and phenotypic analyses performed at the WHO TB Supranational Reference Laboratory in Copenhagen, Denmark, for TB/HIV coinfected patients. Subsequently, DST results were related to treatment regimen and outcome. *Methods.* Thirty TB/HIV coinfected patients from Minsk were included and descriptive statistics applied. *Results.* Based on results from Minsk, 10 (33%) TB/HIV patients had drug-sensitive TB. Two (7%) had isoniazid monoresistant TB, 8 (27%) had multidrug-resistant (MDR) TB, 5 (17%) preextensive drug-resistant (preXDR) TB, and 5 (17%) had extensive drug-resistant (XDR) TB. For the first-line drugs rifampicin and isoniazid, there was DST agreement between Minsk and Copenhagen for 90% patients. For the second-line anti-TB drugs, discrepancies were more pronounced. For 14 (47%) patients, there were disagreements for at least one drug, and 4 (13%) patients were classified as having MDR-TB in Minsk but were classified as having preXDR-TB based on DST results in Copenhagen. Initially, all patients received standard anti-TB treatment with rifampicin, isoniazid, pyrazinamide, and ethambutol. However, this was only suitable for 40% of the patients based on DST. On average, DR-TB patients were changed to 4 (IQR 3-5) active drugs after 1.5 months (IQR 1-2). After treatment adjustment, the treatment duration was 8 months (IQR 2-11). Four (22%) patients with DR-TB received treatment for >18 months. In total, sixteen (53%) patients died during 24 months of follow-up. *Conclusions.* We found high concordance for rifampicin and isoniazid DST between the Minsk and Copenhagen laboratories, whereas discrepancies for second-line drugs were more pronounced. For patients with DR-TB, treatment was often insufficient and relevant adjustments delayed. This example from Minsk, Belarus, underlines two crucial points in the management of DR-TB: the urgent need for implementation of rapid molecular DSTs and availability of second-line drugs in all DR-TB high-burden settings. Carefully designed individualized treatment regimens in accordance with DST patterns will likely improve patients' outcome and reduce transmission with drug-resistant *Mycobacterium tuberculosis* strains.

1. Introduction

Tuberculosis (TB) continues to be a major public health threat, especially due to drug-resistant TB (DR-TB) [1]. Of special concern are the increasing rates of HIV-associated TB and multidrug-resistant TB (MDR-TB) in eastern Europe. In this region, the rates of MDR-TB are among the highest in the world, ranging from 12-40% among new TB cases to 30-70% among previously treated [1, 2]. Belarus holds some of the highest MDR-TB rates in the region (app. 40% and 70% among new and previously treated patients, respectively) [1, 3]. While the first is an indicator of poor infectious control and ongoing *Mycobacterium tuberculosis* (*Mtb*) transmission, the latter indicates inappropriate management where new or additional resistance develops during treatment.

In eastern Europe, the HIV-positive population is particularly vulnerable to TB acquisition due to overlapping risk groups and a generally higher risk of TB disease due to more pronounced immunodeficiency. As a result, the prevalence of coinfection with *Mtb* and HIV is increasing in this region [1, 4, 5].

Diagnosis of TB and determination of drug-susceptibility patterns using conventional culture-based phenotypic methods (i.e., culture on either solid or liquid media) can be time consuming (up to few months), which may compromise timely initiation of active treatment. This is especially problematic in settings with a high prevalence of MDR-TB. Access to rapid DNA-based genotypic drug-susceptibility tests (DST) may allow for rapid adjustment of therapy according to resistance patterns, potentially helping to improve clinical outcomes and reducing complications for the individual patients, as well as helping to reduce transmission with resistant *Mtb* strains in society.

Treatment outcome for TB/HIV patients in eastern Europe, especially those with MDR-TB, is poor, with a reported one-year mortality rate of approximately 30% and higher [6, 7]. Management of MDR-TB, particularly in the context of HIV infection, can be complicated. It is crucial to design individualized drug-regimens based on specific *Mtb* susceptibility patterns as fast as possible. In situations, where susceptibility patterns are not available and patients are treated empirically, there is a high risk of suboptimal treatment regimens with a limited number of active drugs, which may lead to drug resistance [8].

In this study, we explored the management of TB/HIV patients by comparing DST results from the Republican Scientific and Practical Center for Pulmonology and TB, Minsk, Belarus (Minsk), and the WHO TB Supranational Reference Laboratory (Copenhagen) in Copenhagen, Denmark. We aimed then to assess adequacy of used treatment regimens and patients' survival according to the DST patterns. In addition, we compare phenotypic DST results with rapid DNA-based genotypic DST and whole-genome sequencing (WGS) results and describe the genomic epidemiology of the involved *Mtb* strains.

2. Methods

As part of the international prospective TB:HIV cohort study (https://www.chip.dk), consecutive HIV-positive patients from Minsk with TB diagnosis between 01/01/2011 and 31/12/2013 were identified [9]. Demographic and clinical data were collected on standardized case report forms at the date of TB diagnosis (baseline), and at 6, 12, and 24 months thereafter. Specific information on TB treatment was collected, as were the results of locally performed DSTs for *Mtb*. Participants were followed until two years after TB diagnosis, date of death, or loss to follow-up. Ethical approval was obtained in accordance with local rules and legislations.

2.1. Laboratory Methods. For first-line anti-TB drugs, the DST assays used in Minsk were conventional phenotypic methods on solid Löwenstein-Jensen (LJ) media and liquid Mycobacteria Growth Indicator Tube (MGIT) between 2011 and 2013. For the second-line drugs, DST was performed both phenotypically on MGIT and for some patients genotypically by GenoType MTBDR*sl* (Hain Lifescience, Nehren, Germany) (limited availability in 2011-2015).

The *Mtb* cultures on a solid LJ media were stored locally and subsequently shipped to the SRL according to the international regulations for shipment of class III material (Category A material according to the IATA Dangerous Goods Regulations, https://www.iata.org/en/programs/cargo/dgr/), for phenotypic and genotypic DST. In Copenhagen, all strains were subcultured in Dubos before performing DST. Initially, phenotypic DST performed for the four first-line drugs: isoniazid (H), rifampicin (R), ethambutol (E), and pyrazinamide (Z). Only in case of any first-line resistance was DST for second-line drugs performed. These included aminoglycosides (streptomycin (S), amikacin (Am), kanamycin (Km), and capreomycin (Cm)), fluoroquinolones (moxifloxacin (Mfx), ofloxacin (Ofx)), ethionamide (Eto), and linezolid (Lzd). Phenotypic DST was performed on MGIT 960, and all drugs were provided by the manufacturer. The MGIT 960 SIRE kit (Becton Dickinson) contained lyophilized vials with low (critical) and high concentrations for first-line drugs. For 2nd-line drugs, recommended critical concentrations were used [10]. The results were reported as sensitive or resistant by the system. When a "resistant" result was obtained, the vial was checked for purity and verified by retesting.

The genotypic DST was performed by using the line probe assay (LPA) GenoType MTBDR*plus* and *sl* (Hain Lifescience, Nehren, Germany), the latter if any phenotypic resistance to first-line drugs was detected, or if subculture failed to grow. Analysis and interpretation of results were carried out according to manufacturer's instructions (https://www.hain-lifescience.de/en/). Among first-line drugs, resistance to isoniazid and rifampicin was determined by detection of mutations in inhA/katG genes and in rpoB gene of *Mtb* strains, respectively. Among second-line drugs, resistance to fluoroquinolones was determined by mutations in gyrA and gyrB genes; and resistance to aminoglycosides by was determined by detection of mutations in rrs and eis genes [11].

Whole-genome sequencing (WGS) was performed for all *Mtb* culture samples as previously described [12]. The resulting FastQ files were uploaded to PhyResSe, a Phylo-Resistance Search Engine used to search for mutations conferring resistance (https://bioinf.fz-borstel.de/mchips/phyresse/) [13].

In addition to the mutations listed above, WGS allowed for additional genotypic susceptibility testing for the following drugs: ethambutol (by detection of mutations in the embB gene), pyrazinamide (mutations in the pncA and rpsA genes), streptomycin (mutations in rpsL gene), ethionamide (mutations in the mshA and ethA genes), linezolid (mutations in the rplC gene), and para-aminosalicylic acid (PAS) (mutation in thyA). All strains with a coverage > 25x were included. Sequences have been deposited in the European Nucleotide Archive under project accession number PRJEB38234.

2.2. Statistics and Study Definitions. TB/HIV patients from Minsk ($n = 62$) were stratified according to the availability of *Mtb* culture samples, and descriptive statistics were used to compare baseline demographic and clinical characteristics. Further, the group with *Mtb* samples available ($n = 30$) was characterized in detail according to resistance and treatment patterns (Figure 1). DST results reported from Minsk were compared with phenotypic DST, LPA, and WGS performed in Copenhagen.

Patients were grouped according to the following resistance patterns: drug-sensitive (DS) TB, MDR-TB, preXDR-TB, and XDR-TB (Table 1). In Copenhagen, the *Mtb* in samples were considered resistant if resistance was detected in any of the analyses (either phenotypic, LPA, or WGS). Specific treatment patterns were analysed for each patient and included initial anti-TB treatment and any consecutive changes.

3. Results

A total of 62 patients were enrolled from Minsk. Of those, 55 (89%) were *Mtb* culture positive. Samples from 30 patients (55% of all culture positive) were stored locally and sent to Copenhagen (Figure 1). Table 2 presents baseline clinical and demographic characteristics of patients with/without *Mtb* culture samples and shows that these two groups are comparable. The majority of patients in both groups were young males with a history of injected-drug use (IDU), imprisonment, and/or excessive alcohol consumption. Even though the majority of patients were diagnosed with HIV infection several years before TB diagnosis, only a small proportion were on antiretroviral therapy (ART) at time of TB diagnosis, and the majority had low CD4 cell counts (Table 2).

In Copenhagen, 7 of 30 samples (23%) failed to grow. For samples fully susceptible based on phenotypic DST, genotypic DST was not performed, except for WGS, which was performed for all samples but failed for 8 (27%). For samples where phenotypic resistance was detected, or there was no culture growth, an LPA analysis was performed (Flowchart).

3.1. Drug-Susceptibility Test Patterns. DST results, provided by Minsk and Copenhagen, are presented in Tables 3 and 4. DST results for all four first-line drugs from Minsk were available, except for 11 cases, where DST for pyrazinamide was not reported. DST for second-line drugs in Minsk included aminoglycosides (S, Amk/Km, and Cm), fluoroquinolones (Ofx, Lfx), Eto/Pto, Cs, and PAS. DSTs for Mfx and Lzd were not performed in Minsk during the study period, whereas DST for Lfx, Cs, and PAS were not performed in Copenhagen (Table 3).

Good agreement between the two laboratories was observed comparing the results of the phenotypic DST for first-line drugs (Tables 3 and 4): 18 out of 23 cases with available results were identical (78%). Two patients (PIDs 13 and 14) were found to have MDR-TB in Minsk but DS-TB in Copenhagen, and one patient (PID 26) had discrepancies in rifampicin phenotypic testing: resistant in Minsk and sensitive in Copenhagen. Another patient (PID 18) was found to be infected with *Mtb* resistant to ethambutol and pyrazinamide in Minsk and sensitive in Copenhagen, and PID 15 had *Mtb* resistant to ethambutol in Minsk and sensitive in Copenhagen (Table 3).

Among phenotypic DSTs for second-line drugs, discrepancies were noticed for 7 out of 11 *Mtb* samples, where *Mtb* was sensitive for these drugs in Minsk but resistant in Copenhagen. Few other minor discrepancies were observed in DSTs for aminoglycosides (Table 3).

According to the susceptibility patterns obtained from Minsk, *Mtb* strains from 10 (33.3%) patients were classified as fully DS-TB; 2 (6.7%) as isoniazid monoresistant TB; 8 (26.7%) as MDR-TB; 5 (16.7%) as preXDR-TB, and 5 (16.7%) as XDR-TB (Table 4). In Copenhagen, DS-TB was diagnosed in 12 patients (40.0%, $p = 0.79$).

Comparing results from Minsk and Copenhagen laboratories for patients with drug-resistant TB, MDR-TB was found in 8 of 30 (26.7%) vs. 3 of 30 (10.0%), $p = 0.18$; preXDR-TB was found in 5 of 30 (16.7%) vs. 8 of 30 (30.0%), $p = 0.36$; and XDR-TB was found in 5 of 30 (16.7%) vs. 7 of 30 (13.3%), $p = 1.0$, respectively (Table 4).

3.2. TB Treatment Regimens and Survival. Patterns of anti-TB treatment for each patient are presented in Figure 2. Twenty-eight (93%) patients initiated treatment with a standard four-drug first-line regimen (RHZE), and of these, four (14%) had streptomycin added. All patients with DS-TB according to Minsk results ($n = 10$) were treated with standard first-line anti-TB drugs, but for various durations, including prolonged intensive phases of treatment (Figure 2). Median treatment duration for DS-TB was 9.5 months (IQR 7.3-10.0 months). Three patients with DS-TB died: one within the first month of treatment where TB was indicated as the cause of death, and two due to non-TB related causes after completion of anti-TB treatment.

Among the two patients with isoniazid monoresistant TB, 1 died due to TB 3 days after initiation of the RHZES regimen.

Patients with at least MDR-TB ($n = 18$) according to Minsk data switched from the initial first-line to a second-line treatment after a median of 1 month (IQR 1-2 months). Second-line regimens were standardized and included one fluoroquinolone (Ofx or Lfx), one aminoglycoside (mainly Cm, and to a rarer extent, Am), Cs, Eto, and PAS. Pyrazinamide was also commonly used in second-line regimens despite resistance being reported. Second-line regimens contained a median of 6 drugs. However, the median number of active drugs was 4 (IQR 3-5) according to the national DST

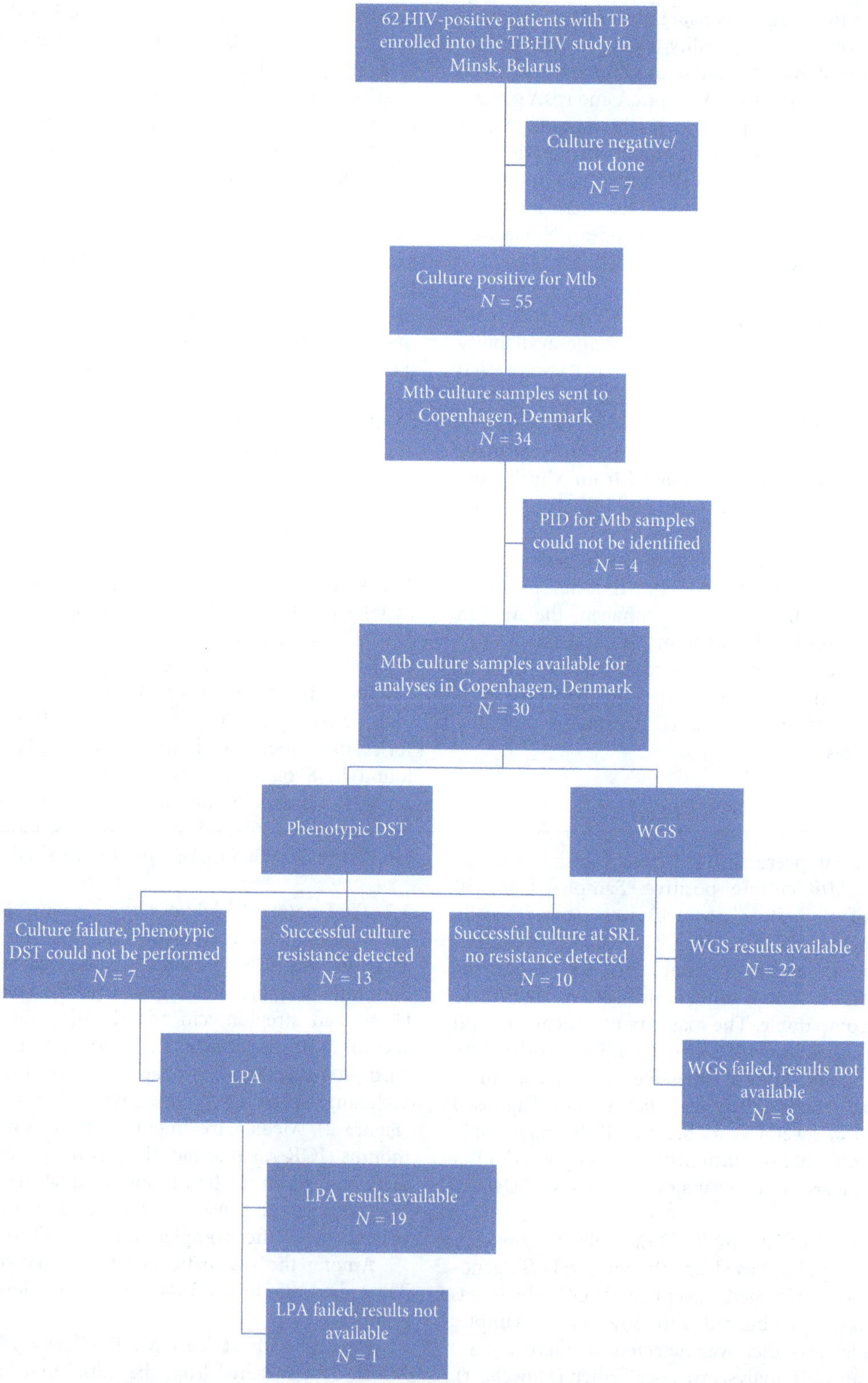

FIGURE 1: Flow chart of TB/HIV patients from Minsk, Belarus, enrolled into the TB : HIV study during 2011-2013, who have *Mycobacterium tuberculosis* (*Mtb*) culture samples available and with various drug susceptibly tests performed on these samples. Abbreviations: DST = drug-susceptibility testing; LPA = line probe assay; WGS = whole-genome sequencing. Patients were enrolled and followed up from the Republican Scientific and Practical Center for Pulmonology and TB, Minsk, Belarus. *Mtb* cultures were sent to the WHO TB Supranational Reference Laboratory, Copenhagen, Denmark, where drug-susceptibility testing was performed using phenotypic, LPA, and WGS methods.

TABLE 1: Definitions for anti-TB drug resistance [29, 30].

Resistance terminology	Definition
Drug-sensitive TB (DS-TB)	*Mtb* sensitive to all first-line anti-TB drugs
Monoresistant TB	*Mtb* resistant to one first-line anti-TB drug only
Drug-resistant TB (DR-TB)	At least MDR-TB, combined terminology for any of the below definitions
Multidrug-resistant TB (MDR-TB)	*Mtb* resistant to at least both isoniazid and rifampicin
Preextensive drug-resistant TB (preXDR-TB)	*Mtb* resistant to isoniazid and rifampicin and either any fluoroquinolone *or* a second-line injectable agent but not both
Extensive drug-resistant TB (XDR-TB)	*Mtb* resistant to isoniazid and rifampicin and to any fluoroquinolone *and* to at least one of three second-line injectable drugs (capreomycin, kanamycin, and amikacin)

Mtb = *Mycobacterium tuberculosis.*

TABLE 2: Baseline characteristics of 62 TB/HIV coinfected patients from Minsk, Belarus, stratified according to availability of *Mycobacterium tuberculosis* (Mtb) culture sample.

Total		Sample yes, *n* (%) 30	Sample no, *n* (%) 32	*p*
Gender	Male, *n* (%)	22 (73)	28 (88)	0.206
Age	Years, median (IQR)	37 (30-41)	35 (32-42)	0.789
TB/HIV risk factors	Ever injecting drug use, *n* (%)	19 (63)	24 (75)	0.319
	History of imprisonment, *n* (%)	5 (17)	12 (38)	0.090
	History of excess alcohol consumption, *n* (%)	19 (63)	15 (47)	0.213
Mtb culture positive	Yes, *n* (%)	30 (100)	25 (78)	0.0015
MDR-TB	Yes, *n* (%)	18 (60)	16 (50)	0.456
TB disease	Disseminated, *n* (%)	12 (40)	6 (19)	0.060
Hepatitis C*	Ever, *n* (%)	24 (80)	23 (72)	0.454
HIV duration prior to TB	Months, median (IQR)	88 (44-136)	67 (25-120)	0.535
Antiretroviral therapy at baseline	Yes, *n* (%)	15 (50)	14 (44)	0.622
CD4 count	Cells/mm^3, median (IQR)	85 (22-171)	126 (57-310)	0.097

Abbreviations: baseline = date of TB diagnosis; IQR = interquartile range; *n* = number; MDR-TB = multidrug-resistant TB; Mtb = *Mycobacterium tuberculosis*; TB = tuberculosis; *Hepatitis C antibody positive.

results, and 3 (IQR 2-4) according to the DST results obtained in Copenhagen. After the first treatment adjustment, 8 patients according to Minsk and 10 patients according to Copenhagen DST results received 3 or less active drugs. Further treatment switches were directed on either exchange drugs within the same drug class (e.g., Ofx to Lfx) or on a reduction in the number of drugs (also a reduction in the number of active drugs) (Figure 2). Median treatment duration with second-line drugs for patients with at least MDR-TB was 12 months (IQR 10-21). Twelve patients (67%) with at least MDR-TB died within 24 months of treatment initiation: 8 (67%) due to TB and 4 (33%) due to some other reasons (Figure 2). For those, who were alive at 24 months ($n = 6$), treatment duration ranged from 10 to 26 months.

3.3. Lineages. Half of the successfully genotyped strains belonged to lineage 2 (Beijing) ($n = 11/22$), and of those, 7 (63%) had at least MDR-TB and 7 died. Among people with other lineages, 4 (36%) had at least MDR-TB and 5 (45%) died. The small numbers did not allow for further analyses.

4. Discussion

Comparing *Mtb* DST between the national laboratory in Minsk, a middle-income MDR-TB high-prevalence setting, and the WHO TB Supranational Reference Laboratory in Copenhagen, we found a good level of concordance for 1st line anti-TB drugs, whereas there was some discordance for second-line drugs. In addition, several issues in the management of TB/HIV patients in Minsk were identified, particularly in the management of patients with DR-TB. In Copenhagen, quality assurance of *Mtb* DST from Minsk included both phenotypic and genotypic tests, namely LPA and WGS. In general, the DST performed in Minsk were reliable and results of phenotypic DSTs for first-line drugs for patients with DS-TB were nearly identical between the two laboratories except for two patients who were reported as having MDR-TB locally, but DS-TB in Copenhagen. For pyrazinamide and ethambutol, phenotypic DST is usually challenging, but DST results for these two drugs were very consistent and similar between laboratories with only few discrepancies [14].

Table 3: Individual results of *Mycobacterium tuberculosis* (Mtb) drug-susceptibility testing performed in two different laboratories (Belarus vs. Denmark) for 30 TB/HIV patients from Minsk, Belarus.

PID	Place of analysis		Isoniazid	Rifampicin	Ethambutol	Pyrazinamide	Streptomycin	Amikacin	Kanamycin	Capreomycin	Moxifloxacin	Ofloxacin	Levofloxacin	E-/prothionamide	Linezolid	Cycloserine	*p*-Amino salicylic acid	Lineage
Drug-sensitive TB																		
1	Minsk		S	S	S		S	S	S	S		S				S	S	
	Copenhagen	Pheno	S	S	S	S												
		LPA																
		WGS	S	S	S	S	S	S	S	S	S	S						Beijing
2	Minsk		S	S	S		R	S	S	S		R		S		S	S	
	Copenhagen	Pheno	S	S	S	S												
		LPA																
		WGS	S	S	S	S	S	S	S	S	S	S						EAS
3	Minsk		S	S	S		S			S		S		S		S	S	
	Copenhagen	Pheno	S	S	S	S												
		LPA																
		WGS	S	S	S	S	S	S	S	S	S	S						Beijing
4	Minsk		S	S	S		S	S	S	S		S		S		S	S	
	Copenhagen	Pheno	S	S	S	S												
		LPA																
		WGS	S	S	S	S	S	S	S	S	S	S						Beijing
5	Minsk		S	S	S	S	S	S	S	S		S		S		S	S	
	Copenhagen	Pheno	S	S	S	S												
		LPA																
		WGS	S	S	S	S	S	S	S	S	S	S						EAS
6	Minsk		S	S	S	S												
	Copenhagen	Pheno	S	S	S	S												
		LPA																
		WGS	S	S	S	S	S	S	S	S	S	S						EAS
7	Minsk		S	S	S	S	S	S	S	S		S		S		S	S	
	Copenhagen	Pheno	S	S	S	S												
		LPA																
		WGS	S	S	S	S	S	S	S	S	S	S						Ural
8	Minsk		S	S	S	S	R	S	S	S		S	S	S		S	S	
	Copenhagen	Pheno	Failed															
		LPA	S	S				S	S	S		S						
		WGS	Failed															
9	Minsk		S	S	S	S		S	S	S			S					
	Copenhagen	Pheno	Failed															
		LPA	S	S				S	S	S	S	S						
		WGS	Failed															
10	Minsk		S	S	S	S	S	S	S	S			S	S		S	S	
	Copenhagen	Pheno	S	S	S	S												
		LPA																
		WGS	S	S	S	S	S	S	S	S	S	S						EAS
Monoresistant TB																		
11	Minsk		R	S	S	S	S	S	S	S		S		S		S	S	
	Copenhagen	Pheno	R	S	S	S	S	S	S	S	S	S		S	S			
		LPA	R	S				S	S	S	S	S						
		WGS	R	S	S	S	S	S	S	S	S	S						Beijing

Table 3: Continued.

PID	Place of analysis		Isoniazid	Rifampicin	Ethambutol	Pyrazinamide	Streptomycin	Amikacin	Kanamycin	Capreomycin	Moxifloxacin	Ofloxacin	Levofloxacin	E-/prothionamide	Linezolid	Cycloserine	p-Amino salicylic acid	Lineage
	Minsk		R	S	S		S	S	S			S						
12	Copenhagen	Pheno	R	S	S	S	S	S	S	S	S	S		S	S			
		LPA	R	S														
		WGS	R	S	S	S	S	S	S	S	S	S						LAM
Multidrug-resistant TB																		
	Minsk		R	R	S		S	S	S									
13	Copenhagen	Pheno	S	S	S	S												
		LPA																
		WGS	S	S	S	S	S	S	S	S	S	S						EAS
	Minsk		R	R	S	S	R	S	S	S			S					
14	Copenhagen	Pheno	S	S	S	S												
		LPA	N/A															
		WGS	Failed															
	Minsk		R	R	R	R	R	S	S	S		S		S		S	S	
15	Copenhagen	Pheno	R	R	S	R	R	S	S	S	S	S		R	S			
		LPA	R	R				S	S	S	S	S						
		WGS	R	R	R	R	R	S	S	S	S	S						Beijing
	Minsk		R	R	R		R	S	S	S			S	S		R	R	
16	Copenhagen	Pheno	R	R	R	R	R	NG										
		LPA	R	R				S	S	S	S	S						
		WGS	R	R	R	S	R	S	S	S	S	S						LAM
	Minsk		R	R	R	R	R	S	S	S		S	S	S		S	S	
17	Copenhagen	Pheno	Failed															
		LPA	R	R				S	S	S	S	S						
		WGS	Failed															
	Minsk		R	R	R	R	R	S	S	S		S		S		S	S	
18	Copenhagen	Pheno	R	R	S	S	R	S	R	S	S	S		R	S			
		LPA	R	R				S	S	S	S	S						
		WGS	R	R	R	S	R	S	S	S	S	S						Beijing
	Minsk		R	R	R		R	S	S	S			S	S		S	S	
19	Copenhagen	Pheno	R	R	R	R	R	S	S	S	S	S		R	S			
		LPA	R	R				R	R	R	S	S						
		WGS	R	R	R	R	R	S	S	S	S	S						LAM
	Minsk		R	R	R	R	R	S	S	S		S		S		S	S	
20	Copenhagen	Pheno	R	R	R	R	R	S	R	S	S	S		R	S			
		LPA	R	R				R	R	R	S	S						
		WGS	R	R	R	R	R	S	S	S	S	S						LAM
Preextensive drug-resistant TB																		
	Minsk		R	R	S	R	R	R	R	R			S	S		R	R	
21	Copenhagen	Pheno	R	R	S	R	R	R	R	R	S	S		S	S			
		LPA	R	R				R	R	R	S	S						
		WGS	Failed															
	Minsk		R	R	S		R	R	R	S		S		S		S	S	
22	Copenhagen	Pheno			Failed													
		LPA	R	R				R	R	R	S	S						
		WGS	Failed															

Table 3: Continued.

PID	Place of analysis		Isoniazid	Rifampicin	Ethambutol	Pyrazinamide	Streptomycin	Amikacin	Kanamycin	Capreomycin	Moxifloxacin	Ofloxacin	Levofloxacin	E-/prothionamide	Linezolid	Cycloserine	*p*-Amino salicylic acid	Lineage
23	Minsk		R	R	R			R	R	S			S	R		R	R	
	Copenhagen	Pheno	Failed															
		LPA	R	NC				R	R	R	S	S						
		WGS	Failed															
24	Minsk		R	R	R		R	S	R	S		S		R		S	R	
	Copenhagen	Pheno	Failed															
		LPA	R	R				R	R	R	S	S						
		WGS	R	R	R	R	R	S	S	S	S	S						LAM
25	Minsk		R	R	R	R	R	S	S	S		R	S	S		S	R	
	Copenhagen	Pheno	R	R	R	R	R	S	R	S	R	R		S	S			
		LPA	R	R				S	S	S	R	R						
		WGS	R	R	R	R	R	S	S	S	R	R						Beijing
Extensive drug-resistant TB																		
26	Minsk		R	R	R	S	R	R	R	R		R		S		S	S	
	Copenhagen	Pheno	R	S	R	S	R	R	R	R	S	S		S	S			
		LPA	R	S				R	R	R	S	S						
		WGS	R	R	R	S	R	R	R	R	S	S						Beijing
27	Minsk		R	R	R	R	R	R	R	R		R		S		S	S	
	Copenhagen	Pheno	R	R	R	R	R	R	R	S	R	R		R	S			
		LPA	R	R				R	R	R	R	R						
		WGS	R	R	R	R	S	R	R	R	R	R						Beijing
28	Minsk		R	R	R	R	R	S	R	S		R	R	R		S	S	
	Copenhagen	Pheno	Failed															
		LPA	R	R				R	R	R	R	R						
		WGS	Failed															
29	Minsk		R	R	R	R	R	R	R			R		S			S	
	Copenhagen	Pheno	R	R	R	R	R	R	R	S	R	R		R	S			
		LPA	R	R				R	R	R	R	R						
		WGS	R	R	R	S	S	R	R	R	R	R						Beijing
30	Minsk		R	R	R	R	R	R	R	R			R	S		S	S	
	Copenhagen	Pheno	R	R	R	R	R	R	R	R	R	R		R	S			
		LPA	R	R				R	R	R	R	R						
		WGS	R	R	R	R	R	R	R	R	R	R						Beijing

Abbreviations: PID = patient's identification number. DST = drug susceptibility testing. LPA = line probe assay. Pheno = phenotypic resistance. R = resistant. S = sensitive. WGS = whole-genome sequencing. Genotypic resistance was determined by detection of mutations in the inhA/katG genes for isoniazid, in the rpoB gene for rifampicin, in the embB gene for ethambutol, and in the pncA gene for pyrazinamide. For second-line drugs, resistance was determined for a drug class by detection of the following mutations: aminoglycosides (amikacin, capreomycin, and kanamycin) in the rrs and eis genes; streptomycin in the rpsL gene; fluoroquinolones (moxifloxacin, levofloxacin, and ofloxacin) in the gyrA and gyrB genes. EAS = Euro-American superlineage, LAM = Latin American-Mediterranean lineage. In Minsk, DST was performed at the Republican Scientific and Practical Center for Pulmonology and TB, Minsk, Belarus. In Copenhagen, DST was performed at the WHO TB Supranational Reference Laboratory, Copenhagen, Denmark. Drug-sensitive TB = *Mtb* sensitive to all first-line anti-TB drugs. Monoresistant TB = *Mtb* resistant to one first-line anti-TB drug only. Multidrug resistant TB = *Mtb* resistant to at least both isoniazid and rifampicin. Preextensive drug resistance = *Mtb* resistant to isoniazid and rifampicin and either to any fluoroquinolone or a second-line injectable agent but not to both. Extensive drug resistance = *Mtb* resistant to isoniazid and rifampicin and to any fluoroquinolone and to at least one of three second-line injectable drugs.

TABLE 4: Type of TB in 30 TB/HIV patients from Minsk according to the DST performed in Belarus and in Denmark, and number of active drugs in treatment regimens.

Type of TB	Minsk* n (%)	Copenhagen** n (%)	*p* value	Number of active drugs initially, median (range)		Number of active drugs after 1st change of treatment regimen, median (range)	
				RSPCPT	SRL	RSPCPT	SRL
DS TB	10 (33,3)	12 (40.0)	0.79	4 (4-4)	4 (4-4)	2 (2-3)	2 (2-3)
Isoniazid-resistant TB	2 (6.7)	2 (6.6)	1.00	4 (3-4)	4 (3-4)	5 (4-5)	5 (4-5)
MDR-TB	8 (26.7)	3 (10.0)	0.18	0 (0-5)	0 (0-0)	5 (1-5)	4 (1-5)
preXDR-TB	5 (16.7)	9 (30.0)	0.36	1 (0-1)	1 (0-1)	4 (1-5)	3 (1-4)
XDR-TB	5 (16.7)	4 (13.3)	1.00	0 (0-1)	0 (0-1)	3 (2-3)	3 (1-4)

In Minsk, drug-susceptibility testing (DST) was performed at the Republican Scientific and Practical Center for Pulmonology and TB, Minsk, Belarus. In Copenhagen, DST was performed at the WHO TB Supranational Reference Laboratory, Copenhagen, Denmark. DST = drug-susceptibility test. DS TB = drug-sensitive TB; *Mycobacterium tuberculosis* sensitive to all first-line anti-TB drugs. MDR-TB = multidrug-resistant TB; *Mycobacterium tuberculosis* resistant to both isoniazid and rifampicin. preXDR-TB = preextensive drug-resistant TB; Mycobacterium tuberculosis resistant to isoniazid and rifampicin and either to any fluoroquinolone or a second-line injectable agent but not to both. XDR-TB = extensive drug resistance; *Mycobacterium tuberculosis* resistant to isoniazid and rifampicin and to any fluoroquinolone and to at least one of three second-line injectable drugs. *As reported. **According to the results of combined phenotypic DST, line probe assay (LPA), and whole-genome sequencing (WGS). In case of discrepancies, the worst result was considered.

All patients with DS-TB were treated with four first-line drugs during intensive phase, followed by 2-3 drugs in the continuation phase, generally in concordance with local guidelines recommending longer treatment duration in case of HIV coinfection at that time.

At the time of data collection, phenotypic DST for the main second-line drugs (fluoroquinolones and aminoglycosides) was available and was performed for all 30 patients in Minsk. Although phenotypic DST for second-line drugs was not performed in Copenhagen for patients with DS-TB, DST results from Minsk were very consistent with WGS results in Copenhagen. The discrepancies in resistance patterns for second-line drugs were therefore observed among patients with DR-TB, but these also included discrepancies between phenotypic, LPA, and WGS internally within the Copenhagen laboratory. This discrepancy between different methods in Copenhagen was primarily, but not exclusively, observed for aminoglycosides. While LPA, and to some extent WGS, predominately include well-documented mutations, there might be less known mutations that are expressed phenotypically, but not yet captured by the genetic analyses. In addition, novel mutations continue to arise or are discovered/described.

In our study, the majority of patients with DR-TB spent at least one month on empirical RHZE-containing treatment prior to switching to a second-line regimen. Despite DST availability for both first- and second-line drugs, all patients with DR-TB received standard second-line treatment, including those with (pre)XDR. Thus, treatment was suboptimal for many patients with (pre)XDR-TB. Using Copenhagen results, patients with DR-TB received a smaller number of active drugs. Although the number of drugs was sufficient for some patients (i.e., 4 drugs), the regimens seemed to be weak in their effectiveness, and availability of early DST results could potentially have allowed avoidance of ineffective and more toxic drugs [15]. Another important observation is that despite of DST patterns becoming available during treatment, patients were not switched to a more effective regimen. This could reflect reduced drug availability at the time of study and may have subsequently improved [16, 17]. Bedaquiline, for example, was not available at the time of the study, but it is now.

At the time of data collection, the recommended treatment duration for MDR-TB was 18-24 months [18]. The median duration of treatment of MDR-TB in our study was difficult to assess, as the majority of patients died while on treatment. More recently, shorter treatment durations have become a possibility for some patients with MDR-TB only, which underlines the importance of rapid DSTs for second-line drugs to rule out (pre)XDR-TB [19, 20].

DST is essential in the management of TB patients in settings with a high prevalence of DR-TB. Ideally, DST should be performed prior to initiation of TB therapy, especially in patients with a previous history of TB or known exposure for DR-TB, to guide clinical management. The use of rapid molecular assays reduces the time for drug resistance diagnostic to just a few days, and may help not only to guide treatment but also to control the ongoing TB transmission. This is of particular importance in settings with a high prevalence of MDR-TB, where rapid DST for second-line drugs can help to exclude resistance and allow for treatment adjustments.

In a few cases, we observed a discrepancy between the phenotypic and genotypic resistance patterns. This is a phenomenon, which has been described previously and underlines the need for both methods at present [14, 21]. This is because not all molecular mechanisms of drug resistance are known, and new genes conferring resistance are continuously being described [12, 22, 23]. On the other hand, several studies have documented that some clinically relevant resistance mutations could be overlooked in phenotypic DSTs [21, 24]. Thus, while rapid molecular DSTs for *Mtb* is now paramount in TB diagnostics, especially in settings with high prevalence of DR-TB, phenotypic DST still plays an important role in the management of TB, especially for second-line and new drugs.

PID	Type of TB according to DST in Minsk	Type of TB according to DST in Copenhagen	Initial treatment: Duration of treatment and drugs used	Initial treatment: Number of active drugs Minsk (Copenhagen)	Treatment changes and duration: Duration of treatment and drugs used	Treatment changes and duration: Number of active drugs Minsk (Copenhagen)	Vital status at 24 months after TB treatment initiation
Drug-sensitive (DS) TB							
1	DS	DS	4 R, H, Z, E	4 (4)	6 R, H, E	3 (3)	Alive
2	DS	DS	9 R, H, Z, E	4 (4)	2 R, H	2 (2)	Alive
3	DS	DS	1 R, H, Z, E	4 (4)			Death due to TB
4	DS	DS	4 R, H, Z, E	4 (4)	7 R, H	2 (2)	Alive
5	DS	DS	5 R, H, Z, E	4 (4)	4 R, H	2 (2)	Alive
6	DS	DS	4 R, H, Z, E	4 (4)	6 R, H	2 (2)	Death due to non-TB AIDS
7	DS	DS	3 R, H, Z, E	4 (4)	5 R, H 2-months break 11 Z, Lfx, Amk, Cs, Eto, PAS	2 (2) 5 (5)	Alive
8	DS	DS	2 R, H, Z, E	4 (4)	5 R, H	2 (2)	Alive
9	DS	DS	3 R, H, Z, E	4 (4)	7 R, H, E	3 (3)	Alive
10	DS	DS	3 R, H, Z, E	4 (4)	3 R,H	2 (2)	Death due to malignancy
Monoresistant TB							
11	H-res	H-res	R, H, Z, E, S	4 (4)			Death due to TB
12	H-res	H-res	1 R, H, Z, E	3 (3)	4 R, Z, E, Ofx, Amk 4-months break 11 R, Z, E, Ofx	5 (5) 4 (4)	Alive
Multidrug-resistent (MDR) TB							
13	MDR	DS	1 R, H, E	1 (3)			Death due to alcohol intoxication
14	MDR	DS	1 R, H, Z, E	2 (4)			Death due to TB
15	MDR	MDR	1 R, H, Z, E, S	0 (0)	3 Z, Ofx, Cm, Cs, Eto, PAS 5 Ofx, Amk, Cs, Eto, PAS	5 (4) 4 (5)	Death due to TB
16	MDR	MDR	2 R, H, Z, E	0 (0)	3 Z, Lfx, Cm, Cs, Eto, PAS	3 (3)	Death due to TB
17	MDR	MDR	2 R, H, Z, E	0 (0)	14 Z, Lfx, Cm, Cs, Eto, PAS 12 Z, Lfx, Cs, Eto, PAS	5 (5) 4 (4)	Alive
18	MDR	preXDR	2 Z, Lfx, Cm, Cs, Eto, PAS	5 (5)			Death due to TB
19	MDR	preXDR	2 R, H, Z, E	0 (0)	1 Z, Lfx, Cm, Cs, Eto, PAS 9 Z, Lfx, Amk, Cs, Eto, PAS	5 (3) 5 (3)	Alive
20	MDR	preXDR	1 R, H, Z, E	0 (0)	11 Z, Lfx, Cm, Cs, Eto, PAS 11 Z, Lfx, Cs, Eto, PAS	5 (3) 4 (3)	Alive
PID	Type of TB according to DST in Minsk	Type of TB according to DST in Copenhagen	Initial treatment: Duration of treatment and drugs used	Initial treatment: Number of active drugs Minsk (Copenhagen)	Treatment changes and duration: Duration of treatment and drugs used	Treatment changes and duration: Number of active drugs Minsk (Copenhagen)	Vital status at 24 months after TB treatment initiation
Preextensive drug-resistant (preXDR) TB							
21	preXDR	preXDR	4 R, H, Z, E, S	1 (1)	3 R, H, Z, E 4-months break 1 R, H, Z, E, S 1 Z, E, Lfx, Amk, Cs, Eto 4-months break 1 Z, E, Lfx, Cm, Cs, Eto, PAS, Amx-Clv 5 Z, Lfx, Cm, Cs, Eto, PAS, Amx-Clv 2 Lfx, Cm, Cs, Eto, PAS, Amx-Clv 10 Lfx, Cs, Eto, PAS, Amx-Clv	1 (1) 1 (1) 3 (3) 3 (3) 2 (2) 2 (2) 2 (2)	Alive
22	preXDR	preXDR	1 R, H, Z, E, S	1 (1)	1 Ofx, Cm, Cs, Eto, PAS 8 E, Lfx, Amk, Cs, Eto 2 E, Lfx, Cs, Eto	5 (4) 4 (4) 4 (4)	Death due to TB
23	preXDR	preXDR	2 R, H, Z, E	1 (1)	3 Z, Lfx, Cm, Cs, Eto, PAS 6-months break 8 Z, Lfx, Amk, Cs, Eto, PAS	3 (2) 2 (2)	Death due to unknown reason
24	preXDR	preXDR	1 R, H, Z, E	0 (0)			Death due to HCV
25	preXDR	XDR	1 R, H, Z, E	0 (0)	9 Z, Lfx, Cm, Cs, Eto, PAS 2 E, Lfx, Cm, Cs, PAS 3 E, Lfx, Cs, PAS	4 (3) 3 (2) 2 (1)	Death due to unknown reason
Extensive drug-resistant (XDR) TB							
26	XDR	preXDR	2 R, H, Z, E	1 (1)	1 Ofx, Amk, Cs, Eto, PAS 8 Lfx, Cm, Cs, Eto, PAS, Amx-Clv 2 Z,Lfx, Cs, Eto, Amx-Clv	3 (4) 4 (4) 4 (4)	Alive
27	XDR	XDR	1 R, H, Z, E	0 (0)	2 Z, E, Ofx, Cm, Cs, Eto, PAS 6 Ofx, Cm, Cs, Eto, PAS, Amx-Clv 4-months break 4 Z, Lfx, Cm, Cs, Eto, clarithromycin	3 (2) 3 (2) 2 (1)	Death due to TB
28	XDR	XDR	2 R, H, Z, E	0 (0)	2 Mfx, Cm, Cs, Eto, PAS, Amx-Clv	2 (3)	Death due to TB
29	XDR	XDR	3 R, H, Z, E	0 (0)	10 Z, Lfx, Cm, Cs, Eto, PAS 16 Z, Lfx, Amk, Cs, Eto	3 (2) 2 (1)	Alive
30	XDR	XDR	1 R, H, Z, E	0 (0)	12 Z, Lfx, Cm, Cs, Eto, PAS, Amx-Clv 7 MXF, Cm, Cs, Eto, PAS, Amx-Clv	3 (2) 3 (2)	Death due to TB

FIGURE 2: Individual TB treatment patterns and vital status at 24 months after TB diagnosis for 30 TB/HIV patients from Minsk, Belarus according to the results of *Mycobacterium tuberculosis* (*Mtb*) drug-susceptibility testing performed at two different laboratories (Belarus vs. Denmark). Abbreviations: Am = amikacin; Amx-Clv = amoxicillin-clavulanic acid; Cm = capreomycin; Cs = cycloserine; E = ethambutol; Eto = ethionamide; H = isoniazid; Km = kanamycin; Lfx = levofloxacin; Lzd = linezolid; Mfx = moxifloxacin; Ofx = ofloxacin; PAS = *p*-aminosalicylic acid; Pto = prothionamide; R = rifampicin; S = streptomycin; Z = pyrazinamide; PID = patient's identification number. In Minsk, DST was performed at the Republican Scientific and Practical Center for Pulmonology and TB, Minsk, Belarus. In Copenhagen, DST was performed at the WHO TB Supranational Reference Laboratory, Copenhagen, Denmark. Number in front of drug combination means number of months the drug combination was used. A drug was included in the analysis, if it was used for >15 days. Green = *Mtb* was sensitive to a drug. Red = *Mtb* was resistant to a drug. Orange = *Mtb* was sensitive to a drug by DST analysis in Minsk and resistant in Copenhagen. Blue = *Mtb* was resistant by DST analysis in Minsk and sensitive in Copenhagen. In case of discrepancies between phenotypic and genotypic tests within laboratory in Copenhagen, the worst result (i.e. resistance) was considered. DS = Drug sensitive TB; *Mtb* sensitive to all first-line anti-TB drugs. Mono-resistant TB = *Mtb* resistant to one first-line anti-TB drug only. MDR-TB = multidrug resistant TB; *Mtb* resistant to at least both isoniazid and rifampicin. preXDR-TB = preextensive drug resistance; *Mtb* resistant to isoniazid and rifampicin and either to any fluoroquinolone or a second-line injectable agent but not to both. XDR-TB = extensive drug resistance; *Mtb* resistant to isoniazid and rifampicin and to any fluoroquinolone and to at least one of three second-line injectable drugs.

Patients in our study initiated their TB treatment between 2011 and 2013. At that time, WHO guidelines already recommended rapid molecular DSTs, such as GeneXpert and LPA, to determine susceptibility for rifampicin and isoniazid prior to treatment initiation [18]. However, this was not yet implemented in Minsk. Currently, WHO recommends GeneXpert as the primary diagnostic tool, and if rifampicin resistance is detected, LPA for second-line drugs should be performed.

In recent years, new molecular methods applicable directly on primary specimens have become available. For example, we now have FlouroType MTBDR (Hain Lifescience, Nehren, Germany) and Deeplex Myc-TB (GenoScreen, Lille, France). These may help to further reduce the time until targeted personalized treatment can be initiated [25].

Half of the *Mtb* strains successfully genotyped in our study were of the Beijing spoligotype, a lineage 2 strain (11/22), which is in accordance with previous results from Minsk [26]. It has been speculated that some lineages, including linage 2, may be more virulent than others [27]. As none of the study strains were identical, we saw no indications of recent *Mtb* transmission between patients (data not shown).

Regarding study limitations, the sample size was small resulting in limited statistical power. However, our data on the prevalence of MDR-TB is representative for Belarus (and Minsk), where the prevalence of MDR-TB is approximately 40% [1]. In addition, all patients in the study were TB/HIV coinfected; thus, it was not possible to assess the influence of HIV on *Mtb* transmission and development of resistance. It is also worth to noting that MDR-TB treatment guidelines in Belarus have recently been revised, and they are now recommending oral regimens and avoidance of the most toxic drugs, particularly aminoglycosides. Further, new drugs (e.g., linezolid, clofazimine, bedaquiline, and delamanid) have now become available in Belarus.

To the best of our knowledge, this is the first study providing detailed description of anti-TB treatment for individual TB patients according to *Mtb* drug resistance patterns. It is a good example for TB clinicians elsewhere on the importance of rapid DSTs and concordance between resistance patterns and timely prescribed adequate anti-TB treatment. Overall, outcomes of patients with DR-TB are known to be poor, with a success rate of approximately 50-60% [1, 5]. Studies have shown that treatment success improves essentially when adequate treatment regimens (in terms of efficacy and number of effective drugs) are used [28].

In conclusion, we found some discordances between phenotypic DST results in Belarus and an international reference laboratory in Copenhagen. This was especially true for second-line drugs, compromising early identification and initiation of individualized treatment of patients with DR-TB. Our results advocate for wide implementation and validation of rapid DSTs in all DR-TB high-burden areas with simultaneous wide availability of drugs for the treatment of drug-resistant TB. Future studies are encouraged to follow-up on resistance and treatment patterns, drugs tolerability, and patient outcomes.

Consent

Written informed consent was obtained as per local regulations.

Authors' Contributions

DNP, DBF, OK, TL, and JDL developed the study concept and design, had full access to all the data in the study, and took responsibility for the integrity of the data and the accuracy of the data analysis. DNP and DBF did the statistical analysis and wrote the first draft of the report under the supervision of OK and TL. DBF was responsible for the laboratory part of the project (culturing of *Mtb* and performing DST and WGS). HH and IK were responsible for study performance in Minsk, Belarus. AS, AV, DK, and AS coordinated the study in Minsk, Belarus and collected data. JDL was the study leader and had overall responsibility. All authors interpreted data and critically reviewed and commented on the draft report. All authors have approved the final version of the report. Daria N. Podlekareva and Dorte Bek Folkvardsen shared first authorship and contributed equally to this work. Ole Kirk and Troels Lillebaek shared last authorship and contributed equally to this work.

Acknowledgments

We thank the patients who participated in the study and the staff involved at the participating hospitals in the TB : HIV Study Group. The TB : HIV Study Group in Minsk, Belarus is composed of staff from the Belarusian State Medical University, Department of Infectious Disease (I. Karpov (PI), A. Vassilenko) and the Republican Scientific and Practical Center for Pulmonology and Tuberculosis (A. Skrahina (PI), H. Hurevich, D. Klimuk, A. Skrahin, O. Kondratenko, and A. Zalutskaya). We thank Aase Bengaard Andersen, MD (D.M.Sc), and Joanne Reekie, senior statistician, PhD, for reading the manuscript and providing critical review. This study was funded by the European Union's Seventh Framework Programme for research (FP7/2007–2013), technological development and demonstration under EuroCoord grant agreement number 260694, the Danish Council for Independent Research, the Danish National Research Foundation (grant 126), Augustinus Fonden (Denmark), and the A.P. Moeller Fund (Denmark).

References

[1] WHO, *Global Tuberculosis Report 2020*, World Health Organization, Geneva, 2020, Licence: CC BY-NC-SA 3.0 IGO. https://www.who.int/publications/i/item/9789240013131.

[2] A. Skrahina, H. Hurevich, A. Zalutskaya et al., "Alarming levels of drug-resistant tuberculosis in Belarus: results of a survey in Minsk," *The European Respiratory Journal*, vol. 39, no. 6, pp. 1425–1431, 2012.

[3] A. Skrahina, H. Hurevich, A. Zalutskaya et al., "Multidrug-resistant tuberculosis in Belarus: the size of the problem and associated risk factors," *Bulletin of the World Health Organization*, vol. 91, no. 1, pp. 36–45, 2013.

[4] J. DeHovitz, A. Uuskula, and N. El-Bassel, "The HIV epidemic in Eastern Europe and Central Asia," *Current HIV/AIDS Reports*, vol. 11, no. 2, pp. 168–176, 2014.

[5] European Centre for Disease Prevention and Control/WHO Regional Office for Europe, *Tuberculosis Surveillance and Monitoring in Europe 2020–2018 Data*, ECDC, Stockholm, 2020, https://www.ecdc.europa.eu/sites/default/files/documents/TB-Surveillance-report_24March2020.pdf.

[6] D. N. Podlekareva, A. M. Efsen, A. Schultze et al., "Tuberculosis-related mortality in people living with HIV in Europe and Latin America: an international cohort study," *The Lancet HIV*, vol. 3, no. 3, pp. e120–e131, 2016.

[7] A. Khaliaukin, A. M. Kumar, A. Skrahina et al., "Poor treatment outcomes among multidrug-resistant tuberculosis patients in Gomel Region, Republic of Belarus," *Public Health Action*, vol. 4, no. 2, pp. 24–28, 2014.

[8] A. M. W. Efsen, A. Schultze, R. F. Miller et al., "Management of MDR-TB in HIV co-infected patients in Eastern Europe: results from the TB:HIV study," *The Journal of Infection*, vol. 76, no. 1, pp. 44–54, 2018.

[9] A. M. Efsen, A. Schultze, F. Post et al., "Major challenges in clinical management of TB/HIV co-infected patients in Eastern Europe compared with Western Europe and Latin America," *Journal of the International AIDS Society*, vol. 17, 4, Supplement 3, p. 19505, 2014.

[10] WHO, *Technical Report on Critical Concentrations for Drug Susceptibility Testing of Medicines Used in the Treatment of Drug-Resistant Tuberculosis*, World Health Organization, Geneva, 2018, (WHO/CDS/TB/2018.5). Licence: CC BY-NC-SA 3.0 IGO.

[11] D. Hillemann, S. Rusch-Gerdes, and E. Richter, "Feasibility of the GenoType MTBDRsl assay for fluoroquinolone, amikacin-capreomycin, and ethambutol resistance testing of *Mycobacterium tuberculosis* strains and clinical specimens," *Journal of Clinical Microbiology*, vol. 47, no. 6, pp. 1767–1772, 2009.

[12] D. B. Folkvardsen, A. Norman, A. B. Andersen, E. M. Rasmussen, T. Lillebaek, and L. Jelsbak, "A major *Mycobacterium tuberculosis* outbreak caused by one specific genotype in a low-incidence country: exploring gene profile virulence explanations," *Scientific Reports*, vol. 8, no. 1, p. 11869, 2018.

[13] S. Feuerriegel, V. Schleusener, P. Beckert et al., "PhyResSE: a web tool delineating mycobacterium tuberculosis antibiotic resistance and lineage from whole-genome sequencing data," *Journal of Clinical Microbiology*, vol. 53, no. 6, pp. 1908–1914, 2015.

[14] J. Heyckendorf, S. Andres, C. U. Köser et al., "What is resistance? Impact of phenotypic versus molecular drug resistance testing on therapy for multi- and extensively drug-resistant tuberculosis," *Antimicrobial Agents and Chemotherapy*, vol. 62, no. 2, 2018.

[15] A. Van Deun, T. Decroo, A. Piubello, B. C. de Jong, L. Lynen, and H. L. Rieder, "Principles for constructing a tuberculosis treatment regimen: the role and definition of core and companion drugs," *The International Journal of Tuberculosis and Lung Disease*, vol. 22, no. 3, pp. 239–245, 2018.

[16] M. Mansfeld, A. Skrahina, L. Shepherd et al., "Major differences in organization and availability of health care and medicines for HIV/TB coinfected patients across Europe," *HIV Medicine*, vol. 16, no. 9, pp. 544–552, 2015.

[17] A. Bentzon, V. Mitsura, E. Borodulina et al., "Health care delivery for HIV-positive people with tuberculosis in Europe," in *17th European AIDS Conference in Basel*, Switzerland, 2019Abstract PE1/3. 2019.

[18] World Health Organization, *Guidelines for the Programmatic Management of Drug-Resistant Tuberculosis—2011 Update*, WHO, 2011.

[19] K. J. M. Aung, A. Van Deun, E. Declercq et al., "Successful "9-month Bangladesh regimen" for multidrug-resistant tuberculosis among over 500 consecutive patients," *The International Journal of Tuberculosis and Lung Disease*, vol. 18, no. 10, pp. 1180–1187, 2014.

[20] A. J. Nunn, P. P. J. Phillips, S. K. Meredith et al., "A trial of a shorter regimen for rifampin-resistant tuberculosis," *The New England Journal of Medicine*, vol. 380, no. 13, pp. 1201–1213, 2019.

[21] D. B. Folkvardsen, V. O. Thomsen, L. Rigouts et al., "Rifampin heteroresistance in *Mycobacterium tuberculosis* cultures as detected by phenotypic and genotypic drug susceptibility test methods," *Journal of Clinical Microbiology*, vol. 51, no. 12, pp. 4220–4222, 2013.

[22] M. R. Farhat, R. Sultana, O. Iartchouk et al., "Genetic determinants of drug resistance in *Mycobacterium tuberculosis* and their diagnostic value," *American Journal of Respiratory and Critical Care Medicine*, vol. 194, no. 5, pp. 621–630, 2016.

[23] T. M. Walker, M. Merker, T. A. Kohl, D. W. Crook, S. Niemann, and T. E. Peto, "Whole genome sequencing for M/XDR tuberculosis surveillance and for resistance testing," *Clinical Microbiology and Infection*, vol. 23, no. 3, pp. 161–166, 2017.

[24] L. Rigouts, M. Gumusboga, W. B. de Rijk et al., "Rifampin resistance missed in automated liquid culture system for *Mycobacterium tuberculosis* isolates with specific rpoB mutations," *Journal of Clinical Microbiology*, vol. 51, no. 8, pp. 2641–2645, 2013.

[25] D. Hillemann, C. Haasis, S. Andres, T. Behn, and K. Kranzer, "Validation of the FluoroType MTBDR assay for detection of rifampin and isoniazid resistance in *Mycobacterium tuberculosis* complex isolates," *Journal of Clinical Microbiology*, vol. 56, no. 6, p. e00072, 2018.

[26] K. R. Wollenberg, C. A. Desjardins, A. Zalutskaya et al., "Whole-genome sequencing of mycobacterium tuberculosis provides insight into the evolution and genetic composition of drug-resistant tuberculosis in Belarus," *Journal of Clinical Microbiology*, vol. 55, no. 2, pp. 457–469, 2017.

[27] M. Coscolla and S. Gagneux, "Does _M. tuberculosis_ genomic diversity explain disease diversity?," *Drug Discovery Today: Disease Mechanisms*, vol. 7, no. 1, pp. e43–e59, 2010.

[28] S. D. Ahuja, D. Ashkin, M. Avendano et al., "Multidrug resistant pulmonary tuberculosis treatment regimens and patient outcomes: an individual patient data meta-analysis of 9,153 patients," *PLoS Medicine*, vol. 9, no. 8, article e1001300, 2012.

[29] WHO, *Definitions and Reporting Framework for Tuberculosis—2013 Revision*, WHO Library Cataloguing-in-Publication Data, 2013.

[30] WHO, *Consolidated Guidelines on Drug-Resistant Tuberculosis Treatment*, World Health Organization, Geneva, 2019, Licence: CC BY-NC-SA 3.0 IGO.

Comparison of Interferon-Gamma Release Assay and Tuberculin Skin Test for the Screening of Latent Tuberculosis in Inflammatory Bowel Disease Patients: Indian Scenario

Alok Kumar Mantri,[1] Priti Meena,[2] Amarender Singh Puri,[1] Ajay Kumar,[1] Sanjeev Sachdeva,[1] Siddharth Srivastava,[1] K. Arivarasan,[3] and Shivakumar Varakanahali[4]

[1]*Department of Gastroenterology, G. B. Pant Institute of Postgraduate Medical Education and Research (GIPMER), New Delhi, India*
[2]*Institute of Renal Science, Sir Gangaram Hospital, New Delhi, India*
[3]*Kauvery Hospital Trichy, Tennur, India*
[4]*Narayana Multispeciality Hospital, HSR Layout, Bangalore, India*

Correspondence should be addressed to Priti Meena; pritimn@gmail.com

Academic Editor: Jos R. Lapa e Silva

Background. In a country like India, where the prevalence of tuberculosis is very high, the role of screening tools for detection of latent tuberculosis infection (LTBI) like TST and IGRA is still unclear, especially in inflammatory bowel disease (IBD) patients. Our study is aimed at comparing the interferon-gamma release assay (IGRA) and tuberculin skin test (TST) to determine the prevalence of LTBI in IBD patients in the Indian subset of the population. *Methods.* It was a prospective observational analysis. A total of 257 participants were included in the study. Both TST and IGRA were performed in consecutive patients diagnosed with IBD (131 patients) and in 126 healthy individuals. Both tests were performed on the same day. LTBI diagnosis was considered if any one of TST or IGRA was found to be positive. *Results.* Out of 131 IBD patients, 121 patients had ulcerative colitis and 10 patients had Crohn's disease. 29% of the IBD patients and 22% of the control subjects had LTBI. The study demonstrated concordance between TST and IGRA. Agreement test kappa value for IBD patients was 0.656 (CI 0.50-0.81), with a p value of <0.001, suggestive of a fair agreement. Mean IFN-γ release was lower in the immunosuppressed group as compared to non-immunosuppressed individuals (0.26 ± 0.17 vs. 0.45 ± 0.07, $p = 0.02$). Cohen's kappa coefficient values in IBD cases and control subjects were 0.66 and 0.79, respectively. TST was found to be negatively correlated to BMI. *Conclusion.* Agreement between TST and IGRA was fair in IBD patients. For LTBI screening in IBD patients, TST and IGRA are complementary methods.

1. Introduction

Inflammatory bowel disease (IBD) currently represents a substantial economic burden affecting nearly 4 million people worldwide [1]. Crohn's disease (CD) and ulcerative colitis (UC) are the most common idiopathic IBD [2]. The mainstay of treatment includes anti-inflammatory agents, immunosuppressive drugs, and antitumor necrosis factor (anti-TNF) therapy [3]. While biologicals have been shown to improve prognosis, increased utilization and earlier administration of these therapies have led to a growing concern about the risk of opportunistic infections. Of particular concern is the potential reactivation of latent tuberculosis infection (LTBI), which in this clinical scenario often presents in an aggressive and disseminated fashion. LTBI is defined as a state of persistent bacterial viability, immune control, and no evidence of clinically manifested active tuberculosis (TB) [4, 5]. Currently, it is not possible to directly diagnose LTBI in humans.

So, the diagnosis of LTBI is based on information gathered from the medical history, tuberculin skin test (TST) or interferon-gamma release assay (IGRA) result, chest radiograph, physical examination, and in certain circumstances, sputum examinations. Although several studies assessed performances of IGRA and TST in western populations, there is very limited data in populations with high background rates of TB and bacille Calmette-Guerin (BCG) vaccination. In a country like India, where the prevalence per lakh for tuberculosis is as high as 230 and the prevalence of LTBI is nearly 50%, the role of TST and IGRA is still unclear, especially in IBD patients [6, 7]. Our study is aimed at comparing the interferon-gamma release assay and tuberculin skin test to determine the prevalence of latent tuberculosis in inflammatory bowel disease patients in the Indian subset of patients.

2. Material and Methods

The study was conducted in the Department of Gastroenterology, Maulana Azad Medical College and Associated G.B. Pant Hospital, New Delhi, which is one of the largest tertiary care centers located in north India, catering to a huge population from several neighboring states. It was a prospective observational analysis. The study was approved by the ethical committee of the institute. Informed consent was taken from all the patients and controls after the nature and possible consequences of the study were explained before enrollment in the study. A total of 257 patients were included in the study. One hundred thirty-one consecutive patients with diagnosed inflammatory bowel disease attending the outpatient department (opd) or admitted to the wards were enrolled, and a control group of one hundred twenty-six healthy controls was also included in the study. Most of the controls recruited were healthy relatives of IBS (irritable bowel syndrome) and IBD patients. Patients age 18 to 70 years old were included in the study. Patients with active tuberculosis, any history of diagnosed tuberculosis, and chest radiograph suggestive of old or active tuberculosis were excluded from the study.

Detailed history regarding the course and treatment of all the patients was recorded. History of flare-ups, extraintestinal manifestations, the presence of familial IBD, and smoking habits had been collected in a uniform format. Previous and concomitant medical therapy (steroid and/or immunosuppressive, or biological therapy) was registered. Clinical activity in CD was defined by Crohn's Disease Activity Index (CDAI) and in UC by a Clinical/partial Mayo Score (CMS). A patient was considered to be under an immunosuppressive therapy if any of the following criteria were fulfilled: intake of steroids for a period equal or superior to two weeks; intake of thiopurines, methotrexate, or cyclosporine for a period equal or superior to 2 months; prescription of anti-TNF-α; and intake of any two or three immunosuppressors associated with or in the absence of a concomitant anti-TNF-α prescription. Patients' medical history was screened for predefined TB risk factors including active malignant diseases, active hematological or oncological diseases, disease phenotype, duration of immunosuppressive therapy, number of immunosuppressive therapies, contact person in the daily life of the patient, workplace risk for infection, and previous TB infection. We also recorded the presence of a BCG scar as a sign of BCG vaccination.

Table 1: Various demographic and clinical characteristics of IBD patients.

Patient characteristics	Ulcerative colitis	Crohn's disease
n	**121**	**10**
Male/female	**70/51**	**2/8**
Age (mean ± SD)	**36.5 ± 12.6**	**29.8 ± 8.4**
BMI (kg/m^2) (mean ± SD)	**22.2 ± 4.4**	**23.5 ± 2.8**
Duration (months) mean ± SD)	**46.6 ± 24**	**36.8 ± 16**
Disease extent		
E1	**15 (12.4%)**	
E2	**32 (26.4%)**	
E3	**74 (61.2%)**	
Clinical Mayo Score (mean ± SD)	**4.3 ± 2.5**	
Disease location		
L1		**2**
L2		**1**
L3		**7**
L4		—
CDAI (med/range)		**276 (126-420)**
Immunosuppression	**89/121 (73.6%)**	**10/10**
Steroid	**89**	**2**
AZA	**56**	**10**
IFX	**38**	**6**
ADA	**1**	
Smoking	**37/121 (30.6%)**	**0**
BCG scar	**30/121 (25%)**	**0**
TST+ve	**33/121 (27.2%)**	**1/10**
IGRA+ve	**25/121 (20.7%)**	**1/10**
IGRA (test-nil) (mean ± SD)	**0.30 ± 0.1**	**0.23 ± 0.1**
TST MM (mean ± SD)	**5.9 ± 3.1**	**4.1 ± 2.3**

Blood samples for IGRA were collected during routine laboratory testing on the same day when TST was performed. Prior to the tests, written informed consent was taken from all participants. Whole-blood interferon-γ (IFN-γ) release assay (QuantiFERON-TB Gold in tubes, Cellestis, Carnegie, Australia) based on specific peptides ESAT-6, CFP-10, and TB7.7 was performed and evaluated according to the manufacturer's recommendations [8, 9]. Standard TST was performed by Tuberculin PPD RT23 SSI (Staten Serum Institute, Denmark), which consists of an intradermal injection of tuberculin RT23 purified protein derivative (PPD) in 0.1 ml solution for injection into the inner surface of the forearm. A positive Mantoux reaction was defined with a predefined cut-off rate as a skin induration diameter at 72 hours after a skin test. A TST reaction of ≥10 mm of induration was considered positive. In special circumstances, a TST reaction of ≥5 mm of induration was considered positive like (a)

Table 2: Comparison between IBD group and control subjects.

	IBD patients ($n = 131$)	Control group ($n = 126$)	p value (IBD vs. control)
Age, mean (SD)	**36.0 (12.5)**	**45.9 (9.6)**	**0.001**
SEX (male) n (%)	**72 (55%)**	**82 (65%)**	NS
BMI (kg/m^2) (SD)	**22.3 (4.3)**	**24.8 (3.4)**	**0.001**
BCG scar, n (%)	**30 (23%)**	**39 (31%)**	NS
Smoking, n (%)	**37 (28%)**	**30 (55%)**	NS
QFT test-nil (SD)	**0.3 (0.4)**	**0.3 (0.4)**	**0.06**
TST in mm (SD)	**5.9 (1.6)**	**5.8 (1.6)**	NS
HB (SD)	**10.5 (2.3)**	**14.4 (8.9)**	**0.001**
TLC (SD)	**8187.9 (2980.3)**	**8469.0 (1780.2)**	NS
Platelet (SD)	**280612 (114245)**	**275493 (114163)**	NS
Total protein gm/l (SD)	**6.8 (1.0)**	**7.6 (0.6)**	**0.001**
Albumin gm/l (SD)	**3.7 (2.7)**	**4.4 (0.4)**	**0.01**

Table 3: Distribution of QFT-GIT and TST in IBD cases and controls.

QFT-GIT in IBD cases and controls		Frequency	Percent	p value (χ^2 test)
IBD patients	Positive	**26**	**19.8%**	**0.60**
	Negative	**99**	**75.6%**	
	Indeterminate	**6**	**4.6%**	
Control subjects	Positive	**22**	**17.5%**	
	Negative	**99**	**78.6%**	
	Indeterminate	**5**	**4%**	
TST in IBD cases and controls				
IBD patients	Positive	**34**	**26%**	**0.31**
	Negative	**97**	**74%**	
Control subjects	Positive	**26**	**20.6%**	
	Negative	**100**	**79.4%**	

patients with immunosuppression (including patients taking the equivalent of ≥15 mg/day of prednisone for 1 month or more or those taking TNF-α antagonists), (b) human immunodeficiency virus- (HIV-) infected persons, (c) recent contacts of a person with infectious TB disease, and (d) administration and measurement of the tuberculin skin test [5, 10].

2.1. Data Analysis. Categorical variables were described through absolute and relative frequencies, and continuous variables were described through the mean and standard deviation, or median and interquartile range (IQR), whenever appropriate. The prevalence of LTBIs was estimated with 95% confidence intervals (CIs) using QFT and TST. The concordance between these two tests was evaluated using the kappa (κ) statistic. The κ statistics were interpreted as follows: $\kappa > 0.75$ was considered to indicate excellent agreement, $\kappa < 0.40$ to indicate poor agreement, and κ between 0.40 and 0.75 to indicate fair to good agreement. Multivariate linear regression was used to compare groups to control confounding. To know the dependence, Pearson's correlation was calculated. All the reported p values were two-sided, and p values of <0.05 were considered statistically significant. The sample size was calculated using the latent TB prevalence of 40% with population correction, which showed the requirement of 120 subjects required in each group. All data were arranged, processed, and analyzed with SPSS v.23 (Statistical Package for Social Sciences).

3. Results

The study has recruited a total of 257 subjects including 131 IBD patients and 126 healthy controls. Table 1 shows various demographic and clinical characteristics of the IBD patients. Among the IBD patients, most of the patients were in the age group of 18-40 years. The mean ages of the IBD patients and healthy controls included were 36.03 years (SD ± 12.5) and 46 years (SD ± 9.6), respectively. The majority of the study subjects were males, 65.1% in the IBD group and 55% in the control group. Out of the 131 IBD patients, 121 patients had ulcerative colitis and 10 patients had Crohn's disease. In the IBD patients, mean duration of illness of IBD was 46 ± 25 months. 23% in the IBD patient group and 31% in the control group had a BCG scar. Out of the 121 included UC patients, most patients (61.2%) had pancolitis (Montreal extent E3). According to the Clinical Mayo Score, at the time of evaluation, 31% of the ulcerative colitis patients had severe

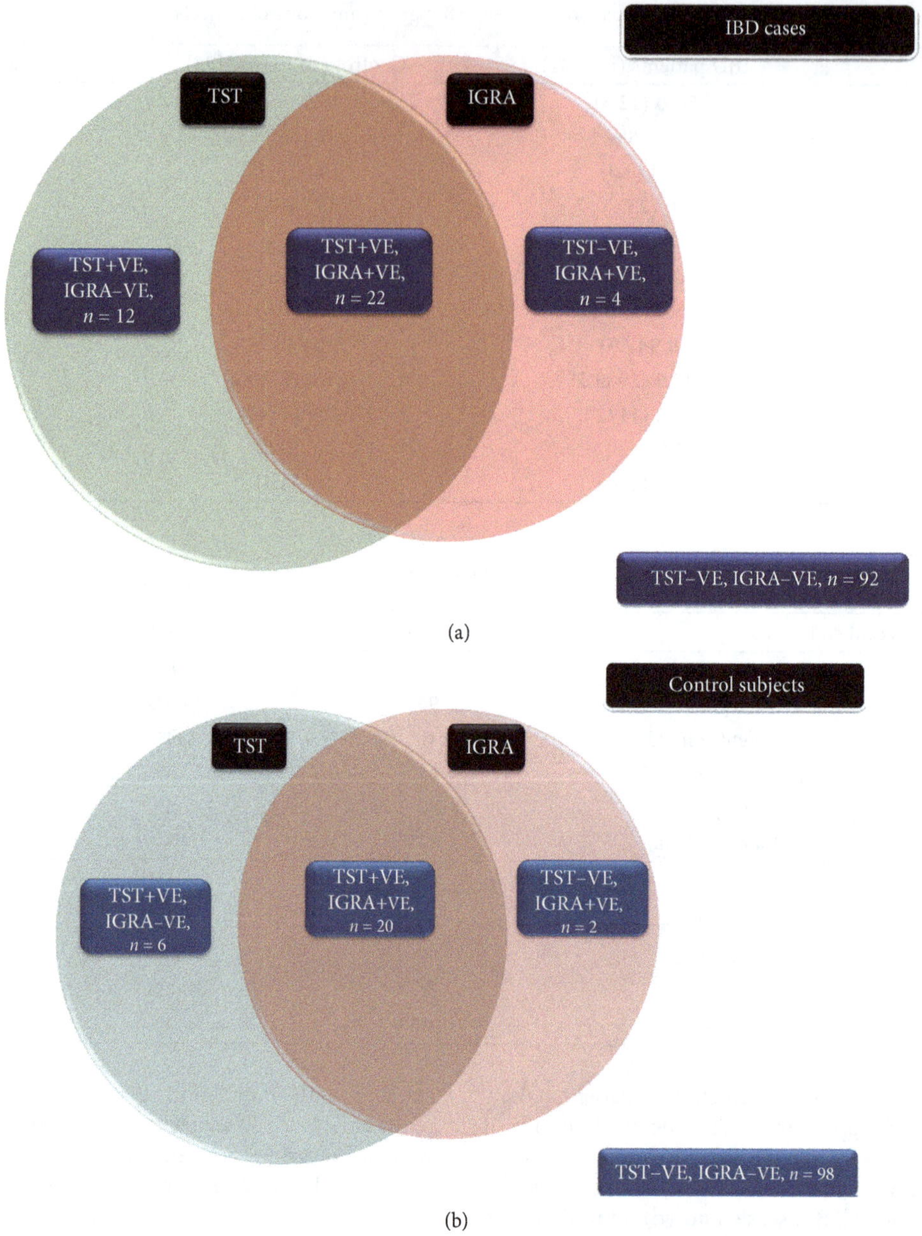

FIGURE 1: (a) Venn diagram shows the distribution of LTBI among IBD patients. (b) Venn diagram shows the distribution of LTBI among control subjects.

activity. Most of the parameters were comparable between the two groups (see Table 2); however, IBD patients had low hemoglobin and body mass index (BMI) as compared to control subjects.

3.1. Latent Tuberculosis Screening. LTBI diagnosis was considered if any one of TST or IGRA was found to be positive. Out of a total of 257 participants, 66 (25.7%) were detected to have LTBI. 38 (29%) of the IBD patients and 28 (22%) of the control subjects had LTBI. The distribution of QFT-GIT and TST in IBD cases and controls is shown in Table 3 and Figures 1(a) and 1(b). Mean TST in IBD patients was 5.9 (± 1.6); in IBD patients with positive TST, mean TST was -5.9 (±1.8), whereas it was 5.8 mm (±1.6) in control subjects (p value = NS) (Figure 2).

In BCG-vaccinated IBD patients, the TST and IGRA positivity rates were 22.4% and 18.7%, respectively, whereas the positivity rates were 19% and 16%, respectively, in healthy controls.

3.2. Agreement between TST and IGRA. We found that Cohen's kappa coefficient in IBD cases and control subjects was 0.66 and 0.79, respectively, which is indicative of a fair agreement (see Table 4 and Figure 3). Agreement test kappa

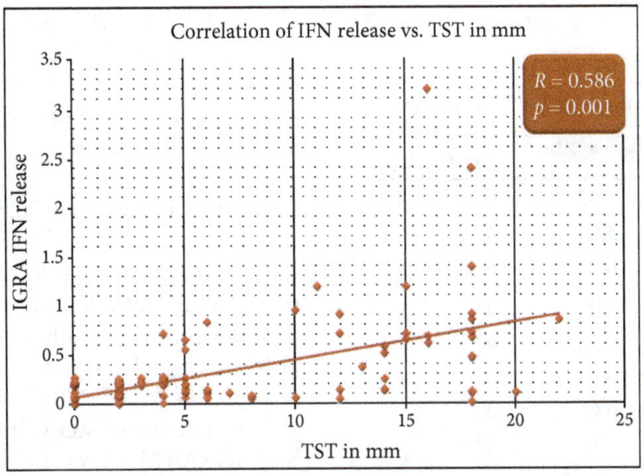

FIGURE 2: Correlation of IGRA: IFN release and TST measured in mm.

TABLE 4: Pearson's correlation of TST and IGRA.

		QFT test-nil	TST (mm)	BMI (kg/m^2)	Age	Albumin	HB
QFT test-nil	Pearson's correlation	—	**0.55**	-0.03	0.16	-0.05	0.15
	p value	—	**0.001**	0.71	0.08	0.58	0.09
TST in mm	Pearson's correlation	**0.55**	—	**-0.34**	-0.06	-0.06	0.13
	p value	**0.00**	—	**0.001**	0.51	0.49	0.13

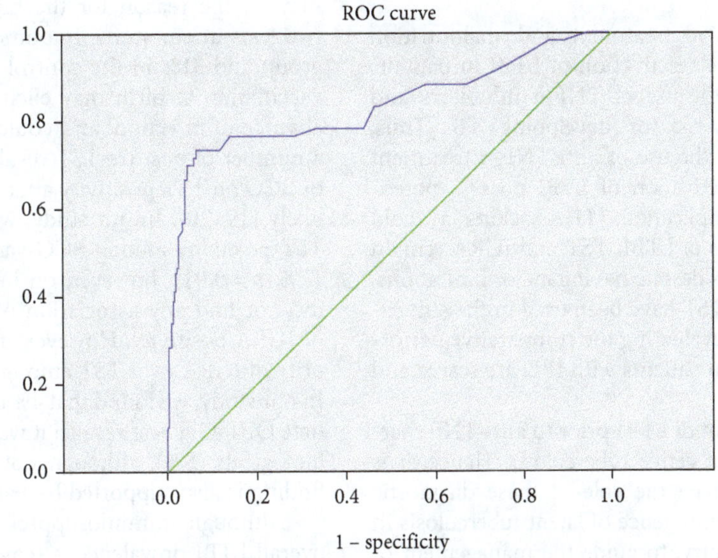

FIGURE 3: ROC curve for TST in mm with IGRA positivity.

value for IBD patients was 0.656 (CI 0.50-0.81), with a *p* value of <0.001. Analysis suggested that TST and IGRA were concordant tests. TST was found to be negatively correlated to BMI. Table 5 shows logistic regression for factors affecting IGRA and TST positivity. Binary logistic regression showed that smoking and TST predict IGRA positivity.

Effect of immunosuppressive agents and biological use on both TST and IGRA results were evaluated (see Tables 6(a) and 6(b)). There was no statistically significant difference concerning the mean TST values between the two groups. Quantitative IFN-γ release was assessed by quantity of IFN − γ test tube − nil tube and compared between two groups of IBD according to immunosuppression and biological use (Table 6). It was found that the mean IFN-γ released by the immunosuppressed group was significantly lower than that of the patients who were not immunosuppressed. We found that the mean IFN-γ released by a group of patients on biologicals was less than that of patients not on biologicals, although the difference was not statistically significant. Figures 4(a) and 4(b) show the comparison of IFN-γ release according to immunosuppression use and biological use, respectively.

TABLE 5: Logistic regression for factors affecting IGRA and TST positivity.

Logistic regression for factors affecting IGRA positivity				
	p value	ODD's ratio	95% C.I. for OR Lower	Upper
Age (years)	0.63	1.02	0.93	1.12
Sex (male)	0.16	2.33	0.71	7.67
BCG vaccination	0.53	0.65	0.16	2.54
Smoker (yes)	0.001	0.06	0.01	0.34
BMI (kg/m^2)	0.68	0.97	0.86	1.11
TST (mm)	0.001	0.68	0.61	0.75
Immunosuppression	0.94	0.92	0.11	7.72
Biological treatment	0.87	1.18	0.15	9.40
Age (yrs)	0.77	0.98	0.85	1.13
Sex (male)	0.40	0.48	0.09	2.67
BCG vaccination	0.08	7.56	0.82	70.14
Smoker (yes)	0.19	4.59	0.47	45.11
BMI (kg/m^2)	0.02	0.78	0.63	0.95
Immunosuppression	0.46	4.69	0.08	2.55
Biological treatment	0.21	12.41	0.25	6.20

4. Discussion

requent immunosuppressive treatment and malnutrition increase the chances of the reactivation of LTBI in patients with IBD. In particular, the use of TNF-α inhibitors and biologicals increases the risk of developing TB. Thus, screening for LTBI before the use of anti-TNF-α treatment is necessary since the reactivation of LTBI poses a potentially life-threatening complication [11]. Lacking a "gold standard" for the diagnosis of LTBI, TST and IGRA remain the primary screening tools despite having major limitations. An innovative IGRA and TST have been used in the surveillance of LTBI, but studies evaluating the comparative performance of TST and IGRA in patients with IBD are scarce and limited [12].

Detection and treatment of LTBI prior to anti-TNF therapy decrease the chance of active tuberculosis. Hence, it is equally important to evaluate the role of these diagnostic methods according to the prevalence of latent tuberculosis in a particular region or country, to guide the management of LTBI before immunosuppressive therapy. In our study, we compared these diagnostic methods in a large patient cohort and controls in a country with a high incidence of both latent and active tuberculosis. In our study, 257 subjects were analyzed including 131 IBD patients (121 were diagnosed with ulcerative colitis and 10 were diagnosed with Crohn's disease) and 126 healthy controls. Due to the lower prevalence rate of CD in India, our study had a lesser number of CD patients compared to other studies [13, 14]. As per the European Crohn's and Colitis Organisation (ECCO) guidelines for the management of opportunistic infections in IBD [11], LTBI diagnosis was considered if any one of TST or IGRA is found to be positive. According to these criteria, in our study, 66 (25.7%) of 257 participants were found to have LTBI. 38 (29%) of the 131 IBD patients and 28 (22%) among the 126 control subjects had LTBI. Studies by other authors have shown a prevalence rate between 15 and 24% [15]. Table 7 shows a comparison of various studies on the prevalence of LTBI in IBD patients.

No significant difference in LTBI was found between IBD cases and controls ($p = 0.23$). A previous study from India showed a prevalence of LTBI in 31% of healthy individuals. Joshi et al. showed that 51% of healthcare workers had LTBI, which could be explained by the higher exposure to infection in India [6, 7]. A study from South Korea which included only healthy adults, not an at-risk population, found only a 15% prevalence of LTBI [16].

In the current study, TST positivity was slightly higher than IGRA (23.3% vs. 19%). We found that the use of biologicals was associated with lower TST positivity (34% vs. 14%, $p = 0.02$); we did not find any significant difference in TST positivity among the immunosuppressed and non-immunosuppressed groups ($p = 0.34$). This may be explained by the defective T-cell function in patients on biologicals, a result that is supported by other studies with a similar conclusion [17, 18]. Our study demonstrated a fair agreement between TST and IGRA (kappa 0.656, 90.2% overall agreement). We found that agreement between both tests was similar between cases and controls and was not affected by immunosuppression status. The higher prevalence of LTBI may be the reason for the higher agreement between the two tests in our study. In our study, 23% in the IBD patient group and 31% in the control group had a BCG scar. BCG vaccination at birth may elicit a positive TST result in the absence of infection, and could therefore be responsible for a number of positive TST results. However, a relevant effect of BCG on TST positivity after a period of 15-20 years is less likely [19, 20]. In our study, we found that there was more TST positivity among BCG-vaccinated individuals (34% vs. 17%, $p = 0.01$); however, on logistic regression analysis, we did not find any association of BCG vaccination with TST or IGRA positivity. However, our study supports the superiority of IGRA over TST among BCG-vaccinated individuals. In our study, we found that 4% of participants had indeterminate QFT-GIT test results; it was higher among patients with biologicals (8%), although not statistically significant. This finding is also supported by Papay et al. [21].

Although immunosuppression was not found to affect overall LTBI prevalence, a major finding in our study is the negative impact of immunosuppressive therapy on the TST results and total IFN-γ released. Mean IFN-γ release was lower in the immunosuppressed group as compared to non-immunosuppressed individuals (0.26 ± 0.17 vs. 0.45 ± 0.07, $p = 0.02$). This is consistent with findings from a recent meta-analysis and other studies from Europe [21–24]. IGRA relies on the cell-mediated immunity to produce interferon-γ after stimulation with TB antigens; hence, any condition that alters the T-cell immunity may have an impact on the IGRA results. Immunosuppressive drugs may reduce the interferon-γ released by T cells, resulting in a reduced rate of positive result [28].

Our study is the first study from India to evaluate the prevalence of LTBI among IBD patients. Furthermore, the

TABLE 6

(a) Comparison of TST according to immunosuppression and biological use

	Immunosuppression	TST according to immunosuppression n	Mean ± SD (mm)	p value (independent sample unpaired t-test)
TST	Yes	**99**	**5.8 ± 1.34**	**0.08**
	No	**32**	**5.8 ± 1.5**	
IFN-γ release according to biological use				
TST	Yes	**38**	**5.6 ± 1.2**	**0.07**
	No	**93**	**5.8 ± 1.4**	

(b) Comparison of IFN-γ release according to immunosuppression and biological use

	Immunosuppression	IFN-γ release according to immunosuppression n	Mean ± SD	p value (independent sample unpaired t-test)
QFT-GIT (test-nil tube)	Yes	**99**	**0.26 ± 0.17**	**0.02**
	No	**32**	**0.45 ± 0.07**	
IFN-γ release according to biological use				
QFT-GIT (test-nil tube)	Yes	**38**	**0.23 ± 0.13**	**0.06**
	No	**93**	**0.34 ± 0.07**	

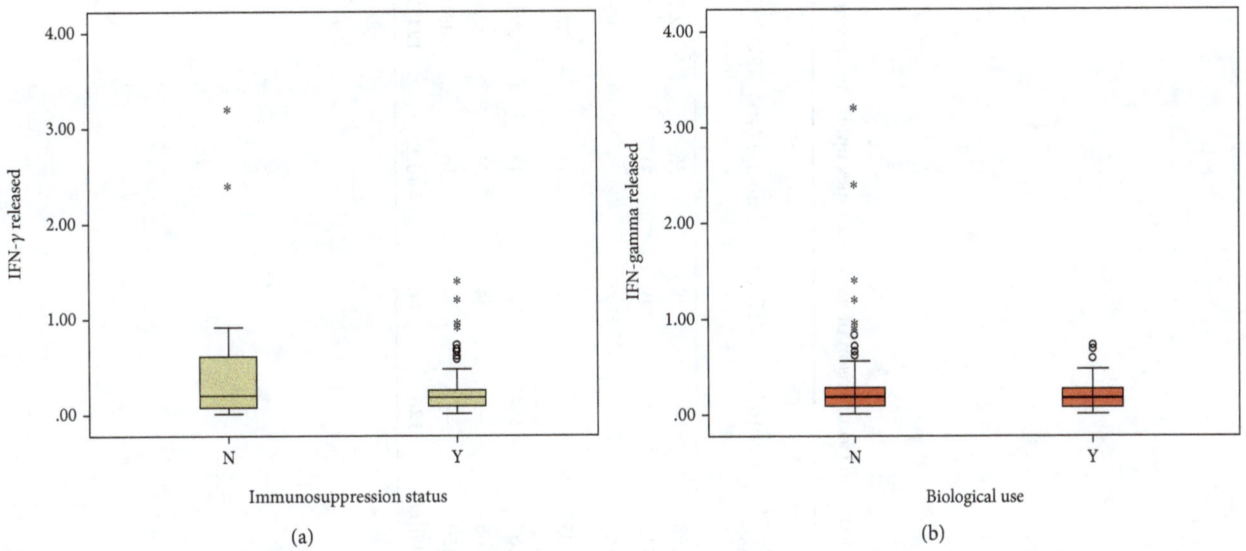

FIGURE 4: (a) Box plot comparing IFN-γ release according to immunosuppression. (b) Comparison of IFN-γ release according to biological use.

study included a well-matched control population to ascertain factors affecting the result of testing for LTBI. A well-characterized and diverse study population, with a fairly large sample size, and the measurement of TST and IGRA using a standardized technique are the strengths of our study. However, there are certain limitations in our study: (1) the study was not designed to follow the patients with latent TB for the development of active tuberculosis; [2] the inexistence of a gold standard reference test to diagnose LTBI, which would enable the identification of false positive and false negative results; and [3] we did not repeat the tests with negative results.

5. Conclusion

Our study is one of the few studies from a country like India where tuberculosis is highly prevalent that is aimed at evaluating the actual prevalence of LTBI among IBD patients and healthy controls. The study shows a prevalence of 25.7% of latent TB infection in IBD patients which is not significantly different from the control group. There was a fair agreement between TST and IGRA (91%, kappa value = 0.66). Although immunosuppression was not found to affect overall LTBI prevalence, it has a negative impact on the TST results and total IFN-γ released.

Table 7: Comparison of various studies upon the prevalence of LTBI in IBD patients.

Study	Country	No. of patients (n)	Control (n)	Male (%)	Mean age (yrs)	IBD UC/CD	BCG (%)	TST+ve (%)	IGRA +ve (%)	IGRA method	Indeterminant IGRA (%)	Kappa (κ) concordance/ agreement TST/IGRA
Papay et al., 2011 [21]	Austria	208	—	49	36	152/56	—	12.5	7.2	QFT-GIT	7.7	0.21
Schoepfer et al., 2008 [12]	Switzerland	212	44	49	31	44/114	70	18	8.3	QFT-GIT	3	0.029
Andrisani et al., 2013 [15]	Italy	92	50	39.6		60/32	—	15.2	14.1	QFT-TST	0.9	0.51
Arias-Guillen et al., 2014 [25]	Spain	205	—	50	44	157/48	—	26.8	7.8	QFT-GIT, TSPOT	8.4	0.34
Wong et al., 2014 [20]	China	268	234	160	43	128/136	95	9.9	20.6	QFT-GIT	4	0.19
Kurti et al., 2015 [26]	Hungary	166	—	54	24	122/44	—	21	8.4	QFT-GIT	0.6	0.41
Abreu et al., 2016 [27]	Portugal	250	—	44	36	81/19	—	23	10	QFT-GIT	2.2	0.22
Our study	India	**131***IBD*	**126**	**60**	**40.1**	**121/10**	**26**	**23.3**	**18.9**	*QFT-GIT*	**4.3**	**0.66**

Screening of latent TB before the commencement of immunosuppressive therapy particularly in IBD patients pre-anti-TNF-α therapy is suggested. TST and IGRA tests are complementary methods.

Authors' Contributions

The authors have contributed in the conception, study design, acquisition of data, analysis and interpretation of data, and drafting of the manuscript.

References

[1] A. P. Yu, L. A. Cabanilla, E. Q. Wu, P. M. Mulani, and J. Chao, "The costs of Crohn's disease in the United States and other Western countries: a systematic review," *Current Medical Research and Opinion*, vol. 24, no. 2, pp. 319–328, 2008.

[2] M. D. Kappelman, S. L. Rifas-Shiman, K. Kleinman et al., "The Prevalence and Geographic Distribution of Crohn's Disease and Ulcerative Colitis in the United States," *Clinical Gastroenterology and Hepatology*, vol. 5, no. 12, pp. 1424–1429, 2007.

[3] C. Mowat, A. Cole, A. Windsor et al., "Guidelines for the management of inflammatory bowel disease in adults," *Gut*, vol. 60, no. 5, pp. 571–607, 2011.

[4] H. Getahun, A. Matteelli, R. E. Chaisson, and M. Raviglione, "Latent *Mycobacterium tuberculosis* infection," *The New England Journal of Medicine*, vol. 372, no. 22, pp. 2127–2135, 2015.

[5] U. Mack, G. B. Migliori, M. Sester et al., "LTBI: latent tuberculosis infection or lasting immune responses to *M. tuberculosis*? A TBNET consensus statement," *The European Respiratory Journal*, vol. 33, no. 5, pp. 956–973, 2009.

[6] K. B. Gupta, "Challenges in diagnosis and treatment of latent tuberculosis infection," *The Indian Journal of Tuberculosis*, vol. 59, no. 1, pp. 1–5, 2012.

[7] R. Joshi, U. Narang, A. Zwerling et al., "Predictive value of latent tuberculosis tests in Indian healthcare workers: a cohort study," *The European Respiratory Journal*, vol. 38, no. 6, pp. 1475–1477, 2011.

[8] M. Pai, L. W. Riley, and J. M. Colford Jr., "Interferon-γ assays in the immunodiagnosis of tuberculosis: a systematic review," *The Lancet Infectious Diseases*, vol. 4, no. 12, pp. 761–776, 2004.

[9] A. Lalvani and M. Pareek, "Determinaciones de la liberacion de interferon gamma: principios y practica," *Enfermedades Infecciosas y Microbiología Clínica*, vol. 28, no. 4, pp. 245–252, 2010.

[10] D. P. de León, E. Acevedo-Vásquez, A. Sánchez-Torres et al., "Attenuated response to purified protein derivative in patients with rheumatoid arthritis: study in a population with a high prevalence of tuberculosis," *Annals of the Rheumatic Diseases*, vol. 64, no. 9, pp. 1360-1361, 2005.

[11] J. F. Rahier, S. Ben-Horin, Y. Chowers et al., "European evidence-based consensus on the prevention, diagnosis and management of opportunistic infections in inflammatory bowel disease," *Journal of Crohn's & Colitis*, vol. 3, no. 2, pp. 47–91, 2009.

[12] A. M. Schoepfer, B. Flogerzi, S. Fallegger et al., "Comparison of interferon-gamma release assay versus tuberculin skin test for tuberculosis screening in inflammatory bowel disease," *The American Journal of Gastroenterology*, vol. 103, no. 11, pp. 2799–2806, 2008.

[13] A. N. Ananthakrishnan, "Epidemiology and risk factors for IBD," *Nature Reviews. Gastroenterology & Hepatology*, vol. 12, no. 4, pp. 205–217, 2015.

[14] A. K. Jain, S. Sircar, M. Jain, S. Adkar, and C. Waghmare, "Inflammatory bowel disease in Central India: a single centre experience over five years," *Tropical Doctor*, vol. 42, no. 4, pp. 198-199, 2012.

[15] G. Andrisani, A. Armuzzi, A. Papa et al., "Comparison of Quantiferon-TB Gold versus tuberculin skin test for tuberculosis screening in inflammatory bowel disease patients," *Journal of Gastrointestinal and Liver Diseases*, vol. 22, no. 1, pp. 21–25, 2013.

[16] D. H. Jung, K.-W. Jo, and T. S. Shim, "Prevalence of latent tuberculosis infection among medical students in South Korea," *Tuberculosis and Respiratory Diseases*, vol. 73, no. 4, pp. 219–223, 2012.

[17] M. F. Greaves, "Biological effects of anti-immunoglobulins: evidence for immunoglobulin receptors on "T" and "B" lymphocytes," *Transplantation Reviews*, vol. 5, no. 1, pp. 45–75, 1970.

[18] J. Zuniga, D. Torres-Garcia, T. Santos-Mendoza, T. S. Rodriguez-Reyna, J. Granados, and E. J. Yunis, "Cellular and humoral mechanisms involved in the control of tuberculosis," *Clinical & Developmental Immunology*, vol. 2012, article 193923, 2012.

[19] M. Legesse, G. Ameni, G. Mamo, G. Medhin, G. Bjune, and F. Abebe, "Community-based cross-sectional survey of latent tuberculosis infection in Afar pastoralists, Ethiopia, using QuantiFERON-TB Gold In-Tube and tuberculin skin test," *BMC Infectious Diseases*, vol. 11, no. 1, p. 89, 2011.

[20] S. H. Wong, M. Ip, W. Tang et al., "Performance of interferon-gamma release assay for tuberculosis screening in inflammatory bowel disease patients," *Inflammatory Bowel Diseases*, vol. 20, no. 11, pp. 2067–2072, 2014.

[21] P. Papay, A. Eser, S. Winkler et al., "Predictors of indeterminate IFN-γ release assay in screening for latent TB in inflammatory bowel diseases," *European Journal of Clinical Investigation*, vol. 41, no. 10, pp. 1071–1076, 2011.

[22] T. S. Shim, "Diagnosis and treatment of latent tuberculosis infection in patients with inflammatory bowel diseases due to initiation of anti-tumor necrosis factor therapy," *Intestinal Research*, vol. 12, no. 1, pp. 12–19, 2014.

[23] Y. J. Jung, H. I. Woo, K. Jeon et al., "The significance of sensitive interferon gamma release assays for diagnosis of latent tuberculosis infection in patients receiving tumor necrosis factor-α antagonist therapy," *PLoS One*, vol. 10, no. 10, p. e0141033, 2015.

[24] S. H. Wong, Q. Gao, K. K. Tsoi et al., "Effect of immunosuppressive therapy on interferon γ release assay for latent tuberculosis screening in patients with autoimmune diseases: a systematic review and meta-analysis," *Thorax*, vol. 71, no. 1, pp. 64–72, 2016.

[25] N. N. Andersen and T. Jess, "Risk of infections associated with biological treatment in inflammatory bowel disease," *World Journal of Gastroenterology*, vol. 20, no. 43, pp. 16014–16019, 2014.

[26] Z. Kurti, B. D. Lovasz, K. B. Gecse et al., "Tuberculin skin test and Quantiferon in BCG vaccinated, immunosuppressed patients with moderate- to-severe inflammatory bowel dis-

ease," *Journal of Gastrointestinal and Liver Diseases*, vol. 24, pp. 467–472, 2020.

[27] C. Abreu, F. Magro, J. Santos-Antunes et al., "Tuberculosis in anti-TNF-α treated patients remains a problem in countries with an intermediate incidence: analysis of 25 patients matched with a control population," *Journal of Crohn's & Colitis*, vol. 7, no. 10, pp. e486–e492, 2013.

[28] M. Arias-Guillén, S. Riestra, R. de Francisco et al., "T-cell profiling and the immunodiagnosis of latent tuberculosis infection in patients with inflammatory bowel disease," *Inflammatory Bowel Diseases*, vol. 20, no. 2, pp. 329–338, 2014.

25

Time to Develop and Predictors for Incidence of Tuberculosis among Children Receiving Antiretroviral Therapy

Fassikaw Kebede,[1] Tsehay Kebede,[2] Birhanu Kebede,[3] Abebe Abate,[4] Dube Jara,[4] Belete Negese,[5] and Tamrat Shaweno[6]

[1]*Woldia University, College of Health Science, School of Public Health, Department of Epidemiology & Biostatics, Ethiopia 2021*
[2]*Bahir Dare University, Faculty of Social Science, Department of Geography & Environmental Studies, Ethiopia 2021*
[3]*Pawe Woreda Agriculural Inpute and Production Team Leaders, Metekel Zone, Pawe Woreda, North West, Ethiopia*
[4]*Debre Markos University, College of Medicine and Health Sciences, Department of Public Health 2021, Debre Markose, Ethiopia*
[5]*Debre Birhan University, College of Medicine and Health Sciences, Department of Nursing 2021, Debre Birhan, Ethiopia*
[6]*Jimma University Institute of Health Science, Faculty of Public Health, Department of Epidemiology 2021, Jimma, Ethiopia*

Correspondence should be addressed to Fassikaw Kebede; fassikawk@yahoo.com

Academic Editor: Karl Drlica

Infection by the human immune deficiency virus (HIV) is the strongest risk factor for latent or new infection of tuberculosis (TB) through reduction of CD4 T-lymphocytes and cellular immune function. Almost one-third of deaths among people living with HIV are attributed to tuberculosis. Despite this evidence, in Ethiopia, there is a scarcity of information regarding the incidence of tuberculosis for children living with HIV. Thus, this study assessed time to develop and predictors for incidence of tuberculosis in children attending HIV/AIDS care in public hospitals: North West Ethiopia 2021. *Methods.* A facility-based retrospective cohort study was conducted among 421 seropositive children on antiretroviral therapy in two hospitals between January 1, 2011 and December 31, 2020. EPI-DATA version 3.2 and STATA/14 software were used for data entry and analysis, respectively. Tuberculosis-free survival time was estimated using the Kaplan-Meier survival curve. Bivariate and multivariable Cox regression model was fitted to identify predictors at a P value <0.05 within 95% CI. *Results.* In the final analysis, a total of 421 seropositive children were included, of whom, 64 (15.2%) developed tuberculosis at the time of follow-up. The mean (±SD) age of the children was 10.62 ± 3.32 years, with a median (IQR) time to develop TB that was 23.5 (IQR = ±19) months. This study found that the incidence of tuberculosis was 5.9 (95% CI: 4.7; 7.6) per 100 person-years (PY) risk of observation. Cases at baseline not taking cotrimoxazol preventive therapy (CPT) (AHR = 2.5; 95% CI, 1.4-4.7, $P < 0.021$), being severely stunted (AHR = 2.9: 95% CI, 1.2-7.8, $P < 0.03$), and having low hemoglobin level (AHR = 4.0; 95% CI, 2.1-8.1, $P < 0.001$) were found to be predictors of tuberculosis. *Conclusion.* A higher rate of tuberculosis incidence was reported in our study as compared with previous studies in Ethiopia. Cases at baseline not taking cotrimoxazol preventive therapy (CPT), being severely stunted, and having low hemoglobin (≤10 mg/dl) levels were found to be at higher risk to developed TB incidence.

1. Introduction

The human immune deficiency virus (HIV) is the strongest risk factor for latent or new infection of tuberculosis (TB) through reduction of CD4 T-lymphocytes and cellular immune function [1].

The coinfections of TB/HIV are bidirectional, and the diseases reinforce each other, in that HIV sustains the progression of latent tuberculosis bacilli into active TB, while tuberculosis accelerates the progression of HIV disease to its advanced clinical stage [1, 2]. In 2019, there were an estimated 10.1 million new cases of TB and 1.7 million new deaths, making TB the leading cause of death from a single infectious agent (ranking above HIV/AIDS) [3]. In fact TB is responsible for one–third of TB/HIV-associated deaths for children living with HIV [4, 5]. The burden of this disease is higher in sub-Saharan Africa, where HIV remains a significant problem with inadequate coverage with antiretroviral drugs [6]. Globally, about 36.7 million patients were living with HIV/AIDS, and 2.1 million people became newly infected in 2015. The sub-Saharan Africa countries account for the largest proportion, with 25.6 million people living with HIV [1, 3]. Likewise, in 2018, there were about 251,000 deaths from TB among PLWHIV, which accounts for 33% of total deaths associated with HIV, which is much higher than the case fatality rate expected by WHO, which is ≤5% [1, 7]. Despite different interventions, TB incidence rate in children on ART is high in different settings at different times. Notably, 0.28 per 100 person-years reported in Latin America [8], 1.9 per 100 person-years reported in Zambia [9], 4.0 and 21.1 per 100 person years in South Africa [10], and 17.4 in East Africa [11]. Often in resource-limited settings, estimates of TB in children have been based on extrapolation from adult data [4], but children with TB differ significantly from adult TB patients in their immunological and pathophysiological responses [7].

The Ethiopian Federal HIV and AIDS Prevention and Control Office estimated that the single national HIV/AIDS is among the top ten high burden counties with an incidence rate of 341/100,000 of which 31% of TB patients are living with HIV [5, 7]. Still now, TB/HIV coinfection is the leading cause of death in people living with HIV/AIDS [12]. Although the incidence of TB among adult HIV patients has been exhaustively studied, it is overlooked for HIV-positive children receiving antiretroviral therapy. So, this study was intended to determine the incidence rate and predictors for the time to developed TB among HIV-positive children receiving antiretroviral therapy in North West, Ethiopia 2021.

2. Methods

2.1. Study Design, Area, and Populations. Facility-based retrospective cohort study was employed among 421 seropositive children from 1st January 2011 to December 31/2020 in two (Assosa and Pawe) general hospitals. Both are located in the Benishangul Gumuz region, Northwest of Ethiopia [13]. Apart from other services, these hospitals have been providing ART follow-up care services since 2007. In the hospital, the recorded number of HIV-positive people starting ART care was 2968, of who were 447 HIV-positive children files were there since January 1, 2011 and December 31, 2020 (Figure 1).

2.2. Sample Size Determination and Sampling Techniques. The sample size was calculated by using the formula for survival analysis by [14] considering two-sided significance level ($\alpha = 5\%$), $Z_a/2 = Z$ value at 95%confidence interval = 1.96, power $(Z_B) = 80\%$, and $P = \%$cumulative occurrence of TB incidence, 1.65 HR [15].

$$\text{The final sample size} \quad (n) = \frac{\text{Event}}{P(\text{Event})} = \frac{(Z_{a/2} + Z_B)2}{\theta^2 p(1-p)} = \frac{(za/2 + ZB)}{p(1-p)(\ln\text{HR})2}, \quad \theta = \ln(\text{HR}), \quad \text{HR} = e^{\theta}, \tag{1}$$

where alpha is $(a) = 0.05$, beta is $(\beta) = 0.2$, AHR is the hazard ratio, E is the number of event, and N is the (sample size) $= E/P(E)$, where $P(E)$ = probability of event, and P is the cumulative occurrence of treatment failure using values from reference for sample size calculation from two [16]. The final sample size was determined as 430 after adding 10% contingency for incompleteness. From 1st January 2011 to December 31/2020 in the two general hospitals, 447 children started ART care. We included all without any sampling procedure.

Exclusion criteria: patients taking anti-TB treatment at the time of HIV/AIDS enrolment were excluded from the study.

2.3. Outcome Ascertainment. The new incidence of TB considered as an event of interest, which is defined as the occurrence of TB in HIV-positive children during successive follow-up at any time after enrollment in the pediatrics HIV care clinic. Children who were lost, died, transferred out, or did not develop the events until the last visit were considered censored, whereas variables including sociodemographic such as age, sex, residence, family size, parental history of TB contact, plus clinical factors like WHO clinical stage, baseline cluster of differentiation (CD4 count), Hgb, functional status, and nutritional status like (stunting, wasting, underweight, MUAC) were considered as independent variables.

2.4. Operational Words. Smear-positive pulmonary tuberculosis: at least one sputum smear examination is positive for acid fast bacilli (AFB) by direct microscopy. Smear-negative pulmonary tuberculosis: sputum specimens negative for AFB and radiographical abnormalities were consistent with active TB and the decision by a clinician to treat with a full course of antituberculosis chemotherapy. Extra Pulmonary TB: defined as tuberculosis outside the lung usually results from hematogenous dissemination. Sometimes infection directly extends from an adjacent organ. Symptoms vary by site but generally include fever, malaise, and weight loss. Diagnosis is most often by sputum smear and culture and, increasingly, by rapid molecular-based diagnostic test. Serpositive children: children who had human immune deficiency virus (HIV) in their blood and catgories under age less than 15 years.

2.5. Data Collection Instruments and Quality Assurance. A structured English version checklist was developed and used for data extraction from the patients' medical records sheet and Federal Ministry of Health Pediatrics antiretroviral therapy (ART) follow-up form [17]. Four diploma nurses and two degree nurses were recruited for data collection and supervision. One day of training was given for data collection and supervision procedures. A pretest was conducted on 5% of the final sample size at Felege Selam health center to check the reliability of the checklist. After the pretest, necessary modification of the data collection tool was made. Strict follow-up and supervision were carried out during data collection by the principal investigators, and feedback was given daily.

2.6. Data Processing and Analysis. EPI-DATA version 3.2 and STATA/14 software were used for data entry and analysis, respectively. Proportional hazard assumption was checked for each variable, and no variable was found with

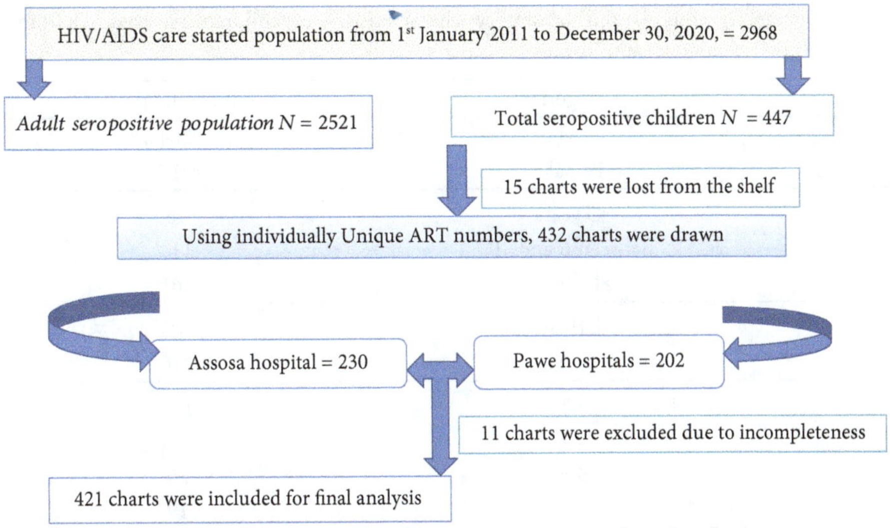

FIGURE 1: Schematic presentation of sampling procedure from the two general hospitals.

Schoenfeld residual test < 0.05. Categorical variables at bivariable Cox regression were assessed for candidates transferred at P value <0.25 for final multivariable Cox regression models, and variables associated with TB incidence in 95% CI at $P < 0.005$ were claimed as the predictor.

2.7. Ethical Approval and Consent of Participants. Ethical clearance and ethical approval were obtained from the research institute review board (IRB) of Debre Markose University with reference (Refill no: DMU IRB-984/118/13). A formal letter was submitted to all three hospitals for permission to be done. Debra Markose University waived consent from caregivers in addition to the national research, and ethical review guide waived consent for secondary files.

3. Results

3.1. Baseline Sociodemographic and Clinical Characteristics. After excluding 11 individuals' files due to incompleteness, we reviewed a total of 421 charts registered from 1st January 2011 to December 31, 2020 as depicted (Figure 1). The mean (± SD) age of study participant was 10.6 ± 3.3 years. More than three-fifths of 261 (62%) participant children were aged ≥11 years, and the majority 219 (52%) of them were from the rural area. About 57.5% of participant had both parents (Table 1).

3.2. Baseline Clinical, Hematological, and Laboratory Characteristics. Of the total, 128 (30%) and 89 (21%) of participant children were found to be in clinical world health organization stages (WHO) I and III, respectively. Nearly two-thirds, 263 (62%), of the children had hemoglobin ≥ 10 mg/dl, whereas the majority, 317 (75%), of participants had CD4 cell count ≥ 201 cell/mm^3. Moreover, 316 (75%) of children took cotrioxzol prophylaxis (CPT). Nearly two in five, 168 (39%), participant children missed isoniazid preventive therapy. Nearly one in five, 81 (19%), study participants shifted baseline ART regimens. The frequent reason was due to toxicity and TB incidence (24/81) and (22/81), respectively. Thirty nine percent of the children had an opportunistic infection. Bacterial pneumonia 53 (35.9%) and PCP 27 (21.6%) were the commonest. Of the total, 147 (35%) had hemoglobin ≤ 10 mg/dl, and more than two-thirds 276 (66%) children vaccinations. Majority, 338 (80%), of cases were in the appropriate developmental stage, while 56 (13.4%) children had poor ART adherence (Table 1).

3.3. Baseline Nutritional Status of HIV-Infected Children. Of the total, 33 (8%) and 72 (17%) cases had severe stunting and moderate wasting, respectively. However, 303 (72.3%) participants were on normal percentiles of weight for age > −2 Z score (Table 2).

3.4. Time to Developed Tuberculosis. In this study, a total of 421 study participants were followed for a different period, contributing a cohort of 1043.1 PY of observation with minimum and maximum of observation 4 to 98 months.

During the follow-up period, 64 (15.2%) individuals were devloped new tuberculosis. this makes the overall incidence density rate(IDR) particicpant children was found 5.9 (95% CI: 4.7; 7.7) per 100 person-years of risk observation. Majority, 44 (70%), of new cases occurred after ART that started 3 years later. About 44 (69%) cases were EPTB, and the remaining 19 (30%) were PTB (Table 3).

At the end of follow-up, 357 (85%) participant children were censored (excluded), among these 199 (47%) were on follow-up, 91 (21.6%) transferred into adult cohort, and 12 (4.7%) cases died (Figure 2).

3.5. Kaplan Meier TB Free Probability. The median duration of TB-free probability time was found 35 (IQR = ±29) months. The mean TB-free survival time of the entire follow up was 74.5 months (95% CI: 73.8, 84.3 months). Tuberculosis-free survival probability by the end of the follow-up was determined as 28.5% (95% CI; 22.3-36.9%) (Figures 3–5).

3.6. Predictors for Tuberculosis Incidence. In the final multi-Variabel Cox regression model, only three variables found

Table 1: Baseline sociodemographic, clinical, and laboratory characteristics of children received ART in two public hospitals (between = 2009 and 2018).

Variables	Categories	Numbers (total = 421)	Percent
Sex	Male	204	49
	Female	217	51
Age	≤5 years	46	11
	Between 6 and 10	114	27
	≥11 years	261	62
Residence	Urban	205	48
	Rural	216	51
Family size	≤2	133	31
	3-4	219	52
	5-6	50	11
	≥7	19	5
Hemoglobin	>10 mg/dl	263	63
	≤10 mg/dl	158	38
WHO	Stage I	128	30
	Stage II	147	35
	Stage III	89	21
	Stage IV	57	13
CD4 count	<100	30	7
	101-200	74	7
	≥201	317	75
Functional status	Working	307	72
	Ambulatory	72	17
	Bedridden	42	10
Adherence	Good	224	59
	Fair	121	29
	Poor	56	13
Isoniazid	Took	258	61
	Missed	163	38
Cocotrimoxazole	Took	321	76
	Missed	100	23
Opportunistic infections	Present	126	29
	Absent	295	70
Vaccination	Completed	276	66
	Not updated	76	18
	Defaulted	69	16
TB contact history	Yes	135	32
	No	286	68
Change of AR regiment	Present	85	20
	Absent	336	79
Parental status	Both parent alive	242	57
	Paternal orphan	115	27
	Maternal orphan	38	9
	Both parent orphan	26	6

TABLE 2: Baseline nutritional status of seropositive children attending HIV/AIDS care in two public hospitals North West Ethiopia 2021 ($N = 421$).

Nutritional parameter	Frequency	Percent	$chi^2(2)$	$P < 0.05$
Weight for height (WFH) normal (>-2 Z score)	304	72		
Moderate wasting $\leq -2-3\,Z$ score	71	17	7.5724	0.023
Severe wasting $\leq -3\,Z$ score	46	11		
Height for age (HFA) normal (>-2 Z score)	284	68		
Moderate stunting $\leq -2-3\,Z$ score	104	5	5.9262	0.052
Severe stunting $\leq -3\,Z$ score	33	8		
Weight for age(WFA) normal (>-2 Z score	277	66		
Moderate underweight $\leq -2-3\,Z$ score	115	27	9.1780	0.010
Severe underweight $\leq -3\,Z$ score	29	7		

TABLE 3: Time to developed TB incidence for seropositive children attending HIV/AIDS care in public hospitals between January 2011 and December 31/2020, North West Ethiopia ($N = 421$).

Years	No. of children at started	Withdrawn during year	At risk children	No. of TB case (63)	TB incidence	Cumulative probability	Survival rate	95% CI
>1 year	421 (100)	13 (20.6)	408(96.9%)	13 (20.6)	13 (3.1%)	13 (20.6%)	96.7%	94.5-98.1
2 years	408 (96.9%)	18 (28.5%)	390(92.6%)	18 (28.5%)	18 (4.3%)	31 (49.2%)	90.5%	86.5-93.2
3 years	390 (92.6%)	8 (12.6%)	382(90.7%)	8 (12.6%)	8 (1.99%)	39 (61.8%)	86.3%	81.5-89.9
4 years	382 (90.7%)	5 (7.93%)	377(89.5%)	5 (7.93%)	5 (1.15%)	44 (69.7%)	82.5%	76.5-87.1
5 years	377 (89.5%)	12 (19.0%)	365(86.6%)	12 (19.0%)	12 (2.8%)	56 (88.7%)	61.9%	49.5-72.8
6 years	365 (86.6%)	4 (6.34%)	361(85.7%)	4 (6.34%)	4 (0.98%)	60 (95.1%)	38.9%	29.1-57.5
7 years	361 (85.7%)	2 (3.17%)	359(85.2%)	2 (3.17%)	2 (0.047%)	62 (98.2%)	29.9%	26.5-46.4
End of follow	358 (84.8%)	1 (1.72%)	358(84.8%)	1 (1.72%)	1 (0.023%)	63 (100)	28.5%	22.3-36.9
Total		63 (100)	—	63 (100)	—	100	—	—

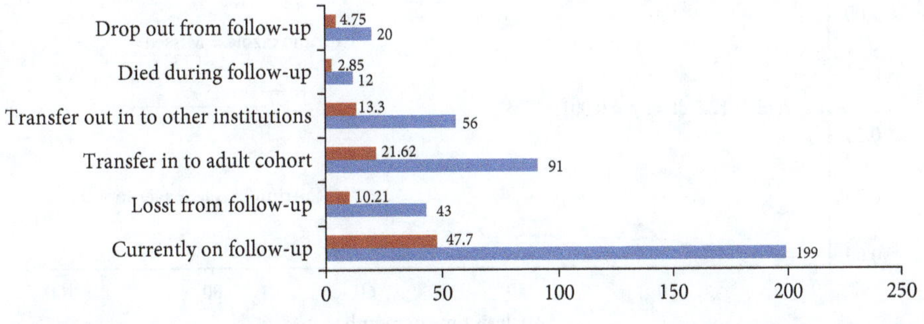

FIGURE 2: Seropositive children started HIV/AIDS care status in two public hospitals during data collection in public January 2011 to December 31/2020, North West Ethiopia ($N = 421$).

significantly associated with time to developed TB. Of this, the risks of developing TB for children who were not taking cotrimoxazole preventive therapy (CPT) were nearly three times higher as compared participant children who took CPT (AHR = 2.5: 95% CI,1.84-4.74, $P < 0.021$). Likewise, the risks of acquiring TB infection for seropositive children being nutritionally curve (height for age (HFA) $\leq -3\,Z$ score) or being severely stunted were three times (AHR = 2.9: 95% CI,1.2-7.8, $P < 0.03$) higher than as compared with participant children having normal percentiles (HFA, $> -2\,Z$ score). Hemoglobin levels had a high predictive value for incident TB; indeed, baseline hemoglobin ≤ 10 mg/dl was four times increase the hazard of developing TB as compared to children having ≥ 10 mg/dl (AHR = 4.02: 95% CI, 2.1-8.1, $P < 0.001$) (Table 4).

4. Discussion

This study is aimed at assessing TB incidence rate and its predictors in children on ART. Accordingly, at the end of

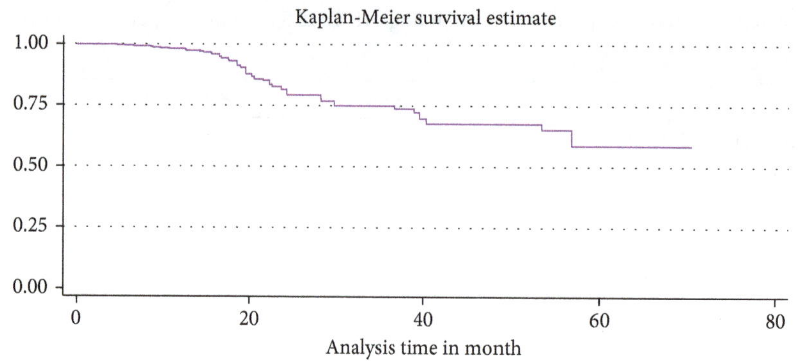

FIGURE 3: Overall Kaplan Meier survival estimate for all HIV/AIDS care seropositive children care started in two hospitals between 2011 and 2020 North West Ethiopia 2021 ($N = 421$).

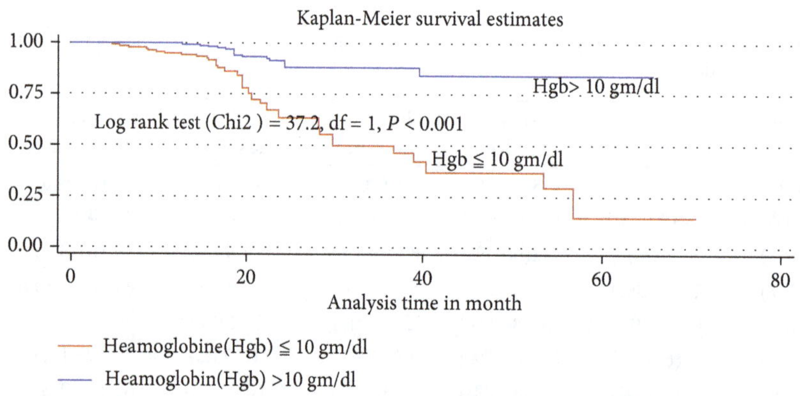

FIGURE 4: Kaplan Meier estimate of tuberculosis-free survival probability based on levels of hemoglobin for seropositive children, North West Ethiopia 2021.

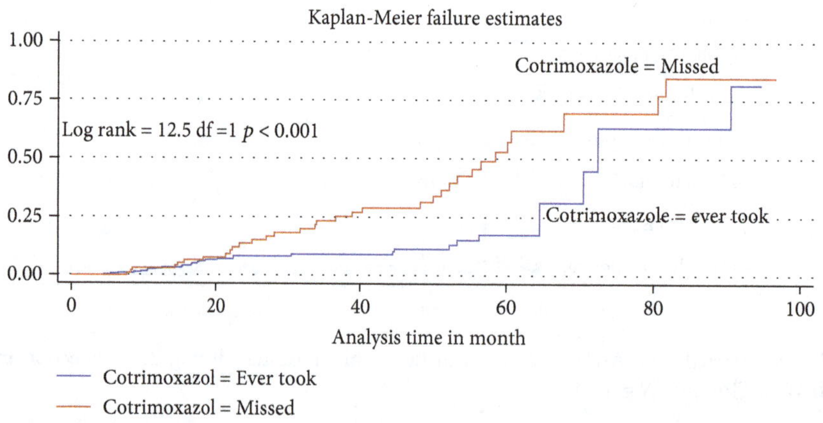

FIGURE 5: Difference in hazard for tuberculosis incidence in children not taking CPT seropositive children received ART care in two hospitals North West Ethiopia 2021.

the study period, 63 (15%) participants developed new TB incidence, making the overall incidence density rate 5.9 cases per 100 person-years (95% CI: 4.68; 7.68). This is higher than reported from Southern Ethiopia 2.6/100 PYs [18], Debre Markos 2.63/100 PYs [19], Northern Ethiopia 4.2/100 PYs [16], and Gonder 4.9/100 PYOs [20] but lower than findings in Adama hospitals 6.03/100 PYs [21] and South Africa 21.1/100 PYO [10]. This difference might be due to the higher burden of tuberculosis in resource-limited settings [1]. HIV was the immune system and acceleration viral replication responsible depletion of CD4 count [7] and associated

TABLE 4: Bi-variable and multivariable Cox-proportional hazard regression for predictors of TB among children treated on HIV/AIDS care in two public hospitals 2021 ($N = 421$).

Variables	Categories	COR 95% CI	AOR=95% CI	P< 0.05
Age of children	< =5 years	1	1	
	6-10 years	3.4 (1.09 - 5.5)	0.92 (0.28 ; 2.94)	0.82
	>=11 years	3.6.(1.7 - 5.6)	1.2 (0.32; 2.8)	0.12
IPT	Given	1	1	
	Missed	2 .6(2.1 - 8.3)	1.3(0.79 - 2.2)	0.08
CPT	Given	1	1	
	Missed	3.7(2.8- 7.8)	2.5(1.28; 5.3)	0.021
TB history of contact	Yes	1.2(1.08 - 3.4)	1.09 (0.8 - 2.2)	0.11
	No	1	1	
Vaccination	Complete	1	1	
	Not updated	2.1 (0.9 - 2.7)	1.2(0.72 ; 1.5)	0.40
	Defaulted	1.7(1.2- 2.8)	1.3(0.8; 1.9),	0.12
Adherence	Good		1	
	Fair	2.1(1.7 – 4.1)	1.8(0.87 ; 2.9),	0.11
	Poor	3.1(2.05 -6.3)	1.2 (0.93- 2.7)	0.06
HFA>-2 Z score	No stunting	1	1	
	Moderate stunting	2.1(1.5 – 2.8)	1.2(0.8 ; 2.7)	0.17
	Sever stunting	3.9(3.8 –5.1)	2.9(1.2; 7.8)	0.03
WHO clinical	stage I&II	1	1	
	Stage III&IV	9.1(4.9 16.4)	1.3 (0.73-2.5)	0.12
Hemoglobin	> 10 mg/dl	1	1	
	≤10 mg/dl	9.62(5.13 18.0)	4.02(2.1- 8.1)	0.001

with precipitation of new episode for opportunistic infections. This can be reduced early by addressing CPT and IPT, which are inexpensive and highly effective for reducing loads of endogenous reactivation of latent TB [22]. However, being seropositive children who missed CPT were significantly associated with risks of developed TB incidence. This finding is comparable with those reported in Gonder hospital [16] and Adam hospital [20]. The finding of this research also indicated that HIV-infected children having severe stunting were independently associated with the incidence of TB as compared with HIV-infected children who have no stunting. This is in line with the finding in Adama [21], Tanzania [23], Uganda, and Zimbabwe [9]. This might be due to HIV infection increasing nutrient malabsorption due to metabolic alterations that culminate in weight loss and stunting with time leading to early exposure for opportunistic infections [24]. Similarly, the existence of rapid viral replication consumed body energy and creates an arena for the incidence of TB [25, 26]. This finding also showed that children having hemoglobin ≤ 10 mg/dl were independently associated with TB incidence as compared with HIV-infected children having hemoglobin levels > 10 mg/dl. This is in line with the study finding in Adama hospital [21], Gonder hospital [20], Northern Ethiopia [16], Dar es Salaam, Tanzania [23], and England [27]. In fact, this is due to hemoglobin levels having a high predictive value for incident TB and death. TB incidence is directly associated with severe anemia [28]. Regardless of ART, moderate or severe anemia during ART follow-up can be an independent predictor for TB [28, 29].

4.1. Limitation of the Study. The retrospective nature of this study is one of the limitations of this study. Due to this, some of the clinically important predictor variables that have been independently associated with the incidence of TB occurrence in other studies, like the educational status of children and economic status of the family, were not included in this study.

5. Conclusion

Tuberculosis incidence was high among seropositive children attending HIV/AIDS care, especially in the first three years after ART initiated as compared with that of subsequent years, since more than half of 44 (69%) new cases of TB occurred. Levels of hemoglobin, missed cotrimoxazole preventive therapy, and nutritionallysevere stunting (HFA = ≤ −3 Z score) were significantly associated with the incidence of tuberculosis. Besides, intensified screening for provisions of isoniazid preventive therapy to children living with HIV/AIDS is highly recommended.

Abbreviations

HIV: Human immune deficiency syndrome
TB: Tuberculosis
AHR: Adjusted hazard ratio
PLWHIV: People living with HIV
WFH: Weight for height
WFA: Weight for age
HFA: Height for age
PYOs: Person years of observations
LLH: Log likely hood ratio.

Consent

There is no consent for this study.

Disclosure

In the role the funders took in the study, funders had no role in this study as I am a ph.D. candidate in the abovementioned university, and funders have no role except giving stay for their students on the time of research.

Authors' Contributions

FK, TG, and TK were equally contributing to the work reported, conception, study design, execution, analysis, and interpretation and writing the manuscript, and finally, all authors approved for submission.

Acknowledgments

Our final heartfelt thanks goes to Tamirate Shewan (Assistance Professor of Epidemiology), for his unreserved cleaning, editing, and rewriting of this manuscript for final submission. This study material and financial support are from Debre Markose University's Post-Graduate School as a Ph.D. student research support fund.

References

[1] FMOH, *Ethiopia-National guidelines for TB, DR-TB and Leprosy in Ethiopia-Sixth Edition*, 2017.

[2] K. A. Alene, K. Viney, H. C. Moore, M. Wagaw, and A. C. A. Clements, "Spatial patterns of tuberculosis and HIV co-infection in Ethiopia," *PLoS One*, vol. 14, no. 12, article e0226127, 2019.

[3] WHO, *GLOBAL TUBERCULOSIS REPORT 2020*, 2020.

[4] WHO, *GLOBAL TUBERCULOSIS REPORT 2019*, 2019.

[5] Z. Dawit, S. Abebe, S. Dessu, M. Mesele, S. Sahile, and D. Ajema, "Incidence and predictors of mortality among children co-infected with tuberculosis and human immunodeficiency virus at publichospitals in Southern Ethiopia," *PloS ONE*, vol. 16, no. 6, article e0253449, 2021.

[6] A. Alemu, A. Yesuf, B. Zerihun, M. Getu, T. Worku, and Z. W. Bitew, "Incidence and determinants of tuberculosis among HIV-positive individuals in Addis Ababa, Ethiopia: A retrospective cohort study," *International Journal of Infectious Diseases*, vol. 95, no. 95, pp. 59–66, 2020.

[7] FMOH, *NATIONALCONSOLIDATED GUIDELINES FOR COMPREHENSIVE HIV PREVENTION, CARE AND TREATMENT. Manuel Accesed septemebr 2021*, 2018.

[8] K. R. Ravichandra, B. R. Praharaj, and S. Agarwalla, "Opportunistic infections in HIV infected children and its correlation with CD4 count," *International Journal of Contemporary Pediatrics*, vol. 4, no. 5, pp. 1743–1747, 2012.

[9] And The ARROW Trial Team, A. Crook, A. Turkova et al., "Tuberculosis incidence is high in HIV-infected African children but is reduced by co-trimoxazole and time on antiretroviral therapy," *BMC Medicine*, vol. 14, no. 1, pp. 2–11, 2016.

[10] N. A. Martinson, H. Moultrie, R. Van Niekerk et al., "HAART and Risk of tuberculosis in HIV-infected South African children: a multi-site retrospective cohort," *International Journal of Tuberc and Lung Disuberc Lung Diseas*, vol. 13, no. 7, pp. 862–867, 2009.

[11] A. Ciaranello, Z. Lu, S. Ayaya et al., "Incidence of World Health Organization stage 3 and 4 events, tuberculosis and mortality in untreated, HIV-infected children enrolling in care before 1 year of Age," *The Pediatric Infectious Disease Journal*, vol. 33, no. 6, pp. 623–629, 2014.

[12] F. Kebede, B. Kebede, T. Kebede, and M. Agmasu, "Effect of isoniazid preventive therapy on the incidence of tuberculosis among seropositive children attending HIV/AIDS care in two general hospitals, Northwest Ethiopia, 2021," *Journal of Tropical Medicine*, vol. 2021, Article ID 9996953, 9 pages, 2021.

[13] F. Kebede, N. Eticha, B. Negese, M. Giza, T. Tolossa, and B. Wakuma, "Predictors for a cure rate of severe acute malnutrition 6-59 month children in stabilizing center at Pawe General Hospital, Northwest Ethiopia: retrospective cohort study," *International Journal of Child Health and Nutrition*, vol. 10, no. 1, pp. 34–43, 2021.

[14] M. T. Beshir, A. H. Beyene, K. G. Tlaye, and T. M. Demelew, "Incidence and predictors of tuberculosis among HIV-positive children at Adama Referral Hospital and Medical College, Oromia, Ethiopia: a retrospectivefollow-up study," *Epidemiology and Health*, vol. 41, article e2019028, 2019.

[15] D. F. Moore and D. F. Moore, *Applied survival analysis using R. Piscataway*, Springer Nature, NJ, USA, 2015.

[16] Y. M. Alemu, G. Andargie, and E. Gebeye, "High incidence of tuberculosis in the Absence of Isoniazid and Cotrimoxazole preventive therapy in children living with HIV in Northern Ethiopia: a retrospective follow-up study," *PLoS ONE*, vol. 11, no. 4, article e0152941, 2016.

[17] FMOH, *Ethiopian Federal democratic republic of Ethiopia: Ministry of Health National consolidated guidelines for comprehensive HIV prevention, care and treatment*, 2014, https://aidsfree.usaid.gov/sites/default/files/ethiopia_natl_gl_2014.pdf:145.

[18] K. D. Yirdaw, D. Jerene, Z. Gashu et al., "Beneficial effect of isoniazid preventive therapy and antiretroviral therapy on the incidence of tuberculosis in people living with HIV in Ethiopia," *PLoS One*, vol. 9, no. 8, article e104557, 2014.

[19] N. Eahet, "Incidence of tuberculosis in children on antiretroviral therapy: a retrospective cohort study," *BMC Research Notes*, vol. 11, 2018.

[20] S. G. Ayalaw, K. A. Alene, and A. A. Adane, "Incidence and predictors of tuberculosis among HIV positive children at University of Gondar Referral Hospital, Northwest Ethiopia: a retrospective follow-up study," vol. 2015, Article ID 307810, pp. 1–6, 2015.

[21] M. T. Beshir, A. H. Beyene, K. G. Tlaye, and T. M. Demelew, "Incidence and predictors of tuberculosis among HIV-positive children at Adama Referral Hospital and Medical College, Oromia, Ethiopia: a retrospective follow-up study," *Epidemiology and Health*, vol. 41, article e2019028, 2019.

[22] N. Gopalan, P. Chandrasekaran, S. Swaminathan, and S. Tripathy, "Current trends and intricacies in the management of HIV-associated pulmonary tuberculosis," *AIDS Research and Therapy*, vol. 13, no. 1, p. 34, 2016.

[23] N. Li, K. P. Manji, D. Spiegelman et al., "Incident tuberculosis and risk factors among HIV-infected children in Tanzania," *Aids*, vol. 27, no. 8, pp. 1273–1281, 2013.

[24] FMOH, *National Guidelines for Comprehensive HIV Prevention, CARE AND TREATMENT. GUIDELINE*, 2017.

[25] J. O. Alarcón, L. Freimanis-Hance, M. Krauss et al., "Opportunistic and other infections in HIV-infected children in Latin America compared to a similar cohort in the United States," *Aids Research and Human Retroviruses*, vol. 28, no. 3, pp. 282–288, 2012.

[26] World Health Organizations, *Antiretroviral therapy for HIV infection in infants and children: towards universal access*, WHO Library Cataloguing-in-Publication Data, 2010.

[27] A. T. Brennan, R. Bonawitz, K. Schnippel et al., "Incident tuberculosis in HIV-positive children, adolescents andadults on antiretroviral therapy in South Africa," *The International Journal of Tuberculosis and Lung Disease*, vol. 20, no. 8, pp. 1040–1045, 2016.

[28] A. Mocroft, O. Kirk, S. E. Barton et al., "Anaemia is an independent predictive marker for clinical prognosis in HIV-infected patients from across Europe," *Aids*, vol. 13, no. 8, pp. 943–950, 1999.

[29] A. D. Kerkhoff, R. Wood, F. G. Cobelens, A. Gupta-Wright, L. G. Bekker, and S. D. Lawn, "The predictive value of current haemoglobin levels for incident tuberculosis and/or mortality during long-term antiretroviral therapy in South Africa: a cohort study," *BMC Medicine*, vol. 13, no. 1, p. 70, 2015.

26

Contact Screening and Isoniazid Preventive Therapy Initiation for Under-Five Children among Pulmonary Tuberculosis-Positive Patients in Bahir Dar Special Zone, Northwest Ethiopia

Netsanet Fentahun,[1] **Yosef Wasihun**,[1] **Abebe Mamo**,[2] **and Lakew Abebe Gebretsadik**[2]

[1]*School of Public Health, College of Medicine and Health Science, Bahir Dar University, Bahir Dar, Ethiopia*
[2]*Department of Health, Behavior and Society, Institutes of Health, Jimma University, Jimma, Ethiopia*

Correspondence should be addressed to Netsanet Fentahun; netsanet.fentahun@bdu.edu.et

Academic Editor: José R. Lapa e Silva

Background. Children are highly susceptible to *Mycobacterium tuberculosis* infection, and about 70% of children living in the same households with pulmonary tuberculosis-positive patients will become infected. However, pulmonary positive tuberculosis is a common phenomenon and the implementation of the recommended contact screening and initiation of isoniazid preventive therapy is very low. Therefore, this study is aimed at assessing contact screening practice and initiation of isoniazid preventive therapy of under-five children among pulmonary tuberculosis-positive patients in Bahir Dar, northwest Ethiopia. *Methods.* A facility-based cross-sectional study was conducted from March 1 to 30, 2016. A total of 267 pulmonary tuberculosis-positive patients were included in this study. To identify independent predictors of contact screening and isoniazid preventive therapy initiation, we performed multivariable logistic regression analyses using SPSS version 20 with CI of 95% at p value < 0.05. *Results.* A total of 230 (90.2%) pulmonary tuberculosis-positive patients had single contacts with their under-five children. One hundred nine (64.8%) children were screened. From those screened, 11 (7.4%) developed tuberculosis disease and started antituberculosis treatment. Forty-four (31.9%) children started isoniazid preventive therapy. Sex of the participants, place of service delivery, relationship with contacts, HIV status, and attitude of PTB+ cases were significant predictors of contact screening ($p < .05$). Participant's knowledge, attitude of participants, and relationship of the child with participant were significant predictors of isoniazid preventive therapy initiation ($p < 0.05$). *Conclusion.* Contact screening practice and isoniazid preventive therapy initiation of children under the age of 5 in Bahir Dar zone were very low. Intimate family contact with pulmonary tuberculosis-positive patients, place of service delivery, and attitude towards screening are the key factors of contact screening. Participant's knowledge, attitude of participants, and relationship of the child with participant are the key factors of isoniazid preventive therapy initiation. Therefore, household contact screening and isoniazid preventive therapy initiation should be paid attention to reduce transmission.

1. Introduction

Tuberculosis (TB) is a chronic necrotizing disease caused by Mycobacterium tuberculosis complex. The species commonly involved are *M. tuberculosis*, *M. bovis*, *M. africanum*, and *M. microti* [1]. Worldwide, an estimated 10 million people fall ill with TB and about 1.5 million cases died in 2018. From these 10 million cases, about 1.1 million (11%) occurred in children (0-14 years) and there were 205,000 child deaths due to TB in 2018 [2]. The World Health Organization (WHO) reported that a number of new TB cases occurred in Southeast Asia (44%), Africa (24%), and Western Pacific (18%) globally in 2018 [2]. Almost 90% of cases each year are in 30 high TB burden countries, and eight countries account for two-thirds of the total [3].

In Ethiopia, TB is one of the leading infectious diseases, and in 2014/2015, 135,831 TB cases (all forms) were reported; of these, 35% were bacteriologically confirmed pulmonary TB cases [4].

TB ranks among the top causes of childhood morbidity and mortality in developing countries but neglected for years in children [5]. Children living in close contact with PTB+ are at high risk of TB infection. One cough can produce 3,000 and a sneeze up to a million droplet nuclei in which the infectious dose of TB is 1 to 10 bacilli [6].

Contact screening and providing treatment are important and a simple strategy to implement at the primary health care setting [7]. Various studies demonstrated screening as an effective strategy in early identification of children eligible for isoniazid preventive therapy (IPT) and preventing susceptible children from developing the disease who had household contacts with PTB+ patients [8–10]. WHO and CDC reported that IPT is effective for about 93% of under-five children and 59% among children aged 15 years or younger and IPT is recommended in a daily basis for at least 6 months [11–13].

Rates for the initiation of IPT in eligible children ranging from 1.3% to 26% are reported in settings where tuberculosis is endemic [14]. High-burden countries have reported extremely poor compliance with screening and initiation of IPT because of limited awareness of its benefits and inability to perform screening tests by health care providers. Interruption of INH supply and distance from health facilities affect uptake of the service in different settings [15].

Contact tracing, investigation, and prophylaxis of childhood contacts of adult TB cases are widely recommended but rarely practiced in developing countries [16]. Ethiopia is also one of the 22 high-burden countries for TB, and childhood TB is still a major cause of hospital admission and death [17]. In 2014, of the new cases notified in Ethiopia, fourteen percent were pediatric TB cases. Even this could be an underestimate due to difficulty in confirmation of diagnosis of TB in children [18]. Ethiopia has accepted and implemented the WHO's recommendation of a six-month course of IPT as one strategy for prevention, care, and control of TB [19]. Ethiopia also developed a national TB prevention and treatment guideline which emphasizes on contact screening and IPT for under-five children who have a history of contact with PTB+ patients. Clinical assessment alone is conducted to decide whether the contact is eligible for IPT initiation or not. But for symptomatic contacts, further diagnosis like chest radiograph and ESR is conducted to rule out active TB [8, 20].

However, it has been evident that the implementation of the recommended contact screening is very low and IPT initiation has been largely ignored in Ethiopia [8, 15]. In addition, there is limited information regarding suboptimal contact screening and noninitiation of IPT. These indicated that there is a huge gap in implementing the recommended strategies. Hence, identifying and understanding the factors that affect the implementation of contact screening and IPT initiation are crucial to address the challenges. Therefore, the objective of this study was to assess the contact screening and INH prophylaxis practices of under-five children among PTB+ patients in Bahir Dar special zone, northwest Ethiopia.

2. Methods and Materials

2.1. Study Design and Settings. This study used a facility-based cross-sectional study design to assess household contact screening and INH prophylaxis of under-five children who had contact with PTB+. We conducted this study in Bahir Dar special administration zone, with 221,991 predominantly urban populations, Amhara regional state of Ethiopia. It is located around 565 km northwest of Addis Ababa, the capital of Ethiopia. In this zone, there were around 989 TB patients of all forms and 460 were PTB+ patients. The special zone has 18 governmental health facilities (4 hospitals and 14 health centers), which were giving directly observed treatment (DOT) services in the first quarter of 2016.

2.2. Study Participants and Procedures. The study population was all PTB+ patients who had under-five children and registered their household contacts during November 2015–March 2016. These participants were interviewed during DOTS program at health facilities from March 1 to 30, 2016. As per guidelines [8], all diagnosed PTB+ patients are expected to be recorded in the contact investigation register. So, we used the data routinely recorded in the contact investigation register at all health facilities (4 hospitals and 14 health centers) providing DOT services in the study areas. From these health facilities, there were around 460 PTB+ patients, and 267 of them were listed on TB treatment registration book as PTB+ patients who had under-five children and we included all 267 of them as census. Every day, we gathered all PTB+ patients in the morning and selected those who had under-five children at home for interview. Patients' TB treatment cards were used for identification of those PTB+ patients. During data collection, those children who were screened and started IPT and anti-TB treatment were cross-checked from IPT and anti-TB treatment registration books, respectively.

The Ethiopian National TB Program recommends the following groups of persons to be given priority for identification through contact tracing and undergo clinical evaluation: symptomatic contact of the index patient, contacts who are living with HIV, contacts who are under-five children, and contact of an index case with presumed/confirmed DR-TB. Contact tracing is initiated by the TB focal person as soon as the index case is registered to receive TB treatment. The TB focal person communicates with the health extension workers to conduct identification of contacts at the household/community level, do symptom-based TB screening, and refer those who require detailed evaluation and investigation at the health facility level. The initial identification and evaluation of identified contacts for active TB are conducted using symptom-based TB screening questions and may be conducted at the community level by health extension workers and/or at a health facility by trained health care workers.

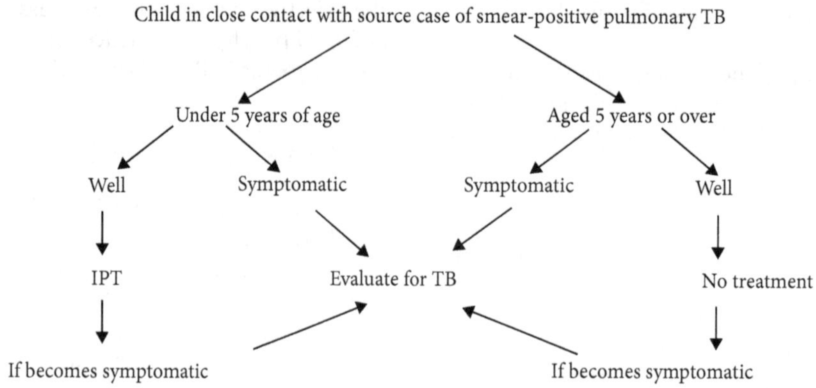

FIGURE 1: Approach contact management of children in Ethiopia.

In Ethiopia, we have two modalities for TB contact tracing. The first modality is contact tracing at the community level: as part of the community TB care package, health extension workers are practicing household contact tracing during routine home visits and upon receiving the request from the catchment health facility. The health extension workers are preferred to identify those at high risk of developing TB and symptomatic ones and bring them to the health facility for clinical evaluation and subsequent management. The second modality is contact tracing at the health facility level: the health care worker at the TB clinic should initiate contact tracing and investigation for close/household contacts upon registering a new index TB patient for treatment (Figure 1).

2.3. Data Collection and Measurements. PTB+ patients with child contacts were interviewed in Amharic (local language) using a pretested, structured, and interviewer-administered questionnaire. The questionnaire is developed by reviewing different literatures [21–24] and prepared in English first and translated into the local language. The questionnaire included sociodemographic variables, knowledge, and attitude of PTB+ patients on tuberculosis, contact screening, and INH prophylaxis and health worker-related questions. The questionnaire was pretested in Merawi district which is found 32 km far from the study area. The data were collected by four college completed BSc nurses and one health officer as a supervisor. Training was given for data collectors about the data collection tool, how to collect data, and taking consent to have common understanding.

The knowledge question was assessed using different items including sign and symptoms, cause, mode of transmission, risk groups, prevention mechanism, and treatment of tuberculosis. Study participants were interviewed on all mentioned dimensions regarding tuberculosis with "yes or no" questions, and finally, a composite measure for each aspect was created out of 15 and this weighted score was used for analysis as continuous variable.

The attitude part of the questions consisted of five items in five-point Likert scale. The scores of individuals for each item were summed up and ranged from 5 minimum to 25 maximum total score after reverse coding for negatively worded items, and this was treated as continuous variable for analysis. Reliability test was checked using Cronbach's alpha and the results were 0.87 and 0.74, respectively.

Contact screening was assessed using two items with the responses of "Yes or No" type like "have you ever heard or been informed about contact screening"? Those who responded "Yes" were considered as eligible for the next question and were asked "have your under-five child/children been screened for TB"? Those who responded "Yes" were considered as they were practicing contact screening. Finally, children who were screened and found free from TB were identified and considered as eligible for IPT and assessed using an item, "did your child/children start INH prophylaxis"? Those who responded "Yes" were considered as the children were starting IPT.

2.4. Data Analysis. Data were coded and entered to a computer using EpiData software version 3.1 (EpiData Association, Odense, Denmark) and exported to SPSS program version 20.0 for further analysis. The descriptive result was presented using frequency and proportions for all variables, and we performed bivariate regression analysis to determine association between factors of contact screening and IPT initiation at 95% confidence interval and p value of <0.25. We performed multivariate logistic regressions, and variables with p value < 0.05 are considered to identify the independent predictors of contact screening and IPT initiation. Goodness of fit of the final models was checked using Hosmer and Lemeshow test of goodness fit for contact screening and IPT, and the results were 0.86 and 0.26, respectively.

3. Result

3.1. Sociodemographic Characteristics. Overall, 267 PTB+ patients who had household contacts were registered between November 2015 and March 2016. A total of 255 PTB+ patients were interviewed from March 1 to 30, 2016, with a response rate of 95.5%. From the interviewed PTB+ patients, 131 (51.4%) were males, 153 (60%) of them were parents (father or mother) of the contacts, and more than half of the respondents 134 (52.5%) were married. Other sociodemographic characteristics of respondents and related factors are given in Table 1.

TABLE 1: Sociodemographic and related profile of PTB+ patients in Bahir Dar special zone, northwest Ethiopia, March 2016 ($N = 255$).

Variables	Categories	Frequency	Percent
Age in years	<20	36	14.1
	20-29	89	34.9
	30-39	84	32.9
	40-49	32	12.5
	>49	14	5.5
Sex	Male	131	51.4
	Female	124	48.6
Religion	Christian	239	93.7
	Muslim	16	6.3
Residence	Urban	168	65.9
	Rural	87	34.1
Marital status	Married	134	52.5
	Unmarried	101	39.6
	Divorced	7	2.7
	Widowed	13	5.1
Educational status	No formal education	75	29.4
	Primary school educated	100	39.2
	Secondary school educated	71	27.8
	College/university educated	9	3.5
Occupation	Farmer	50	19.6
	Merchant	41	16.1
	Student	36	14.1
	Housewife	32	12.5
	Daily laborer	27	10.6
	Government employee	20	7.8
	No work	26	10.2
	Driver	23	9
Household income	<500 eth birr	106	41.6
	500-1000 eth birr	83	32.5
	>1,000 eth birr	66	25.9
Relationship of the index cases with contacts	Parents	153	60
	Siblings	102	40

3.2. Health Information Related to Contact Screening and IPT Initiation. From the 255 interviewed PTB+ patients, 230 (90.2%) of them informed having under-five contacts (1 under-five contact/PTB+ patient), for a total of 230 under-five children evaluated. Of these 230 under-five children, 149 (64.8%) of them were screened for active TB and 11 (7.4%) were diagnosed with TB disease and started anti-TB treatment. One hundred thirty-eight child contacts who were diagnosed as free from TB disease were considered as eligible for IPT; of whom, 44 (31.9%) started IPT. The mean score of knowledge and attitude was 9.74 (SD ± 3.94) and 17.81 (SD ± 2.59), respectively. Contact screening, initiation of IPT, and other related factors are given in Table 2.

TABLE 2: Health information related to contact screening and IPT initiation of PTB+ patients in Bahir Dar special zone, northwest Ethiopia, March 2016 ($N = 255$).

Variable	Category	Frequency	Percent
Informed about contact screening	Yes	230	90.2
	No	25	9.8
Practice contact screening ($N = 230$)	Yes	149	64.8
	No	81	35.2
Outcome of contact screening	Positive	11	7.4
	Negative	138	92.6
Informed about the presence of IPT	Yes	82	32.2
	No	173	67.8
Started to use IPT ($N = 138$)	Yes	44	31.9
	No	94	68.1
HIV status ($N = 230$)	Positive	34	14.8
	Negative	196	85.2
Place of service provision ($N = 230$)	Health center	190	82.6
	Hospital	40	17.4

IPT: isoniazid preventive therapy; PTB+: smear-positive pulmonary tuberculosis; HIV: human immuno virus.

3.3. Factors Associated with Household Contact Screening of Under-Five Children. After controlling for possible confounding factors through multiple logistic regressions, place of service provided, relationship of the index case with the contact, and attitude of respondents were independent predictors of contact screening. Females who had contact with children were five times more likely to bring their under-five children for contact screening than males (AOR = 5.3, 95% CI (1.2, 23.2)). Participants who received the services from a hospital were 7 times more likely to bring their under-five children for contact screening as compared to those participants who received the services from a health center (AOR = 6.5, 95% CI (1.2, 41.8)). Parents who had a contact with children were 15 times more likely to bring their under-five children for contact screening as compared to siblings (brothers, sisters, and other relatives) (AOR = 14.8, 95% CI (3.2, 69.7)). HIV-positive TB patients were 19 times more likely to bring their under-five children for contact screening as compared to HIV-negative TB patients (AOR = 19, 95% CI (2.1, 16.87)). A unit increase in total score of attitude of the participants in the odds of household contact screening was increased by 2.8 (AOR = 2.8, 95% CI (1.5, 5.2)) (Table 3).

3.4. Factors Associated with Initiation of IPT for Under-Five Children. Multiple logistic regression analysis was performed to identify independent predictors of IPT initiation. Children who have parents as index case were twenty times more likely to start IPT as compared to children who had siblings (AOR = 20.0, 95% CI (2.4, 168.1)). A unit increases of

Table 3: Factors associated with household contact screening of under-five children, about contact screening in Bahir Dar special zone, northwest Ethiopia, March 2016 ($N = 230$).

Variables		Contact screening Yes	No	COR (95% CI)	AOR (95% CI)
Sex	Male	69 (46.3%)	50 (61.7%)	1	1
	Female	80 (53.7%)	31 (38.3%)	1.9 (1.1, 3.2)	**5.3 (1.2, 23.2)**∗
Residence	Rural	29 (19.5%)	40 (49.4%)	1	1
	Urban	120 (80.5%)	41 (50.6%)	4.1 (2.2, 7.3)	1.02 (0.2, 5.5)
Health facility	Health center	114 (76.5%)	76 (93.8%)	1	1
	Hospital	35 (23.5%)	5 (6.7%)	4.7 (1.8, 12.4)	**6.5 (1.2, 41.8)**∗
HIV status	Negative	119 (79.9%)	77 (95.1)	1	1
	Positive	30 (20.1%)	4 (4.9%)	4.9 (1.6, 14.3)	**19 (2.1, 16.87)**∗∗
Relationship of the child with participant	Parents	107 (71.8%)	34 (42%)	3.5 (2, 6.2)	**14.8 (3.2, 69.7)**∗∗
	Sibling[#]	42 (28.2%)	47 (58%)	1	1
∗∗[#]Knowledge score				1.7 (1.5, 1.9)	0.9 (0.6, 1.3)
∗∗[#]Attitude score				3.1 (2.3, 4.2)	**2.8 (1.5, 5.2)**∗∗

∗Continuous variables. AOR: adjusted odds ratio; COR: crude odds ratio; HIV: human immuno virus. [#]Sibling: brothers, sisters, and relatives.

Table 4: Factors associated with initiation of IPT of under-five children, in Bahir Dar special zone, northwest Ethiopia, March 2016 ($N = 138$).

Variable		IPT prophylaxis Started	Not started	COR with 95% CI	AOR with 95% CI
Relationship of the case with contacts	Siblings	2 (4.5%)	37 (39.4%)	1	1
	Parent	42 (95.5%)	57 (60.6%)	13.6 (3.1, 59.7)	**20.0 (2.4, 168.1)**
Age of the child	<1 year	3 (6.8%)	40 (42.6%)	0.07 (0.02, 0.3)	1.9 (0.3, 11.2)
	1-2 years	11 (25%)	26 (27.7%)	0.4 (0.2, 1.0)	1.8 (0.3, 11.2)
	>2 years	30 (68.2%)	28 (29.8%)	1	1
HIV status	Negative	25 (56.8%)	86 (91.5%)	1	1
	Positive	19 (43.2%)	8 (8.5%)	8.2 (3.2, 20.9)	0.4 (0.5, 1.5)
∗Attitude		$\beta = 1.230$		6.8 (3.2, 14.5)	**3.4 (1.1, 10.2)**
∗Knowledge		$\beta = 1.065$		3.1 (1.9, 4.9)	**2.9 (1.6, 5.2)**

∗Continuous variables. AOR: adjusted odds ratio; COR: crude odds ratio; IPT: isoniazid preventive therapy.

attitude of participants; the odds of IPT initiation is increased by 3.4 (AOR, 95% CI 3.4 (1.1, 10.2)). A unit increases of knowledge of the participants; the odds of starting IPT initiation is increased by 2.9 (AOR, 95% CI 2.9 (1.6, 5.2)) (Table 4).

4. Discussion

This study provides insight into the operation of household contact screening and IPT initiation of under-five children in northwest Ethiopia. About 64.8% of child contacts underwent screening for TB in our study, and other studies from Vietnam [25], Malawi [26], and Thailand [27] reported much less screening rates (6-52%), while a study in Western Cape Province of South Africa reported much higher screening rates (91%) [28]. The possible explanation for these differences could be due to the lack of an extensive awareness campaign about TB and its treatment, passive contact screening method, and lack of follow-up of the index cases to bring their under-five children to health facilities by health workers.

In addition to contact screening, this study also found that only 31.9% of children were started with IPT. This finding is lower than a study reported in Indonesia which reported 40% of IPT initiation [29], much lower than a study in India (56.4%) [30], but higher than other study in India (19%) of IPT initiation [21]. Inaccessibility of health facilities, isoniazid stock-outs, and risk perception of participants to start IPT without any sign and symptoms could be the main justifications for low initiation of IPT in our study.

In this study, contact screening and initiation of IPT were more likely among child contacts where index case is parents than siblings. This is consistent with the study findings from Vietnam [25] and Timor Leste [31]. In India, children living with parents were more likely to have initiated on IPT than other household members [32]. This study implies that parents are more concerned for their children's health and well-being and the bond between parents and small children are stronger than other household members. These reasons have also been reported in a study from Thailand [27].

This study also found that household contact screening of under-five children was more likely among hospital users than health center users. Studies from Thailand and Malawi reported that health center-based contact screening was poorly used because different types of laboratory services and tests were not available in the health centers, so the hospital is identified as a better option [27, 33].

This study showed that HIV-positive patients had significant association with contact screening unlike a previous study [22]. This could be because HIV-positive patients had regular visits to a health facility for antiretroviral therapy follow-up which might in turn made them know the benefit of early contact screening than HIV-uninfected patients.

Attitude of tuberculosis patients towards household contact screening without signs and symptoms and starting IPT in eligible under-five children had significant association with contact screening as well as IPT utilization. This finding was coherent with a study in India which revealed that most TB patients like to use screening and initiate IPT and they believed that the use of IPT has contributed to a higher reduction of acquiring tuberculosis [33]. This implies that if people believe in positive outcome, they accept it without trying to prove that the treatment is working or not.

According to this study, we found that knowledge was a major influencing factor for contact screening of under-five children. Per a unit increase in total score of knowledge on preventive mechanisms of TB, the odds of IPT initiation is also increased. A study in Ethiopia explained that 79.3% responded transmission of TB would be preventable and 80% knew that TB can be transmitted from a patient to another person [18]. Different studies justified that high-burden countries have reported extremely poor compliance with initiation of IPT because of limited awareness of its benefits and inability to perform prerequisite screening tests.

Rates for the initiation of IPT in eligible children ranging from 1.3 to 26% have been reported in settings where tuberculosis is endemic [14, 22]. As explained in a health belief model, when the barriers of health action outweigh the benefits in the minds of a given person, the likelihood of taking action decreases [33]. Therefore, certain types of barriers are more or less important for particular cultures or norms. Thus, it is not only knowledge but also attitude and other factors which could be special factors associated with the initiation of IPT among participants. As we conducted this study, there were a few limitations, which relate to the use of self-reported questions on knowledge of patients on tuberculosis, contact screening, and INH prophylaxis, which could lead to social desirability biases. However, as these questions were validated in a similar population, it is expected that this problem is minimal. Again, this study is conducted in one zone of the Amhara region. Whether the findings from this administrative zone are representative of contact screening and IPT of the whole region is unknown. But this special administrative zone has relatively higher number of population than other zones.

5. Conclusion

Household contact screening of under-five children and initiation of IPT in this study were very low. Sex of the participants, place of service delivery, relationship with contacts, HIV status, and attitude of PTB+ cases are the key factors for contact screening. Knowledge of participants, attitude of participants, and relationship with contacts are the key factors of initiation of IPT. The regional health bureau and health facilities should pay attention on contact screening and IPT initiation to narrow the practice gaps in Ethiopia.

Abbreviations

AOR: Adjusted odds ratio
CI: Confidence interval
COR: Crude odds ratio
HIV: Human immuno virus
INH: Isoniazid
IPT: Isoniazid preventive therapy
PTB+: Smear-positive pulmonary tuberculosis
TB: Tuberculosis
SD: Standard deviation
SPSS: Statistical Package for the Social Sciences
WHO: World Health Organization.

Authors' Contributions

YW, LA, NF, and AM contributed to the conceptualization, literature review, design, analysis, and writing of the paper. All authors read and approved the final submitted paper. The authors declare that they have agreed to publish on this journal.

Acknowledgments

We would like to acknowledge the assistance of Jimma University, Institute of Health, and Faculty of Public Health in undertaking this research. We would also like to express our gratitude to the study participants and officials working in Amhara regional state, Bahir Dar special zone administration, which really deserve acknowledgement for their cooperation. Last but not least, our thanks also go to the data collectors, supervisors, and advisors. This research was funded by Jimma University, Institute of Health, and Faculty of Public Health.

References

[1] G. Tizazu and T. Anteneh, *Internal medicine lecture notes for health officers. First edit. Ethiopia Public Health Training Initiative*, The Carter Center, the Ethiopia Ministry of Health, and the Ethiopia Ministry of Education, 2006.

[2] WHO, *Global tuberculosis report*, World Health Organization, Geneva, 2020, https://www.who.int/news-room/fact-sheets/detail/tuberculosis/2020.

[3] WHO, *Global tuberculosis report*, World Health Organization, Geneva, 2019, https://www.who.int/tb/publications/global_report/en/.

[4] EFMoH, *Annual performance report*, Addis Ababa, Ethiopia, 2015.

[5] J. R. Starke, "Improving tuberculosis care for children in high-burden settings," *Pediatrics*, vol. 134, no. 4, pp. 655–657, 2014.

[6] Health department of Republic of South of Africa, *Guidelines for the management of tuberculosis in children*, p. 8, 2014.

[7] Virginia department of Health, *Screening for TB infection and disease in Virginia*, Virginia Health Department, 2013.

[8] EFMoH, *Guidelines for clinical and programmatic management of TB, leprosy and TB/HIV in Ethiopia*, Ethiopian federal Ministery of Health, Addis Ababa, Fifth edition, 2012.

[9] R. Triasih, C. F. Robertson, T. Duke, and S. M. Graham, "A prospective evaluation of the symptom-based screening approach to the management of children who are contacts of tuberculosis cases," *Clinical Infectious Diseases*, vol. 60, no. 1, pp. 12–18, 2014.

[10] WHO, *Guidance for national tuberculosis programmes on the management of tuberculosis in children*, World Health Organization, 2014, https://www.who.int/tb/publications/childtb_guidelines/en/.

[11] World Health Organization Stop TB Partnership Childhood TB Subgroup, "Childhood contact screening and management," *The International Journal of Tuberculosis and Lung Disease*, vol. 11, no. 1, pp. 12–15, 2007.

[12] CDC, "The use of preventive therapy for tuberculous infection in the United States. Recommendations of the Advisory Committee for Elimination of Tuberculosis," *Morbidity and Mortality Weekly Report*, vol. 39, no. 8, pp. 9–12, 1990.

[13] J. Ayieko, L. Abuogi, B. Simchowitz, E. A. Bukusi, A. H. Smith, and A. Reingold, "Efficacy of isoniazid prophylactic therapy in prevention of tuberculosis in children : a meta analysis," *BMC Infectious Diseases*, vol. 14, no. 1, pp. 1–10, 2014.

[14] S. S. van Wyk, A. J. Reid, A. M. Mandalakas et al., "Operational challenges in managing isoniazid preventive therapy in child contacts: a high-burden setting perspective," *BMC Public Health*, vol. 11, no. 1, pp. 1–6, 2011.

[15] Y. Tadesse, N. Gebre, S. Daba et al., "Uptake of isoniazid preventive therapy among under-five children : TB contact investigation as an entry point," *PLoS One*, vol. 11, no. 5, 2016.

[16] M. Bonnet, C. Kyakwera, N. Kyomugasho et al., "Prospective cohort study of the feasibility and yield of household child tuberculosis contact screening in Uganda," *The International Journal of Tuberculosis and Lung Disease*, vol. 21, no. 8, pp. 862–868, 2017.

[17] WHO, *Country profiles for 22 hihg-burded countries*, WHO, 2015.

[18] L. F. Assebe, H. L. Reda, A. D. Wubeneh, W. T. Lerebo, and S. M. Lambert, "The effect of isoniazid preventive therapy on incidence of tuberculosis among HIV-infected clients under pre-ART care, Jimma, Ethiopia: a retrospective cohort study," *BMC Public Health*, vol. 15, no. 1, 2015.

[19] World Health Organization, *Gear up to end TB: introducing the end TB strategy*, World Health Organization, 2015, https://apps.who.int/iris/handle/10665/156394.

[20] WHO, *The end TB strategy*, World Health Organization, Geneva, 2015, http://www.who.int/tb/End_TB_brochure.pdf?ua=1.

[21] H. R. Shivaramakrishna, A. Frederick, A. Shazia et al., "Isoniazid preventive treatment in children in two districts of South India: does practice follow policy?," *The International Journal of Tuberculosis and Lung Disease*, vol. 18, no. 8, pp. 919–924, 2014.

[22] G. B. Gebregergs and W. G. Alemu, "Household contact screening adherence among tuberculosis patients in northern Ethiopia," *PLoS One*, vol. 10, no. 5, 2015.

[23] M. Pothukuchi, S. B. Nagaraja, S. Kelamane et al., "Tuberculosis contact screening and isoniazid preventive therapy in a south Indian district : operational issues for programmatic consideration," *PLoS One*, vol. 6, no. 7, 2011.

[24] S. Jirapaiboonsuk and R. S. Chapman, "Knowledge, Attitude, and Practice Towards Childhood Tuberculosis in Guardians of Patients Visiting the Pediatric out-Patient Department, Sirindhorn Hospital, Bangkok," *Journal of Health Research*, vol. 24, no. 2, pp. 101–106, 2010.

[25] G. J. Fox, L. P. Loan, N. V. Nhung et al., "Barriers to adherence with tuberculosis contact investigation in six provinces of Vietnam: a nested case–control study," *BMC Infectious Diseases*, vol. 15, no. 1, pp. 1–8, 2015.

[26] N. J. M. Claessens, F. F. Gausi, S. Meijnen, M. M. Weismuller, F. M. Salaniponi, and A. D. Harries, "Screening childhood contacts of patients with smear-positive pulmonary tuberculosis in Malawi," *The International Journal of Tuberculosis and Lung Disease*, vol. 6, no. 4, pp. 362–364, 2002.

[27] S. Tornee, J. Kaewkungwal, W. Fungladda, U. Silachamroon, P. Akarasewi, and P. Sunakorn, "Factors associated with the household contact screening adherence of tuberculosis patients," *Southeast Asian Journal of Tropical Medicine & Public Health*, vol. 36, no. 2, pp. 331–340, 2005.

[28] N. Beyers, R. P. Gie, H. S. Schaaf et al., "A prospective evaluation of children under the age of 5 years living in the same household as adults with recently diagnosed pulmonary tuberculosis, South Africa," *The International Journal of Tuberculosis and Lung Disease*, vol. 1, no. 1, pp. 38–43, 2007.

[29] M. E. Rutherford, R. Ruslami, M. Anselmo et al., "Management of children exposed to *Mycobacterium tuberculosis*: a public health evaluation in West Java, Indonesia," *Bulletin of the World Health Organization*, vol. 91, no. 12, pp. 932–941A, 2013.

[30] V. V. Banu Rekha, K. Jagarajamma, F. Wares, V. Chandrasekaran, and S. Swaminathan, "Contact screening and chemoprophylaxis in India's Revised Tuberculosis Control Programme : a situational analysis," *The International Journal of Tuberculosis and Lung Disease*, vol. 13, no. 12, pp. 1507–1512, 2009.

[31] C. Hall, P. Sukijthamapan, R. dos Santos et al., "Challenges to delivery of isoniazid preventive therapy in a cohort of children exposed to tuberculosis in Timor-Leste," *Tropical Medicine & International Health*, vol. 20, pp. 730–736, 2015.

[32] A. R. Singh, A. Kharate, P. Bhat et al., "Isoniazid preventive therapy among children living with tuberculosis patients: is it working? A mixed-method study from Bhopal, India," *Journal of Tropical Pediatrics*, vol. 63, no. 4, pp. 274–285, 2017.

[33] M. Nyirenda, R. Sinfield, S. Haves, E. M. Molyneux, and S. M. Graham, "Poor attendance at a child TB contact clinic in Malawi," *The International Journal of Tuberculosis and Lung Disease*, vol. 10, no. 5, pp. 585–587, 2006.

Chest Radiography and Xpert MTB/RIF® Testing in Persons with Presumptive Pulmonary TB: Gaps and Challenges from a District in Karnataka, India

Manjula Kanakaraju,[1] Sharath Burugina Nagaraja,[2] Srinath Satyanarayana,[3] Yella Ramesh Babu,[4] Akshaya Kibballi Madhukeshwar,[5] and Somashekar Narasimhaiah[6]

[1]*Taluka Health Office, Chikkaballapur, Karnataka, India*
[2]*ESIC Medical College and PGIMSR, Bengaluru, Karnataka, India*
[3]*Center for Operational Research, International Union against Tuberculosis and Lung Disease, New Delhi, India*
[4]*District Tuberculosis Office, Chikkaballapur, Karnataka, India*
[5]*Department of Community Medicine, Yenepoya Medical College, Yenepoya (Deemed to be University), Mangaluru, Karnataka, India*
[6]*National Tuberculosis Institute, Bengaluru, Karnataka, India*

Correspondence should be addressed to Manjula Kanakaraju; manjulakmd@gmail.com

Academic Editor: Isamu Sugawara

Background. In India, as per the latest diagnostic algorithm, all persons with presumptive pulmonary TB (PPTB) are required to undergo sputum smear examination and chest radiography (CXR) upfront. Those with sputum smear positive, sputum smear negative, but CXR lesions suggestive of TB or those with strong clinical suspicion of TB are expected to undergo Xpert MTB/RIF® assay test (also known as CB-NAAT (cartridge-based nucleic acid amplification test)). *Objective.* To assess what proportion of PPTB who are undergoing sputum smear examination at microscopy centers of public health facilities have undergone CXR and CB-NAAT. To explore the barriers for uptake of CXR and CB-NAAT from the public health care provider's perspective. *Methods.* We conducted a sequential explanatory mixed-methods study in Chikkaballapur district of Karnataka State, South India. The quantitative component involved a review of records of PPTB who had undergone sputum smear examination in a representative sample of seven microscopy centers. The qualitative component involved key informant interviews with four medical officers and group interviews with 9 paramedical staff. *Results.* In February and March 2019, about 732 PPTB had undergone smear examination. Of these, 301 (41%) had undergone CXR and 49 (7%) had undergone CB-NAAT. The proportion of PPTB who had undergone CXR varied across the seven microscopy centers (0% to 89%). CB-NAAT was higher in PPTB from urban areas when compared to rural areas (8% vs. 3%) and in those who were smear positive when compared to smear negative (65% vs. 2%). The major barriers for CXR and CB-NAAT were nonavailability of these tests at all microscopy centers and patients' reluctance to travel to the facilities where CXR and CB-NAAT services are available. *Conclusions.* CXR and CB-NAAT of PPTB are suboptimal. RNTCP should undertake measures to address these gaps in implementing its latest diagnostic algorithm.

1. Introduction

India, with an annual incidence of more than 2.8 million tuberculosis (TB) cases in 2017, is the highest TB burden country in the world. India also has the highest burden of multidrug-resistant TB in the world (~130,000 cases per year) [1]. The government of India's Revised National TB Control Programme (RNTCP) has developed a national strategic plan (2017-2025) for eliminating TB in India by 2025 [2]. For TB elimination, it is essential to diagnose all cases early and provide appropriate treatment. Previous studies have shown that though a large proportion of persons with presumptive pulmonary TB (PPTB) seek health care from public health facilities, many are being missed due to inadequate or incorrect use of TB diagnostic tests [3]. In 2017, RNTCP introduced a revised diagnostic algorithm (also called integrated diagnostic algorithm) for early detection of pulmonary TB and rifampicin-resistant TB [4]. According to this algorithm, all PPTB (with the exception of children and HIV-positive individuals) are expected to initially undergo two basic tests—sputum smear microscopy and chest radiography (CXR). Those with sputum smear positive, sputum smear negative but CXR lesions suggestive of TB or those with strong clinical suspicion of TB are expected to undergo Xpert MTB/RIF® assay test (also known as CB-NAAT (cartridge based nucleic acid amplification test)). CB-NAAT has higher sensitivity and specificity for detecting TB, and it also detects rifampicin resistance [5].

As in several other high TB burden countries, in India, within the public health system, sputum smear microscopy, CXR, and CB-NAAT are not available at all the health facilities [6]. Patients with presumptive TB who seek health care from health facilities without any of these diagnostic tests are referred to undergo these tests at the nearest public health facility (where these tests are available) or patients may choose to undergo these tests at private health facilities. Even in health facilities which have these diagnostic tests, patients may not be prescribed with the tests [7]. The diagnostic tests at the public health facilities are free of cost to the patients, whereas patients may incur out-of-pocket expenditure if they undergo these tests at a private health facility. Therefore, there is a potential for loosing PPTB during diagnosis or PPTB may experience inadequate use of diagnostic tests [8].

Given this situation, it is imperative for the RNTCP to routinely assess what proportion of presumptive pulmonary TB patients seeking care at various health facilities is able to undergo the diagnostic tests as per the latest diagnostic algorithm. There have not yet been any recent research studies on this aspect from any part of the country. In addition, the facilitators and barriers for the service providers to get the diagnostic tests done for their patients may or may not be uniform across various types of health facilities in the Indian public health system. Documenting the context-specific gaps in testing, the possible reasons and solutions to address these gaps from health providers' perspective will help the programme managers and policy makers to undertake appropriate corrective measures to address these gaps. Understanding the magnitude and reasons for gaps in diagnostic testing requires a combination of quantitative and qualitative research methods.

We, therefore, undertook an operational research study in Chikkaballapur district in the South Indian state of Karnataka. The objectives of our study are as follows: (a) to assess the uptake of chest radiography and/or CB-NAAT tests in presumptive pulmonary TB patients who were undergoing sputum smear examination and the demographic and clinical characteristics associated with the uptake of these two diagnostic tests and (b) to explore the facilitators and barriers for the uptake of these tests from the health care providers' perspective.

2. Methodology

2.1. Study Design. This is a mixed-methods study (sequential explanatory design) where in phase I, the quantitative part (cohort study design) was followed by phase II, the qualitative part (descriptive study design) (reference).

2.2. Study Setting. Chikkaballapur district has a population of 1.25 million people (2018) [9]. It is a predominantly rural district located in the south eastern part of the Karnataka State. The public health facilities in the district include primary health centers, community health centers, taluka hospitals (secondary level health facilities), and district hospital (tertiary level health facility). At the public health facilities, there are 13 designated microscopy centers (DMCs)—one at the district hospital, four at the taluka level hospitals, and seven at the primary health centers and community health centers. The facilities for chest radiography are available at the district hospital and the 6 taluka hospitals. CB-NAAT facility is available only at the district hospital. Approximately 1200-1500 persons undergo sputum smear microscopy every month at various DMCs in the district.

2.2.1. RNTCP Integrated Diagnostic Algorithm (2017). The integrated diagnostic algorithm is given in Figure 1. As per this diagnostic algorithm, all presumptive pulmonary TB patients (persons who have cough > 2 weeks or fever > 2 weeks or significant weight loss or hemoptysis) are expected to initially undergo both sputum smear microscopy and CXR. If the sputum smear is positive or if the CXR is suggestive of TB or there is a strong clinical suspicion for TB (even if sputum smear is negative for TB bacilli and CXR is not suggestive of TB), then they are expected to undergo CB-NAAT. Patients attending designated microscopy centers at primary health facilities are referred to undergo chest radiography and CBNAAT. Patients have to physically visit the taluk hospitals or district hospitals for chest radiography. For the CB-NAAT, either the patients have to physically visit the district hospital or in some places the sputum was collected and transported in cold chain by health workers to the district hospital CB-NAAT center. People living with HIV (PLHIV) are eligible to undergo CB-NAAT upfront.

2.2.2. Recording and Reporting System. The demographic and clinical details of all PPTB undergoing sputum smear examination are documented in a laboratory register at each DMC. This laboratory register also contains details of patients referred for CB-NAAT. The details of all patients who undergo CB-NAAT are documented at the CB-NAAT registers maintained at the CB-NAAT site.

2.3. Study Population, Study Sites, and Sampling

2.3.1. Quantitative Part. The study population comprised all consecutively enrolled PPTB (aged ≥15 years) who underwent sputum smear microscopy in the months of February and March 2019 at the following seven DMCs: district hospital DMC, two randomly selected Taluka hospital DMCs, and four randomly selected PHC DMCs in the district.

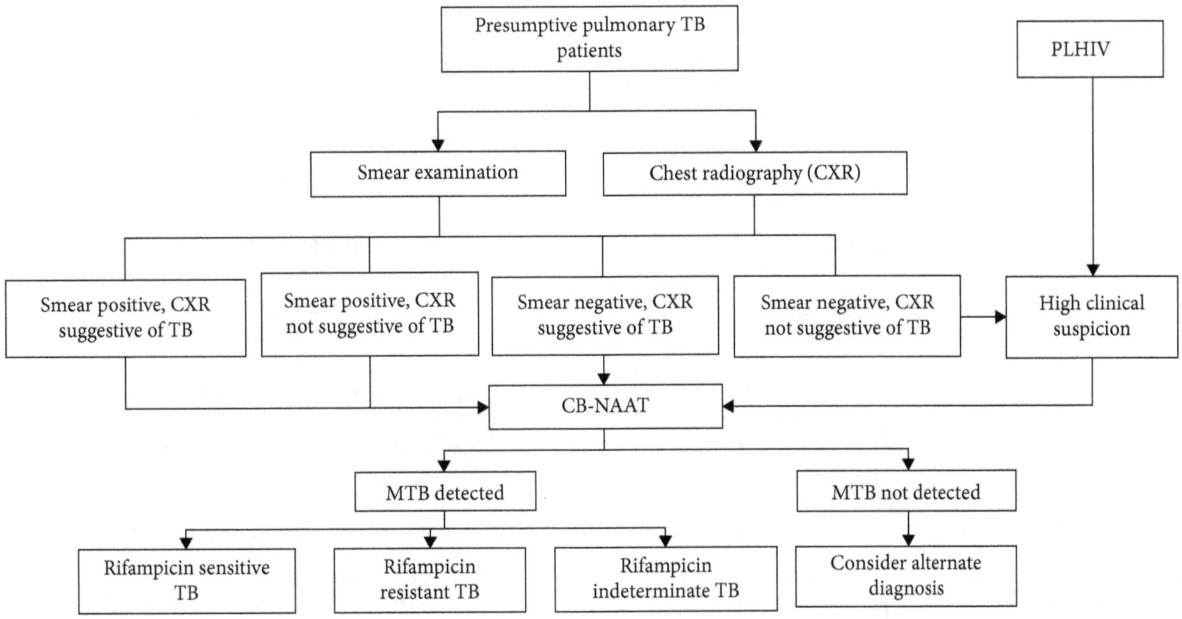

FIGURE 1: Recommendations for chest radiography and CB-NAAT for the evaluation of presumptive pulmonary TB patients as per the integrated diagnostic algorithm of the Government of India's Revised National TB Control Programme (2017).

2.3.2. Qualitative Part. The study population for key informant interviews included one physician at a district hospital, one physician at a taluka level, and two doctors at primary health centers, and one group interview included laboratory technicians of seven DMCs and one RNTCP senior TB laboratory supervisor and one senior treatment supervisor.

2.4. Study Data Collection Tools, Variables, Sources of Data, and Study Investigators

2.4.1. Quantitative Part. The data on all PPTB who underwent sputum smear examination at the seven selected DMCs were collected on a structured pro forma from the laboratory registers. Data on the following variables are routinely recorded in the laboratory register: date of enrolment, name, age, sex, telephone number, name of the referring health facility, whether the patient belongs to any key populations, results of two sputum smear examinations, HIV status, diabetes mellitus status, and CB-NAAT status. During the study period, we requested the laboratory technicians of the seven DMCs to additionally document whether each patient has already undergone CXR: if not, whether the patient was asked to undergo the CXR and, if yes, from which health facility (public/private) the patient underwent CXR. We cross checked the CB-NAAT notification registers to assess whether the information about the CB-NAAT testing status recorded in the laboratory register was correct or not.

2.4.2. Qualitative Part. We conducted key informant interviews with the medical officers and group interviews with the laboratory technicians STLS and STS, to understand the existing practices with respect to chest radiography and CB-NAAT testing and explore the facilitators and barriers in getting these tests done at the various health facilities. The key informant interviews and group interviews were conducted by two investigators (MK and SBN) who were doctors, have masters in community medicine, and have undergone training in qualitative research methods. An interview guide was developed and used for these interviews. The interviews were conducted in local language (Kannada). The interviews were conducted at a date and place convenient to all the participants and after obtaining their informed consent. We audio recorded all the interviews.

2.5. Data Analysis

2.5.1. Quantitative Part. The data collected on a structured format were entered in Epi Data Entry (version 3.1, Epidata Association, Odense, Denmark) and analyzed using Stata Statistical Software (version 15.1, Stata Corporation, College Station, Texas). We described the demographic and clinical characteristics in numbers and proportions. We assessed the number (and proportion) of PPTB who have undergone chest radiography and CB-NAAT. We used the 15th of April 2019 as the cut-off date for assessing the status of whether the PPTB had undergone the chest radiography and CB-NAAT. We used multivariable binomial log models to assess the association between demographic and clinical characteristics with uptake of chest radiography. Since the uptake of CBNAAT was low (<10%), we assessed the association between demographic and clinical characteristics with the uptake of CBNAAT using a chi-squared test or Fischer's exact test (as applicable). A P value of <0.05 was considered statistically significant.

2.5.2. Qualitative Part. For interviews with key informants and group interviews, transcripts were prepared the same day based on the verbatim notes/audio recordings. Manual descriptive content analysis was done by the first author (MK). It was reviewed by other co-authors (SS and AKM)

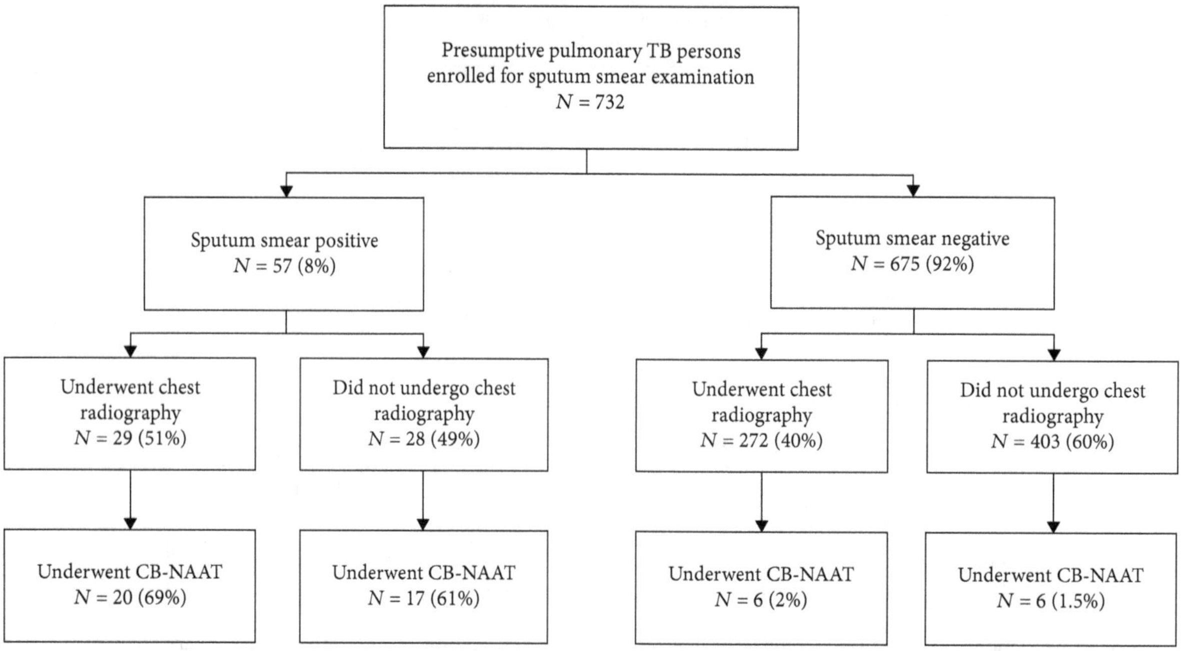

FIGURE 2: Status of chest radiography (CXR) and CB-NAAT tests in presumptive pulmonary TB patients undergoing sputum smear examination at seven selected designated microscopy centres in Chikkaballapur district, February to March, 2019.

to reduce subjectivity in analysis and enhance interpretive credibility. The decision on coding rules and theme generation was done by using standard procedures and in consensus. Any difference between the coauthors was resolved by discussion. The codes/themes were related back to the quantitative data [10], and the findings of the quantitative and qualitative parts of the study have been integrated through narration [11].

3. Ethics

We obtained ethics approval from the Ethics Committee of National Tuberculosis Institute, Bengaluru, India (No. A&C/R.2/2019 dated at the 31st of January 2019) and the Ethics Advisory Group of the International Union against Tuberculosis and Lung Disease, Paris, France (No. 121/18 dated at 30.1.19). For the quantitative component of the study, since it is a record-based study, we obtained waiver from obtaining informed consent. For the qualitative part, written informed consent was obtained from all participants.

4. Results

4.1. Quantitative Part. A total number of 732 PPTB were enrolled during the study period; the status of chest radiography and CBNAAT tests among PPTB who underwent smear examination are shown in Figure 2. Their demographic and clinical characteristics are presented in Table 1. About 85% were enrolled from the district and taluka hospitals. The mean age was 46 years (SD 17). Majority (62%) were men, and 73% were living in urban areas. The predominant symptoms were cough and cough with fever, 84% were HIV seronegative, and 70% did not have diabetes mellitus. About 8% were sputum smear positive for acid fast bacillus.

In this cohort, 301 (41%) had undergone CXR with 290 (96%) undergoing it in public health facilities. The association between demographic and clinical characteristics with undergoing CXR is given in Table 2. There were huge variations in the proportion of patients who had undergone CXR across the health facilities (0% in two PHCs to 89% in one of the taluka hospitals). On bivariable analysis, the type of health facility, age of the study participants, residence in urban areas, and having cough, fever, and/or hemoptysis were associated with undergoing CXR. On multivariable analysis, the type of health facility was the only factor that was independently associated with CXR.

Around 49 (7%) of the total 732 PPTB patients had undergone CB-NAAT, and their demographic characteristics are given in Table 3: PPTB who had their residence in urban areas when compared to rural areas (8% vs. 3%) and in those who were smear positive when compared to smear negative (65% vs. 2%).

4.2. Qualitative Part. We conducted one group interview with nine RNTCP paramedical workers and four key informant interviews with the medical officers. In these interviews, three facilitators, five barriers, and five solutions were suggested to improve the CXR and CB-NAAT testing.

4.2.1. Facilitators. The following three facilitators were identified:

(1) Good awareness about diagnostic algorithm: all lab technicians and senior treatment supervisors and senior Laboratory technician supervisors were aware of the latest diagnostic algorithm

(2) Having chest radiography in the same health facility, same day reporting and sharing of results via mobile

TABLE 1: Characteristics of persons with presumptive pulmonary TB attending seven selected designated microscopy centers in Chikkaballapur District during February-March 2019.

Characteristics	$N = 732$	(%)
Designated microscopy center		
District hospital	243	(33.2)
Taluka hospital 1	249	(34.0)
Taluka hospital 2	125	(17.1)
Primary health center 1	32	(4.4)
Primary health center 2	33	(4.5)
Primary health center 3	17	(2.3)
Primary health center 4	33	(4.5)
Age (in years)		
<25	82	(11.2)
25 to 34	138	(18.9)
35 to 44	106	(14.5)
45 to 54	108	(14.8)
55 to 64	129	(17.6)
> 64	146	(19.9)
Not recorded	23	(3.1)
Gender		
Male	455	(62.2)
Female	276	(37.7)
Transgender	1	(0.1)
Place of residence		
Urban	535	(73.1)
Rural	197	(26.9)
Predominant symptom		
Cough	272	(37.2)
Cough+fever	259	(35.4)
Hemoptysis	1	(0.1)
Not recorded	200	(27.3)
HIV status		
Nonreactive	613	(83.7)
Reactive	3	(0.4)
Not recorded	116	(15.8)
Diabetes mellitus		
Yes	8	(1.1)
No	506	(69.1)
Not recorded	218	(29.8)
Sputum examination results		
Negative	675	(92.2)
Positive	57	(7.8)

application were one of the major facilitators for high chest radiography in one of the taluka level hospitals

"We do X-ray reporting same day and the image is posted in the WhatsApp group of the hospital staff on daily basis... and it helps in same day reporting" (lab technician)

(3) Doctor insistence for these tests was the third major facilitator for the tests. Patients listen to doctors and get investigation done because of trust and opinion

"Doctors should tell , patients to get the X-ray done... otherwise they will not go. They have more respect for them [doctors]" (lab technician)

4.2.2. Barriers. The following five barriers were identified:

(1) Nonavailability of the tests at all health facilities: CBNAAT and CXR facility are available only at the district hospital, while only CXR facility is available at taluka hospitals. So patients have to travel some distance to get these basic investigations done

"In PHC, we don't have x-ray facilities......even we refer for investigation we cannot trace the patients." (senior treatment supervisor)

(2) Patients' reluctance to travel to health facilities or patients have to travel multiple times to get the results: they have to go first to get chest radiography done and then show it to a physician for reporting, and in overcrowded hospitals at taluka and district hospital, it is difficult. Sometimes the concerned doctor (who has to read chest radiology and give reports) may not be available due to other responsibilities of casualty, medicolegal work, and work related to national programmes

"Patients have to travel twice to get x-ray reports, they will lose work and money for these days, they will simply not go." (lab technician at PHC)

"I do ask x-ray investigation but most of them do not get it done,.. they do not even give their sputum for examination till 3 - 5 repeated visits and symptoms have become more." (doctor)

"In some cases when the sputum is negative and I refer the patient for X-ray/CB-NAAT, they don't listen, they say "any ways the sputum test is negative why go so far, we will see later." This is a big obstacle to convince the patient." (doctor)

(3) Long waiting periods: they are long queues at outpatient to consult doctors and followed by waiting at the laboratory for investigations/Chest radiography, reporting and opinion of doctors. Alternate methods of fast tracking PTB patients must be done. Like in some taluka hospitals, they made seals under RNTCP which gives them special access to labs and X-ray labs

'If we send the patients to the X-ray unit also…they are not willing to spend time for the investigations due to the long waiting periods' (lab technician)

It is very cumbersome for the patient who has to travel from peripheral PHC to taluka and district hospital, even If he/she goes there on time they have to endure the long queues starting from registration, consulting the doctors then up-to the investigations, they get very frustrated and do not come back." (doctor)

TABLE 2: Factors associated with undergoing chest radiography in presumptive pulmonary TB persons enrolled for sputum smear examination in seven selected designated microscopy centers in Chikkaballapur District during February-March 2019.

Characteristics	N	n	(%)	RR	(95% CI)	Adj RR	(95% CI)	*P* value
Total	732	301	(41.1)					
Designated microscopy center								
District hospital	243	53	(21.8)	Reference		Reference		
Taluka hospital 1	249	222	(89.2)	4.08	(3.20-5.20)	2.29	(1.01-5.22)	0.047
Taluka hospital 2	125	9	(7.2)	0.33	(0.16-0.64)	0.33	(0.10-1.04)	0.059
Primary health center 1	32	3	(9.4)	0.42	(0.14-1.29)	0.39	(0.12-1.28)	0.122
Primary health center 2	33	0	(0.0)	NE				
Primary health center 3	17	0	(0.0)	NE				
Primary health center 4	33	14	(42.4)	1.94	(1.22-3.09)	1.13	(0.46-2.81)	0.776
Age (in years)								
<25	82	39	(47.6)	0.84	(0.64-1.10)	0.94	(0.64-1.39)	0.775
25 to 34	138	78	(56.5)	Reference		Reference		
35 to 44	106	35	(33.0)	0.58	(0.42-0.79)	0.81	(0.53-1.19)	0.281
45 to 54	108	42	(38.9)	0.68	(0.52-0.90)	1.08	(0.74-1.59)	0.664
55 to 64	129	47	(36.4)	0.64	(0.49-0.84)	0.89	(0.61-1.29)	0.558
> 64	146	54	(37.0)	0.65	(0.50-0.84)	0.94	(0.66-1.34)	0.761
Not recorded	23	6	(26.1)	0.46	(0.22-0.93)	0.95	(0.40-2.25)	0.919
Gender								
Male	455	195	(42.9)	Reference		Reference		
Female	276	105	(38.0)	0.88	(0.73-1.06)	0.92	(0.72-1.18)	0.559
Transgender	1	1	(100.0)	NA				
Place of residence								
Urban	535	257	(48.0)	2.15	(1.63-2.83)	NE		
Rural	197	44	(22.3)	Reference		Reference		
Predominant symptom								
Cough	272	55	(20.2)	Reference		Reference		
Cough+fever	259	225	(86.9)	4.29	(3.37-5.46)	1.91	(0.85-4.30)	0.116
Hemoptysis	1	1	(100.0)	4.94	(3.90-6.26)	4.97	(0.67-36.7)	0.115
Not recorded	200	20	(10.0)	0.49	(0.30-0.79)	0.99	(0.39-2.51)	0.985
Sputum examination results								
Negative	675	272	(40.3)	Reference		Reference		
Positive	57	29	(50.9)	1.26	(0.96-1.65)	1.34	(0.91-2.00)	0.135

NA = not applicable (as outcome predicts exposure perfectly); NE = not estimated due to collinearity with designated microscopy center; RR = relative risk; Adj RR = adjusted relative risk; Reference = strata of data considered as reference population for calculation.

TABLE 3: Factors associated with CB-NAAT in presumptive pulmonary TB enrolled for sputum smear examination in seven selected designated microscopy centers in Chikkaballapur District during February-March 2019.

Characteristics	N	n	(%)	Chi-square test P value
Total	732	49	(6.7)	
Designated microscopy center				
District hospital	243	9	(3.7)	
Taluka hospital 1	249	19	(7.6)	
Taluka hospital 2	125	14	(11.2)	
Primary health center 1	32	3	(9.4)	0.09
Primary health center 2	33	0	(0.0)	
Primary health center 3	17	1	(5.9)	
Primary health center 4	33	3	(9.1)	
Age (in years)				
<25	82	5	(6.1)	
25 to 34	138	10	(7.2)	
35 to 44	106	5	(4.7)	
45 to 54	108	9	(8.3)	0.942
55 to 64	129	10	(7.8)	
>64	146	9	(6.2)	
Not recorded	23	1	(4.3)	
Gender				
Male	455	33	(7.3)	0.336
Female	276	15	(5.4)	
Transgender	1	1	(100.0)	
Place of residence				
Urban	535	43	(8.0)	0.017
Rural	197	6	(3.0)	
Predominant symptom				
Cough	272	12	(4.4)	
Cough+fever	259	18	(6.9)	0.09
Not recorded	200	19	(9.5)	
Hemoptysis	1	0	(0.0)	
Sputum smear results				
Negative	675	12	(1.8)	<0.01
Positive	57	37	(64.9)	
Underwent chest radiography				
Yes	301	26	(8.6)	0.079
No	431	23	(5.3)	

*Fischer's exact test; P value. **Chi-square test; P value.

Charges levied for the chest radiography: at some of the taluka level and district hospitals, they charge INR 100 (~USD 1.5) for any radiographs. This acts as a deterrent for some of the patients to not undergo these tests

"Patients are charged at the big hospital for X-ray...if the patients directly go to OPD they will be charged Rs 100." (lab technician)

(5) Issues with sputum collection and transportation for CB-NAAT tests: the sputum samples produced by patients are of poor quality (i.e., they contain predominantly saliva) or some of them are unable to produce the sputum. Poor quality samples are not accepted for CBNAAT. At times, there were shortages of falcon tubes that can be used for collecting and transporting the sputum specimens

"How many times do I have to get Kappha (sputum)?" "Patients ask us, some say they do not get sputum even after repeated coughing" (lab technician)

"There is shortage of supply of Falcon tubes in the field, so sometimes we are sending in regular sputum cups well packed with ASHA workers, but lab technicians at CBNAAT site are not accepting them" (doctor)

4.2.3. Suggested Solutions to Improve Chest Radiography and CB-NAAT. We identified the following five suggestions to improve the testing process:

(1) Tie-up with private chest radiography centers and CXR vans, to provide CXR facility at PHC level

"The government should set up under RNTCP mobile X ray units like that of that other health related mobile vans from district hospitals/from NGOs or provide at least small and feasible X ray units at PHC it is a basic investigation requirement and decentralize CB-NAAT by providing it at Taluka hospitals." (doctor)

(2) A chest radiography referral slip can be made from PHC so that presumptive pulmonary TB patients have direct/easier access to doctors and laboratory

"A referral slip with a seal has to be made and should be given to all patients referred from PHCs to x-ray centres for free investigation so they can directly go to the labs...." (lab technician)

(3) An additional column to be created in the laboratory register for entering details of chest radiography and its results, similar to the columns that are available for documenting CB-NAAT status. This will help in tracking PPTB to undergo these tests

(4) Establishment of a call center at district TB center for tracking and motivating PPTB to undergo investigations and further follow-up

(5) Innovative and appropriate use of technology like using apps on mobile phone and forming groups of lab technicians and physicians for sharing of PPTB information about CXR and CB-NAAT across various health facilities to minimize delays in obtaining patient reports

5. Discussion

This is the first study from India to assess the CXR and CB-NAAT of persons with presumptive pulmonary TB undergoing sputum smear examination at various levels of the public health facilities in the country after the introduction of the revised diagnostic algorithm in 2017. The major findings of the study are that only 40% and 7% of the persons with presumptive pulmonary TB have undergone chest radiography and CB-NAAT, respectively, in the study setting.

The strengths of the study are the following: (a) this study was done under routine programmatic conditions in a representative sample of public health facilities in this study district. Therefore, the study findings are reflective of ground level realities in this district; (b) we used a mixed-methods study design to understand the facilitators, barriers, and solutions for improving the uptake of chest radiography and CBNAAT. This has helped us to provide further insights to understand the results of the quantitative part of the study.

The major limitations of the study are as follows: (a) we conducted the study in one district of Karnataka. Therefore, the study findings may not be generalisable to the other districts of the state or in the country. Since Chikkaballapur is one of the better performing districts in the State of Karnataka (one of the states with relatively better health systems in India), we expect the results in other districts to be relatively lower than what we found in our study. (b) Though we requested the laboratory technicians to collect information on the radiological reports of CXR, they could not collect this information systematically in all PPTB who had undergone chest radiography. Therefore, we are unable to comment on how many PPTB had normal radiographs and how many had abnormal radiographs. This has limited our ability to provide information about what proportion of PPTB with radiological abnormalities had had undergone CB-NAAT tests. (c) Due to resource constraints, we did not interview patients to understand their perspectives about undergoing these tests. Therefore, the study is deficient on this aspect. (d) We collected data on the demographic and clinical variables of the study participants that are routinely documented in the RNTCP's sputum smear microscopy laboratory register. We did not collect information on several other variables such as socioeconomic status and educational status that are known to influence whether the person undergoes chest radiography and/or CB-NAAT. We are unable to account for the influence of these variables on our study results.

Despite these limitations, the study findings have the following three major implications on policy and practice:

First, only about 40% of the PPTB had undergone CXR despite the RNTCP diagnostic algorithm recommending upfront CXR for all persons with presumptive pulmonary TB. This is higher than 2% that was reported in another similar study that was done in the year 2012 during the era of previous diagnostic algorithm [12]. In PPTB attending health facilities with CXR services (taluka hospitals and district hospital), the proportion of PPTB who had undergone CXR ranged from 7% to 89%, and in persons attending health facilities without CXR services (primary health centers), the proportion who had undergone CXR ranged from 0% to 42%. This strongly indicates that whether a PPTB undergoes chest radiography or not was strongly dependent on other health facility characteristics and not just on whether the facility offered CXR service or not. Our qualitative interviews indicated that the awareness about the current RNTCP diagnostic algorithm was high among health care providers. The qualitative interviews also indicated that if the medical officer requests the patients to undergo CXR, then patients were more likely to undergo CXR. Therefore, the gaps in the proportion of persons who had undergone CXR are likely to be due to the "know-do" gap; i.e., medical officers were aware of the need for CXR but were not prescribing chest radiography for their patients. This type of "know-do" gap is well documented in previous literature [13, 14]. Apart from this, there were also instances where PPTB charged routine user fees of about INR 100/- to undergo CXR at public health facilities and this may have discouraged them from undergoing this. There are clear guidelines from RNTCP that PPTB be excluded from the payment of the user fees. This aspect needs to be reemphasized to the administrative officials of the hospitals which are charging the user fees so that they do not do so in the future and medical officers prescribing the CXR for persons with PPTB must clearly indicate on their prescriptions that these persons must be exempted from the user fees.

Second, only 7% of this cohort of PPTB had undergone CB-NAAT. Even among those who were sputum smear positive, only 65% had undergone CB-NAAT testing. This indicates severe deficiencies in the provision of CB-NAAT services in the district [15, 16]. Our qualitative interviews indicated that knowledge levels about CB-NAAT among health care providers were high. But the major constraint was having only one CB-NAAT machine in the district to cater to the PPTB from all over the district. Either PPTB had to visit this center to undergo the test or their sputum samples had to be collected and transported by the field workers. It appears that there were challenges in operationalising both these activities at the field level. Given these findings, it appears that improving the CB-NAAT services in the district requires interventions at multiple levels. The exact nature of these interventions and understanding whether they will work in this setting is an area for future research.

Third, the qualitative part of the study indicated some good practices and solutions to improve the uptake of CXR. Notable among these were the practice of forming "WhatsApp®" group to share PPTB information and CXR results among the various healthcare providers (medical officer, laboratory technician, and radiography technician) within the health facility. This facilitated high proportion of PPTB to undergo the chest radiography in one of the taluka hospitals. Similar practices can be adopted in other health facilities. Apart from this, there were suggestions of involving private radiography centers for improving uptake of CXR, usage of a "seal" (to indicate that the person is a presumptive pulmonary TB and needs to be fast-tracked without charging any user fees), and suggestions for creating additional columns in the sputum smear microscopy laboratory register to document the CXR status/results of patients. We agree with these suggestions and recommend these measures for improving the provision of CXR at the field level.

Lastly, our study findings may not be unique and may be found in other settings as well. The gaps in implementation shown in our study have the potential to seriously prevent the realisation of the dream of End-TB in India and around the world [2, 17]. The study findings support the "call for action" for public health community involved in TB eradication in India and at the global level to undertake measures to mitigate the gaps in implementing the existing guidelines on TB diagnostic tests in an equitable manner at the field level [18].

In conclusion, this study shows that chest radiography and CB-NAAT are low. The study provides information of facilitators, barriers, and some solutions for addressing the gaps. We call upon RNTCP to take note of these findings and undertake measures to improve the provision of chest radiography and CB-NAAT services for persons with presumptive pulmonary TB in the country.

Disclosure

The funders had no role in the study design, data collection and analysis, decision to publish, or preparation of the manuscript.

Authors' Contributions

MK, SBN, SS, and AKM are assigned to the protocol development. YRB, SBN, SKG, SN, and MK are assigned to the protocol finalization. MK, SBN, and SS collected the data. MK and SBN are responsible for the data entry. MK, SBN, SS, and AKM are responsible for the data analysis and interpretation. MK, SS, and AKM drafted the manuscript. Manuscript review and approval: All investigators reviewed and approved the manuscript.

Acknowledgments

The training programme, within which this paper was developed, was funded by the Department for International Development (DFID), UK. This research was conducted through the Structured Operational Research and Training Initiative (SORT IT), a global partnership led by the Special Programme for Research and Training in Tropical Diseases at the World Health Organization (WHO/TDR). The model is based on a course developed jointly by the International Union Against Tuberculosis and Lung Disease (The Union) and Medécins sans Frontières (MSF/Doctors Without Borders). The specific SORT IT programme which resulted in this publication was jointly developed and implemented by the following: The Union South-East Asia Office, New Delhi, India; the Centre for Operational Research, The Union, Paris, France; Medécins sans Frontières (MSF/Doctors Without Borders), India; Department of Preventive and Social Medicine, Jawaharlal Institute of Postgraduate Medical Education and Research, Puducherry, India; Department of Community Medicine, All India Institute of Medical Sciences, Nagpur, India; Department of Community Medicine, ESIC Medical College and PGIMSR, Bengaluru, India; Department of Community Medicine, Sri Manakula Vinayagar Medical College and Hospital, Puducherry, India; Karuna Trust, Bangalore, India; Public Health Foundation of India, Gurgaon, India; The INCLEN Trust International, New Delhi, India; Indian Council of Medical Research (ICMR), Department of Health Research, Ministry of Health and Family Welfare, New Delhi, India; Department of Community Medicine, Sri Devraj Urs Medical College, Kolar, India; and Department of Community Medicine, Yenepoya Medical College, Mangalore, India. We acknowledge the laboratory technicians for their support in the data collection, Mr. Balakrishna (Senior treatment supervisor), Mrs. Reshma (TBHV), and Dr. Vijay Kumar (former district surgeon, District Hospital, Chikkaballapur) for their technical help.

References

[1] World Health Organization, *Global Tuberculosis Report 2018*, World Health Organization, Geneva, Switzerland, 2018.

[2] Central TB Division, *National Strategic Plan for Tuberculosis Elimination 2017-2025*, Directorate General of Health Services, Ministry of Health and Family Welfare, Government of India, New Delhi, 2017.

[3] R. Subbaraman, R. R. Nathavitharana, S. Satyanarayana et al., "The tuberculosis cascade of care in India's public sector: a systematic review and meta-analysis," *PLoS Medicine*, vol. 13, no. 10, article e1002149, 2016.

[4] A. D. Chaudhuri, "Recent changes in technical and operational guidelines for tuberculosis control programme in India - 2016: a paradigm shift in tuberculosis control," *The Journal of Association of Chest Physicians*, vol. 5, no. 1, pp. 1–9, 2017.

[5] K. R. Steingart, H. Sohn, I. Schiller et al., "Xpert® MTB/RIF assay for pulmonary tuberculosis and rifampicin resistance in adults," *Cochrane Database of Systematic Reviews*, no. 1, article CD009593, 2013.

[6] S. Huddart, E. MacLean, and M. Pai, "Location, location, location: tuberculosis services in highest burden countries," *The Lancet Global Health*, vol. 4, no. 12, pp. e907–e908, 2016.

[7] S. Satyanarayana, R. Subbaraman, P. Shete et al., "Quality of tuberculosis care in India: a systematic review," *The International Journal of Tuberculosis and Lung Disease*, vol. 19, no. 7, pp. 751–763, 2015.

[8] P. MacPherson, R. M. G. J. Houben, J. R. Glynn, E. L. Corbett, and K. Kranzer, "Pre-treatment loss to follow-up in tuberculosis patients in low- and lower-middle-income countries and high-burden countries: a systematic review and meta-analysis," *Bulletin of the World Health Organization*, vol. 92, no. 2, pp. 126–138, 2014.

[9] *Chikkaballapura District*September 2019, https://en.wikipedia.org/wiki/Chikkaballapura_district.

[10] Y. S. Lincoln and E. G. Guba, *Naturalistic Inquiry*, SAGE Publications, Inc, New York, NY, USA, 1985.

[11] M. D. Fetters, L. A. Curry, and J. W. Creswell, "Achieving integration in mixed methods designs-principles and practices," *Health Services Research*, vol. 48, 6, Part 2, pp. 2134–2156, 2013.

[12] V. K. Chadha, P. Praseeja, N. K. Hemanthkumar et al., "Implementation efficiency of a diagnostic algorithm in sputum smear-negative presumptive tuberculosis patients," *The Inter-*

national Journal of Tuberculosis and Lung Disease, vol. 18, no. 10, pp. 1237–1242, 2014.

[13] J. Das, A. Kwan, B. Daniels et al., "Use of standardised patients to assess quality of tuberculosis care: a pilot, cross-sectional study," *The Lancet Infectious Diseases*, vol. 15, no. 11, pp. 1305–1313, 2015.

[14] S. Datta, M. J. Saunders, M. A. Tovar, and C. A. Evans, "Improving tuberculosis diagnosis: better tests or better healthcare?," *PLoS Medicine*, vol. 14, no. 10, article e1002406, 2017.

[15] K. S. Sachdeva, N. Raizada, R. S. Gupta et al., "The potential impact of up-front drug sensitivity testing on India's epidemic of multi-drug resistant tuberculosis," *PLoS One*, vol. 10, no. 7, article e0131438, 2015.

[16] H. Sohn, P. Kasaie, E. Kendall et al., "Informing decision-making for universal access to quality tuberculosis diagnosis in India: an economic-epidemiological model," *BMC Medicine*, vol. 17, no. 1, p. 155, 2019.

[17] K. Lönnroth and M. Raviglione, "The WHO's new end TB strategy in the post-2015 era of the sustainable development goals," *Transactions of the Royal Society of Tropical Medicine and Hygiene*, vol. 110, no. 3, pp. 148–150, 2016.

[18] B. D. Agins, D. J. Ikeda, M. J. A. Reid, E. Goosby, M. Pai, and A. Cattamanchi, "Improving the cascade of global tuberculosis care: moving from the "what" to the "how" of quality improvement," *The Lancet Infectious Diseases*, vol. 19, no. 12, pp. e437–e443, 2019.

Permissions

All chapters in this book were first published by Hindawi Publishing Corporation; hereby published with permission under the Creative Commons Attribution License or equivalent. Every chapter published in this book has been scrutinized by our experts. Their significance has been extensively debated. The topics covered herein carry significant findings which will fuel the growth of the discipline. They may even be implemented as practical applications or may be referred to as a beginning point for another development.

The contributors of this book come from diverse backgrounds, making this book a truly international effort. This book will bring forth new frontiers with its revolutionizing research information and detailed analysis of the nascent developments around the world.

We would like to thank all the contributing authors for lending their expertise to make the book truly unique. They have played a crucial role in the development of this book. Without their invaluable contributions this book wouldn't have been possible. They have made vital efforts to compile up to date information on the varied aspects of this subject to make this book a valuable addition to the collection of many professionals and students.

This book was conceptualized with the vision of imparting up-to-date information and advanced data in this field. To ensure the same, a matchless editorial board was set up. Every individual on the board went through rigorous rounds of assessment to prove their worth. After which they invested a large part of their time researching and compiling the most relevant data for our readers.

The editorial board has been involved in producing this book since its inception. They have spent rigorous hours researching and exploring the diverse topics which have resulted in the successful publishing of this book. They have passed on their knowledge of decades through this book. To expedite this challenging task, the publisher supported the team at every step. A small team of assistant editors was also appointed to further simplify the editing procedure and attain best results for the readers.

Apart from the editorial board, the designing team has also invested a significant amount of their time in understanding the subject and creating the most relevant covers. They scrutinized every image to scout for the most suitable representation of the subject and create an appropriate cover for the book.

The publishing team has been an ardent support to the editorial, designing and production team. Their endless efforts to recruit the best for this project, has resulted in the accomplishment of this book. They are a veteran in the field of academics and their pool of knowledge is as vast as their experience in printing. Their expertise and guidance has proved useful at every step. Their uncompromising quality standards have made this book an exceptional effort. Their encouragement from time to time has been an inspiration for everyone.

The publisher and the editorial board hope that this book will prove to be a valuable piece of knowledge for researchers, students, practitioners and scholars across the globe.

List of Contributors

Assefa Tola
Department of Epidemiology and Biostatistics, College of Health and Medical Sciences, Haramaya University, Harar, Ethiopia

Kirubel Minsamo Minshore and Yohanes Ayele
Department of Clinical Pharmacy, College of Health and Medical Sciences, Haramaya University, Harar, Ethiopia

Abraham Nigussie Mekuria
Department of Pharmacology, College of Health and Medical Sciences, Haramaya University, Harar, Ethiopia

Yibeltal Estemech Ayalew
Department of Medical Nursing, University of Gondar, Gondar, Ethiopia

Fikadu Ambaw Yehualashet
Department of Community Health Nursing, University of Gondar, Gondar, Ethiopia

Worknesh Akanaw Bogale and Mengistu Berhanu Gobeza
Department of Pediatrics and Child Health Nursing, University of Gondar, Gondar, Ethiopia

Eben Godsway Dzodanu and Isaac Dadzie
Department of Medical Laboratory Science, University of Cape Coast, Cape Coast, Ghana

Justice Afrifa
Department of Medical Laboratory Science, University of Cape Coast, Cape Coast, Ghana
Scientific Research Center, The Second Affiliated Hospital of Harbin Medical University, Harbin, China

Desmond Omane Acheampong
Department of Biomedical Sciences, University of Cape Coast, Cape Coast, Ghana

Gambhir Shrestha and Rashmi Mulmi
Department of Cancer Prevention, Control and Research, B.P. Koirala Memorial Cancer Hospital, Bharatpur, Chitwan, Nepal

Deepak Kumar Yadav, Dharanidhar Baral and Paras Kumar Pokharel
School of Public Health and Community Medicine, B.P. Koirala Institute of Health Sciences, Dharan, Sunsari, Nepal

Rabin Gautam
National Tuberculosis Program, Health Research and Social Development Forum, Thapathali, Kathmandu, Nepal

Adwoa Asante-Poku
Noguchi Memorial Institute for Medical Research, University of Ghana, Ghana

Kenneth Mawuta Hayibor
Noguchi Memorial Institute for Medical Research, University of Ghana, Ghana
School of Public Health, University of Ghana, Ghana

Delia Akosua Bandoh and Ernest Kenu
School of Public Health, University of Ghana, Ghana

Habteyes Hailu Tola, Ayinalem Alemu, Bazezew Yenew, Shewki Moga, Desalegn Addise, Zemedu Mohammed, Muluwork Getahun, Mengistu Tadesse, Biniyam Dagne and Misikir Amare
Ethiopian Public Health Institute, Addis Ababa, Ethiopia

Dessie Abera and Kassu Desta
Department of Medical Laboratory Sciences, College of Health Sciences, Addis Ababa University, Addis Ababa, Ethiopia

Getu Diriba
Ethiopian Public Health Institute, Addis Ababa, Ethiopia
Department of Medical Laboratory Sciences, College of Health Sciences, Addis Ababa University, Addis Ababa, Ethiopia

Abebaw Kebede
Ethiopian Public Health Institute, Addis Ababa, Ethiopia
Department of Microbial, Cellular and Molecular Biology, College of Natural and Computational Sciences, Addis Ababa University, Addis Ababa, Ethiopia

Mengistu Fantahun
St. Paul's Hospital Millennium Medical College, Addis Ababa, Ethiopia

Gebeyehu Assefa
Armauer Hansen Research Institute, Addis Ababa, Ethiopia

Lisa Nkatha Micheni
Department of Microbiology, Mbarara University of Science and Technology, Mbarara, Uganda
Department of Microbiology and Immunology, Kampala International University Western Campus, Bushenyi, Uganda

Kennedy Kassaza and Joel Bazira
Department of Microbiology, Mbarara University of Science and Technology, Mbarara, Uganda

Ibrahim Ntulume
Department of Microbiology and Immunology, Kampala International University Western Campus, Bushenyi, Uganda

Hellen Kinyi
Department of Biochemistry, School of Medicine, Kabale University, Kabale, Uganda

Eyram Dogah
Disease Control Unit, Ketu North Municipal Health Directorate, Ghana Health Service, Dzodze, Volta Region, Ghana

Mark Aviisah
Department of Health Policy, Planning and Management, School of Public Health, University of Health and Allied Sciences, Hohoe, Ghana

Da-Ama Mawulom Kuatewo
Hohoe Municipal Health Directorate, Ghana Health Service, Hohoe, Volta Region, Ghana

Godsway Edem Kpene, Sylvester Yao Lokpo and Florence Shine Edziah
Department of Medical Laboratory Sciences, School of Allied Health Sciences, University of Health and Allied Sciences, Ho, Ghana

Abinet Adane
East Hararghe Zone, East Hararghe Zonal Health Office, Harar, Ethiopia

Melake Damena and Hussein Mohammed
School of Public Health, College of Health and Medical Sciences, Haramaya University, Harar, Ethiopia

Fitsum Weldegebreal
Department of Medical Laboratory Sciences, College of Health and Medical Sciences, Haramaya University, Harar, Ethiopia

David A. Oladele and Babatunde L. Salako
Clinical Sciences Department, Nigerian Institute of Medical Research, Lagos, Nigeria

Mobolanle R. Balogun and Kofoworola Odeyemi
Department of Community Medicine and Primary Care, College of Medicine, University of Lagos, Lagos, Nigeria

Siwon Lee, Krisha Lim and Jansel Ferma
International Care Ministries Foundation Inc., Philippines

Lincoln Lau
International Care Ministries Foundation Inc., Philippines
Dalla Lana School of Public Health, University of Toronto, ON, Canada

Donald Cole
Dalla Lana School of Public Health, University of Toronto, ON, Canada

Warren Dodd
School of Public Health and Health Systems, University of Waterloo, ON, Canada

Sailesh Kumar Shrestha
National Academy of Medical Sciences, Bir Hospital, Kathmandu 44600, Nepal

Ratna Bahadur Bhattarai, Lok Raj Joshi, Rajendra Basnet and Kedar Narsingh K. C.
National Tuberculosis Control Center, Bhaktapur 44800, Nepal

Nilaramba Adhikari
Central Department of Public Health, Institute of Medicine, Kathmandu 44600, Nepal

Suvesh Kumar Shrestha
Save the Children/Global Fund, Kathmandu 44600, Nepal

Alois Mandizvidza, Evidence Gaka, Joseph Nembaware, Shepherd Nyambi, Blessing Masunungure and Davison Garauzive
Harare Central Prison, Zimbabwe Prison and Correctional Service, Harare, Zimbabwe

Riitta A. Dlodlo
International Union against Tuberculosis and Lung Disease (The Union), Paris, France

Palanivel Chinnakali
Departments of Preventive and Social Medicine, Jawaharlal Institute of Postgraduate Medical Education & Research (JIPMER), Puducherry, India

Hamufare Dumisani Mugauri
AIDS and TB Unit, Ministry of Health and Child Care, Harare, Zimbabwe

Freeman Dube
National Aids Council (NAC), Harare, Zimbabwe

Rogers Sekibira
Makerere University Lung Institute, College of Health Sciences, Makerere University, Uganda

Joanitah Nalunjogi and Irene Najjingo
Makerere University Lung Institute, College of Health Sciences, Makerere University, Uganda
Clinical Epidemiology Unit, College of Health Sciences, Makerere University, Uganda

Pastan Lusiba, Francis Olweny, Edward Kayongo and Achilles Katamba
Clinical Epidemiology Unit, College of Health Sciences, Makerere University, Uganda

Frank Mugabe
Uganda National Tuberculosis and Leprosy Program, Ministry of Health, Uganda

Joseph Mubiru
Accident and Emergency Unit, Mulago National Referral Hospital, Kampala, Uganda

Bruce Kirenga
Makerere University Lung Institute, College of Health Sciences, Makerere University, Uganda
Division of Pulmonary Medicine, College of Health Sciences, Makerere University, Uganda

Aboma Zewude and Gobena Ameni
Aklilu Lemma Institute of Pathobiology, Addis Ababa University, Addis Ababa, Ethiopia

Amir Alelign
Aklilu Lemma Institute of Pathobiology, Addis Ababa University, Addis Ababa, Ethiopia
College of Natural Sciences, Department of Microbial, Cellular and Molecular Biology, Addis Ababa University, Addis Ababa, Ethiopia
College of Natural and Computational Sciences, Department of Biology, Debrebrhan University, Debrebrhan, Ethiopia

Beyene Petros
College of Natural Sciences, Department of Microbial, Cellular and Molecular Biology, Addis Ababa University, Addis Ababa, Ethiopia

Furaha Lyamuya and Kajiru Kilonzo
Kilimanjaro Christian Medical University College, Moshi, Tanzania

Tamary Henry Leveri
Kilimanjaro Christian Medical University College, Moshi, Tanzania
Kibong'oto Infectious Diseases Hospital, Sanya Juu, Tanzania

Isack Lekule
Kibong'oto Infectious Diseases Hospital, Sanya Juu, Tanzania

Edson Mollel
Kilimanjaro Christian Medical University College, Moshi, Tanzania
Western Zone Blood Transfusion Center, Tabora, Tanzania

Aase Bengaard Andersen
Department of Infectious Diseases, Copenhagen University Hospital, Rigshospitalet, Blegdamsvej 9, 2100 Copenhagen Ö, Denmark

Jens D. Lundgren and Marie Helleberg
Department of Infectious Diseases, Copenhagen University Hospital, Rigshospitalet, Blegdamsvej 9, 2100 Copenhagen Ö, Denmark
Centre of Excellence for Health, Immunity and Infections (CHIP), Copenhagen University Hospital/ Rigshospitalet, Blegdamsvej 9, 2100 Copenhagen Ö, Denmark

Daniel Cho and Christina Ekenberg
Centre of Excellence for Health, Immunity and Infections (CHIP), Copenhagen University Hospital/ Rigshospitalet, Blegdamsvej 9, 2100 Copenhagen Ö, Denmark

Søren Sørensen and Marianne Rix
Department of Nephrology, Copenhagen University Hospital, Rigshospitalet, Blegdamsvej 9, 2100 Copenhagen Ö, Denmark

Finn Gustafsson and Michael Perch
Department of Cardiology, Copenhagen University Hospital, Rigshospitalet, Blegdamsvej 9, 2100 Copenhagen Ö, Denmark

Allan Rasmussen
Department of Surgery C, Copenhagen University Hospital, Rigshospitalet, Blegdamsvej 9, 2100 Copenhagen Ö, Denmark

Peter H. S. Andersen
Department of Infection Epidemiology and Prevention, The State Serum Institute, Artillerivej 5, 2300 Copenhagen S, Denmark

Solomon M. Abay
Department of Pharmacology and Clinical Pharmacy, College of Health Sciences, Addis Ababa University, Addis Ababa, Ethiopia

Dawit A. Ejigu
Department of Pharmacology, St Paul's Hospital Millennium Medical College, Addis Ababa, Ethiopia

Sadick Ahmed Agyare
Ghana Health Service, Atwima Nwabiagya, Ghana

Francis Adjei Osei, Ernest Amanor, Michael Owusu-Ansah and Aliyu Mohammed
Kwame Nkrumah University of Science and Technology, Kumasi, Ghana

Samuel Frimpong Odoom, Nicholas Karikari Mensah and Charles Martyn-Dickens
Komfo Anokye Teaching Hospital, Kumasi, Ghana

Eugene Osei Yeboah
Ghana Health Service, Zuarungu, Ghana

Vasco Ayere Avoka
Department of Epidemiology and Biostatistics, School of Public Health, University of Health and Allied Sciences, Ho, Ghana

Eric Osei
Department of Population and Behavioural Sciences, School of Public Health, University of Health and Allied Sciences, Ho, Ghana

Angella Musiimenta and Aaron T. Mugaba
Mbarara University of Science and Technology, Mbarara, Uganda
Angels Compassion Research and Innovations Centre, Mbarara, Uganda

Wilson Tumuhimbise, Esther C. Atukunda and Conrad Muzoora
Mbarara University of Science and Technology, Mbarara, Uganda

Mari Armstrong-Hough
Uganda Tuberculosis Implementation Research Consortium, Makerere University, Kampala, Uganda
Department of Epidemiology of Microbial Diseases, Yale School of Public Health, New Haven, Connecticut, USA
Pulmonary, Critical Care and Sleep Medicine, Yale School of Medicine, New Haven, Connecticut, USA
New York University College of Global Public Health, New York, New York, USA

J. Lucian Davis
Uganda Tuberculosis Implementation Research Consortium, Makerere University, Kampala, Uganda
Department of Epidemiology of Microbial Diseases, Yale School of Public Health, New Haven, Connecticut, USA
Pulmonary, Critical Care and Sleep Medicine, Yale School of Medicine, New Haven, Connecticut, USA

David Bangsberg
Oregon Health & Science University-Portland State University School of Public Health, USA

Jessica E. Haberer
Harvard Medical School, Boston, MA, USA
Massachusetts General Hospital Center for Global Health, Boston, MA, USA

Santosha Kelamane, Vikas Panibatla and Ramesh Dasari
TB Alert India, Hyderabad, India

Srinath Satyanarayana
Independent Public Health Consultant, New Delhi, India
Center for Operational Research, International Union against Tuberculosis and Lung Disease, New Delhi, India

Rajeesham
State TB Office, Telangana State, Hyderabad, India

Amera Khan
Stop TB Partnership, Geneva, Switzerland

Vishnuvardhan Kamineni
Stop TB Partnership, Geneva, Switzerland Public Health, Bengaluru, India

Daria N. Podlekareva
CHIP, Rigshospitalet, University of Copenhagen, Denmark

Dorte Bek Folkvardsen
International Reference Laboratory of Mycobacteriology, Statens Serum Institut, Copenhagen, Denmark

Anna Vassilenko and Igor Karpov
Belarusian State Medical University, Minsk, Belarus

Aliaksandr Skrahin
Republican Scientific and Practical Center for Pulmonology and TB, Minsk, Belarus
Belarusian State Medical University, Minsk, Belarus

Alena Skrahina, Henadz Hurevich and Dzmitry Klimuk
Republican Scientific and Practical Center for Pulmonology and TB, Minsk, Belarus

Ole Kirk
CHIP, Rigshospitalet, University of Copenhagen, Denmark
Department of Infectious Diseases, Rigshospitalet, University of Copenhagen, Denmark

Troels Lillebaek
International Reference Laboratory of Mycobacteriology, Statens Serum Institut, Copenhagen, Denmark
Global Health Section, Department of Public Health, University of Copenhagen, Denmark

Alok Kumar Mantri, Amarender Singh Puri, Ajay Kumar, Sanjeev Sachdeva and Siddharth Srivastava
Department of Gastroenterology, G. B. Pant Institute of Postgraduate Medical Education and Research (GIPMER), New Delhi, India

Priti Meena
Institute of Renal Science, Sir Gangaram Hospital, New Delhi, India

K. Arivarasan
Kauvery Hospital Trichy, Tennur, India

Shivakumar Varakanahali
Narayana Multispeciality Hospital, HSR Layout, Bangalore, India

Fassikaw Kebede
Woldia University, College of Health Science, School of Public Health, Department of Epidemiology & Biostatics, Ethiopia

Tsehay Kebede
Bahir Dare University, Faculty of Social Science, Department of Geography & Environmental Studies, Ethiopia

Birhanu Kebede
Pawe Woreda Agriculural Inpute and Production Team Leaders, Metekel Zone, Pawe Woreda, North West, Ethiopia

Belete Negese
Debre Birhan University, College of Medicine and Health Sciences, Department of Nursing 2021, Debre Birhan, Ethiopia

Tamrat Shaweno
Jimma University Institute of Health Science, Faculty of Public Health, Department of Epidemiology 2021, Jimma, Ethiopia

Netsanet Fentahun and Yosef Wasihun
School of Public Health, College of Medicine and Health Science, Bahir Dar University, Bahir Dar, Ethiopia

Abebe Mamo and Lakew Abebe Gebretsadik
Department of Health, Behavior and Society, Institutes of Health, Jimma University, Jimma, Ethiopia

Manjula Kanakaraju
Taluka Health Office, Chikkaballapur, Karnataka, India

Yella Ramesh Babu
District Tuberculosis Office, Chikkaballapur, Karnataka, India

Akshaya Kibballi Madhukeshwar
Department of Community Medicine, Yenepoya Medical College, Yenepoya (Deemed to be University), Mangaluru, Karnataka, India

Somashekar Narasimhaiah
National Tuberculosis Institute, Bengaluru, Karnataka, India

Index

www.ingramcontent.com/pod-product-compliance
Lightning Source LLC
LaVergne TN
LVHW082152200926
848484LV00008B/2145
9798887405377